FETAL ALCOHOL SYNDROME

A MEDICAL DICTIONARY, BIBLIOGRAPHY,
AND ANNOTATED RESEARCH GUIDE TO
INTERNET REFERENCES

JAMES N. PARKER, M.D.
AND PHILIP M. PARKER, PH.D., EDITORS

ICON Health Publications
ICON Group International, Inc.
4370 La Jolla Village Drive, 4th Floor
San Diego, CA 92122 USA

Publisher, Health Care: Philip Parker, Ph.D.
Editor(s): James Parker, M.D., Philip Parker, Ph.D.

Publisher's note: The ideas, procedures, and suggestions contained in this book are not intended for the diagnosis or treatment of a health problem. As new medical or scientific information becomes available from academic and clinical research, recommended treatments and drug therapies may undergo changes. The authors, editors, and publisher have attempted to make the information in this book up to date and accurate in accord with accepted standards at the time of publication. The authors, editors, and publisher are not responsible for errors or omissions or for consequences from application of the book, and make no warranty, expressed or implied, in regard to the contents of this book. Any practice described in this book should be applied by the reader in accordance with professional standards of care used in regard to the unique circumstances that may apply in each situation. The reader is advised to always check product information (package inserts) for changes and new information regarding dosage and contraindications before prescribing any drug or pharmacological product. Caution is especially urged when using new or infrequently ordered drugs, herbal remedies, vitamins and supplements, alternative therapies, complementary therapies and medicines, and integrative medical treatments.

Cataloging-in-Publication Data

Parker, James N., 1961-
Parker, Philip M., 1960-

Fetal Alcohol Syndrome: A Medical Dictionary, Bibliography, and Annotated Research Guide to Internet References / James N. Parker and Philip M. Parker, editors
        p.   cm.
Includes bibliographical references, glossary, and index.
ISBN: 0-597-83909-3
1. Fetal Alcohol Syndrome-Popular works.   I. Title.

Disclaimer

This publication is not intended to be used for the diagnosis or treatment of a health problem. It is sold with the understanding that the publisher, editors, and authors are not engaging in the rendering of medical, psychological, financial, legal, or other professional services.

References to any entity, product, service, or source of information that may be contained in this publication should not be considered an endorsement, either direct or implied, by the publisher, editors, or authors. ICON Group International, Inc., the editors, and the authors are not responsible for the content of any Web pages or publications referenced in this publication.

Copyright Notice

Acknowledgements

The collective knowledge generated from academic and applied research summarized in various references has been critical in the creation of this book which is best viewed as a comprehensive compilation and collection of information prepared by various official agencies which produce publications on fetal alcohol syndrome. Books in this series draw from various agencies and institutions associated with the United States Department of Health and Human Services, and in particular, the Office of the Secretary of Health and Human Services (OS), the Administration for Children and Families (ACF), the Administration on Aging (AOA), the Agency for Healthcare Research and Quality (AHRQ), the Agency for Toxic Substances and Disease Registry (ATSDR), the Centers for Disease Control and Prevention (CDC), the Food and Drug Administration (FDA), the Healthcare Financing Administration (HCFA), the Health Resources and Services Administration (HRSA), the Indian Health Service (IHS), the institutions of the National Institutes of Health (NIH), the Program Support Center (PSC), and the Substance Abuse and Mental Health Services Administration (SAMHSA). In addition to these sources, information gathered from the National Library of Medicine, the United States Patent Office, the European Union, and their related organizations has been invaluable in the creation of this book. Some of the work represented was financially supported by the Research and Development Committee at INSEAD. This support is gratefully acknowledged. Finally, special thanks are owed to Tiffany Freeman for her excellent editorial support.

About the Editors

James N. Parker, M.D.

Dr. James N. Parker received his Bachelor of Science degree in Psychobiology from the University of California, Riverside and his M.D. from the University of California, San Diego. In addition to authoring numerous research publications, he has lectured at various academic institutions. Dr. Parker is the medical editor for health books by ICON Health Publications.

Philip M. Parker, Ph.D.

Philip M. Parker is the Eli Lilly Chair Professor of Innovation, Business and Society at INSEAD (Fontainebleau, France and Singapore). Dr. Parker has also been Professor at the University of California, San Diego and has taught courses at Harvard University, the Hong Kong University of Science and Technology, the Massachusetts Institute of Technology, Stanford University, and UCLA. Dr. Parker is the associate editor for ICON Health Publications.

About ICON Health Publications

To discover more about ICON Health Publications, simply check with your preferred online booksellers, including Barnes & Noble.com and Amazon.com which currently carry all of our titles. Or, feel free to contact us directly for bulk purchases or institutional discounts:

ICON Group International, Inc.
4370 La Jolla Village Drive, Fourth Floor
San Diego, CA 92122 USA
Fax: 858-546-4341
Web site: **www.icongrouponline.com/health**

Table of Contents

FORWARD

In March 2001, the National Institutes of Health issued the following warning: "The number of Web sites offering health-related resources grows every day. Many sites provide valuable information, while others may have information that is unreliable or misleading."[1] Furthermore, because of the rapid increase in Internet-based information, many hours can be wasted searching, selecting, and printing. Since only the smallest fraction of information dealing with fetal alcohol syndrome is indexed in search engines, such as **www.google.com** or others, a non-systematic approach to Internet research can be not only time consuming, but also incomplete. This book was created for medical professionals, students, and members of the general public who want to know as much as possible about fetal alcohol syndrome, using the most advanced research tools available and spending the least amount of time doing so.

In addition to offering a structured and comprehensive bibliography, the pages that follow will tell you where and how to find reliable information covering virtually all topics related to fetal alcohol syndrome, from the essentials to the most advanced areas of research. Public, academic, government, and peer-reviewed research studies are emphasized. Various abstracts are reproduced to give you some of the latest official information available to date on fetal alcohol syndrome. Abundant guidance is given on how to obtain free-of-charge primary research results via the Internet. **While this book focuses on the field of medicine, when some sources provide access to non-medical information relating to fetal alcohol syndrome, these are noted in the text.**

E-book and electronic versions of this book are fully interactive with each of the Internet sites mentioned (clicking on a hyperlink automatically opens your browser to the site indicated). If you are using the hard copy version of this book, you can access a cited Web site by typing the provided Web address directly into your Internet browser. You may find it useful to refer to synonyms or related terms when accessing these Internet databases. **NOTE:** At the time of publication, the Web addresses were functional. However, some links may fail due to URL address changes, which is a common occurrence on the Internet.

For readers unfamiliar with the Internet, detailed instructions are offered on how to access electronic resources. For readers unfamiliar with medical terminology, a comprehensive glossary is provided. For readers without access to Internet resources, a directory of medical libraries, that have or can locate references cited here, is given. We hope these resources will prove useful to the widest possible audience seeking information on fetal alcohol syndrome.

The Editors

---

[1] From the NIH, National Cancer Institute (NCI): **http://www.cancer.gov/cancerinfo/ten-things-to-know**.

CHAPTER 1. STUDIES ON FETAL ALCOHOL SYNDROME

Overview

In this chapter, we will show you how to locate peer-reviewed references and studies on fetal alcohol syndrome.

The Combined Health Information Database

The Combined Health Information Database summarizes studies across numerous federal agencies. To limit your investigation to research studies and fetal alcohol syndrome, you will need to use the advanced search options. First, go to **http://chid.nih.gov/index.html** From there, select the "Detailed Search" option (or go directly to that page with the following hyperlink: **http://chid.nih.gov/detail/detail.html**). The trick in extracting studies is found in the drop boxes at the bottom of the search page where "You may refine your search by." Select the dates and language you prefer, and the format option "Journal Article." At the top of the search form, select the number of records you would like to see (we recommend 100) and check the box to display "whole records." We recommend that you type "fetal alcohol syndrome" (or synonyms) into the "For these words:" box. Consider using the option "anywhere in record" to make your search as broad as possible. If you want to limit the search to only a particular field, such as the title of the journal, then select this option in the "Search in these fields" drop box. The following is what you can expect from this type of search:

- **Hearing, Language, Speech, Vestibular, and Dentofacial Disorders in Fetal Alcohol Syndrome**

  Source: Alcoholism: Clinical and Experimental Research. 21(2): 227-237. April 1997.

  Summary: Fetal alcohol syndrome (FAS) is characterized by congenital anomalies traditionally associated with hearing disorders. This article reports on a study that sought to evaluate possible central hearing loss; verify and extend previous observations on sensorineural and conductive hearing losses; evaluate possible vestibular disorders; examine the relationships between hearing, speech, language, vestibular, and dentofacial disorders in FAS patients; and evaluate the influence of patient age, race, and gender on the expression of these morbidities. A biracial group of 22 FAS patients (aged 3 to 26 years) were evaluated by standard hearing, speech, language, and vestibular tests. Dentofacial and other malformations were also assessed. Of the 22 FAS patients, 17 (77 percent) had intermittent conductive hearing loss due to recurrent serous otitis media (ear infections) that persisted from early childhood into adulthood; whereas, 6 (27 percent) had sensorineural hearing loss in addition to conductive hearing loss. Among the 12 patients tested for central hearing function, all (100 percent) were significantly impaired. Among the patients tested for speech and language ability, 18 of 20 (90 percent) had speech pathology, 16 of 21 (76 percent) had expressive language deficits, and 18 of 22 (82 percent) had receptive language deficits. Hearing, speech, and language deficits were not influenced by age, race, or gender. On the vestibular tests, all performed within normal limits with the possible exception of one child (n = 6). High incidences of dentofacial, temporomandibular joint, ocular, cardiac, and skeletal disorders were observed. The authors conclude that these findings offer new evidence of the high prevalence of sensorineural, conductive, and central hearing deficits, the persistence of otitis proneness into adulthood, the existence of temporomandibular joint disorders, and the possible influence of gender or race on dental malocclusions. These disorders can contribute to the learning, behavioral, and emotional difficulties seen in FAS patients and warrant early, aggressive intervention. 2 tables. 74 references. (AA-M).

- **Treating the Patient with Fetal Alcohol Syndrome**

Source: Access. 11(5): 60-63. May-June 1997.

Contact: Available from American Dental Hygienists' Association (ADHA). 444 North Michigan Avenue, Chicago, IL 60611. (800) 243-2342 or (312) 440-8900; Fax (312) 440-8929; E-mail: adha@ix.netcom.com; http://www.adha.org.

Summary: This article familiarizes dental hygienists with fetal alcohol syndrome (FAS), the leading known cause of organic brain damage in the United States. FAS can occur in the fetus when a pregnant woman drinks alcoholic beverages heavily. The author describes the clinical presentation and ongoing impact of FAS. The author notes that FAS is often unrecognized and undiagnosed because it shares so many characteristics with other medical and behavioral conditions. Dental manifestations of FAS include late tooth eruption. Once the teeth erupt, the children are likely to develop malocclusion, due to malpositioning of their teeth, overcrowding of the dentition, poor muscle control, tongue thrusting, and lip licking. Teeth are often crooked and prone to cavities. Combined with the unusual behavior and tissue sensitivity, these factors present a unique challenge to the dental hygienist. The author provides specific suggestions for dental hygienists working with this patient population. The author concludes that children with FAS can have pleasant experiences in the dental office, but much depends on the dental hygienist's concern and sensitivity to their particular needs. 37 references. (AA-M).

Federally Funded Research on Fetal Alcohol Syndrome

The U.S. Government supports a variety of research studies relating to fetal alcohol syndrome. These studies are tracked by the Office of Extramural Research at the National Institutes of Health.[2] CRISP (Computerized Retrieval of Information on Scientific Projects) is

---

[2] Healthcare projects are funded by the National Institutes of Health (NIH), Substance Abuse and Mental Health Services (SAMHSA), Health Resources and Services Administration (HRSA), Food and Drug Administration (FDA), Centers for Disease Control and Prevention (CDCP), Agency for Healthcare Research and Quality (AHRQ), and Office of Assistant Secretary of Health (OASH).

a searchable database of federally funded biomedical research projects conducted at universities, hospitals, and other institutions.

Search the CRISP Web site at **http://crisp.cit.nih.gov/crisp/crisp_query.generate_screen**. You will have the option to perform targeted searches by various criteria, including geography, date, and topics related to fetal alcohol syndrome.

For most of the studies, the agencies reporting into CRISP provide summaries or abstracts. As opposed to clinical trial research using patients, many federally funded studies use animals or simulated models to explore fetal alcohol syndrome. The following is typical of the type of information found when searching the CRISP database for fetal alcohol syndrome:

- **Project Title: A CROSS-CULTURAL LONGITUDINAL ASSESSMENT OF FASD (U24)**

  Principal Investigator & Institution: Foroud, Tatiana M.; Associate Professor; Molecular and Medical Genetics; Indiana Univ-Purdue Univ at Indianapolis 620 Union Drive, Room 618 Indianapolis, in 462025167

  Timing: Fiscal Year 2003; Project Start 30-SEP-2003; Project End 31-AUG-2006

  Summary: (provided by applicant): It has been demonstrated that anthropometric data can accurately distinguish individuals with **Fetal alcohol syndrome** (FAS) from those who were alcohol exposed but do not manifest the full spectrum of clinical features, and those who were not alcohol exposed [2]. A more efficient means to collect such data may be through three-dimensional (3-D) digitizing instruments, which can capture a facial image that can then be used to collect a wide range of known and novel clinical variables. Through the collection of 3-D images from individuals of variable ethnicity, age and exposure histories, it should be possible to identify a series of variables that effectively discriminate individuals who were prenatally exposed to alcohol and the degree to which they were exposed, from those who were not exposed. The goal of this collaboration is to analyze three-dimensional (3-D) facial images from individuals of variable ethnicity, age and history of alcohol exposure. The analyses of 3-D facial imaging will be developed and utilized for more effective clinical diagnosis of FAS, as well as the more broadly defined FASD. In addition, we believe these studies will generate important insight regarding the changes that occur in the face both prenatally and postnatally that produce the clinical features associated with FAS and thereby provide improved understanding of the pathophysiological effects of ethanol on human development. To accomplish these goals we propose the following specific aims: 1) Train and supervise personnel at each recruitment site to ensure collection of standardized data; 2) Analyze the 3-D facial imaging data to identify the measurements that most efficiently differentiate alcohol exposed from control subjects; 3) Utilize algorithms and methods derived from the emerging field of Automated Facial Recognition (AFR) to extract and identify the most discriminating higher order surface features from 3-D facial images, with the goal of developing an automated method of identifying facial features diagnostic of prenatal alcohol exposure; and 4) Combine the results from the direct and higher order measurements derived from the 3-D facial imaging with variables collected from other study domains to improve the power to accurately discriminate alcohol exposed from control subjects and to better understand the pathophysiological effects of ethanol on human development.

  Website: http://crisp.cit.nih.gov/crisp/Crisp_Query.Generate_Screen

- **Project Title: ACUTE BRAIN INJURY, MECHANISMS AND CONSEQUENCES**

  Principal Investigator & Institution: Olney, John W.; Professor; Psychiatry; Washington University Lindell and Skinker Blvd St. Louis, Mo 63130

  Timing: Fiscal Year 2002; Project Start 21-FEB-2002; Project End 31-JAN-2007

  Summary: (Adapted from applicant's abstract): This is an application to support studies aimed at clarifying the role(s) of excitotoxic and /or apoptotic cell death mechanisms in developmental (perinatal) brain injury associated with head trauma and hypoxia/ischemia. In addition to addressing these aims during the application period, the investigator has made the unanticipated discovery that during the synaptogenesis period of development transient ethanol intoxication triggers a massive wave of apoptotic neurodegeneration, deleting millions of neurons from many different regions of the developing rat, mouse, or guinea pig brain. Our findings document that ethanol triggers apoptosis by a dual mechanism - blockade of NMDA glutamate receptors and excessive activation of GABAA receptors. We propose that our findings can help explain the reduced brain mass and lifelong neurobehavioral disturbances associated with the human **fetal alcohol syndrome** (FAS). Significance of this discovery is broadened by accompanying evidence that ethanol's neurotoxic properties are shared by numerous other agents that either block NMDA glutamate receptors or activate GABAA receptors, and many of these agents are drugs of abuse and/or are used regularly in obstetric and pediatric medicine. An important feature of our findings is that within the synaptogenesis period (first 2 weeks after birth for rats and mice, but third trimester and first several years after birth for humans) different neuronal populations have different temporal patterns for responding to the apoptosis-inducing effects of these drugs. Thus, depending on the timing of exposure, different combinations of neuronal groups will be deleted.

  Website: http://crisp.cit.nih.gov/crisp/Crisp_Query.Generate_Screen

- **Project Title: ALCOHOL AND CELL ADHESION**

  Principal Investigator & Institution: Charness, Michael E.; Professor; Neurology; Harvard University (Medical School) Medical School Campus Boston, Ma 02115

  Timing: Fiscal Year 2001; Project Start 01-MAY-2001; Project End 31-JAN-2006

  Summary: (Adapted from the Investigator's Abstract) Ethanol inhibits cell adhesion mediated by the L1 cell adhesion molecule in neural cells and fibroblasts transfected with human L1. Because the brains of children with L1 mutations resemble those of children with **fetal alcohol syndrome**, it is possible that inhibition of L1-mediated cell adhesion contributes to the teratogenic effects of ETOH. Structure activity analysis of a series of straight and branch-chain alcohols demonstrates remarkable structural specificity for alcohol inhibition of cell-cell adhesion. Moreover, we have identified a series of compounds that antagonize the effects of ethanol on L1-mediated cell-cell adhesion, on BMP morphogenesis in cultured neural cells, and on the development of mouse whole embryo cultures. The underlying hypothesis of this proposal is that compounds that antagonize ethanol inhibition of L1-mediated cell-cell adhesion will also antagonize ethanol teratogenesis. The proposed research has three specific aims: 1. To identify the structural determinants of alcohols and related compounds that are required for inhibition of cell-cell adhesion in L1-expressing cells and for antagonism of this inhibition; 2. To characterize regions of L1 that are necessary for alcohol inhibition and for antagonism of ethanol inhibition; 3. To evaluate selective ethanol antagonists for their ability to prevent the teratogenic effects of ethanol in mouse whole embryo culture and during early embryogenesis in C57BL/6J mice. Techniques employed in these studies will include mammalian cell transfection, cell-aggregation assays, mutagenesis of the L1 molecule, mouse whole embryo culture, and macroscopic and microscopic analysis of mice exposed to ethanol in utero. These experiments may lead to a better understanding of how ethanol interacts with neural proteins and may reveal mechanisms whereby ethanol causes birth defects. A major goal of the proposed research is to identify compounds that reduce the teratogenic effects of ethanol.

Website: http://crisp.cit.nih.gov/crisp/Crisp_Query.Generate_Screen

- **Project Title: ALCOHOL AND DEVELOPMENT–EFFECTS ON CEREBELLAR SYSTEMS**

Principal Investigator & Institution: Goodlett, Charles R.; Professor; Psychology; Indiana Univ-Purdue Univ at Indianapolis 620 Union Drive, Room 618 Indianapolis, in 462025167

Timing: Fiscal Year 2001; Project Start 08-SEP-1998; Project End 31-MAY-2003

Summary: (from applicant's abstract) Prenatal exposure to alcohol can damage the central nervous system (CNS) and produce life-long learning disabilities, but there is unexplained variability in the observed effects. Different patterns, durations, and timing of drinking episodes during pregnanc may have major influences on the extent of damage, but systematic analysis still is needed in animal models. There has never been integrated, systematic analysis of alcohol-induced effects on the structural integrity and functional plasticity within a defined neural system that has a known, essential role in mediating associative learning. Such an effort requires a well-defined animal model with control over the alcohol exposure, in which the damage involves a key CNS structure and models human outcomes. The behavioral responses and neuronal correlates of learning must be operationally defined and precisely measured, and the neural circuits mediating the associative learning must be known. The studies proposed in this application fulfill each of these requirements. Binge alcohol exposure of neonatal rats has been extensively characterized as a model of third trimester exposure. Dose-related loss of cerebellar neurons during an early neonatal period of enhanced vulnerability i now well established, and the structural damage is similar to effects seen in MRI studies of prenatally exposed children. Recent studies have found that neonatal binge exposure induces profound impairments in classical conditioning of eyeblink responses. Cerebellar mediation of eyeblink conditioning is one of the best-understood models of mammalian associative learning in neuroscience. The components of the cerebellar-brainstem circuit essential for learned eyeblink responses, i.e., the deep cerebellar nuclei, cerebellar cortex, inferior olive, and pontine nuclei, appear to be targets of alcohol neurotoxicity in development. Five specific aims are proposed to test this by evaluating alcohol-induced deficits in structure, functional plasticity, and behavior. Aim 1 will evaluate the deficits in eyeblink conditioning in juveniles and adults, including an assessment of threshold, dose-response, and will extend the analysis to complex motor learning for adults. Aim 2 will determine the extent of cell loss in the four populations, using the same rats tested in Aim 1. Aim 3 will systematically assess learning-related neuronal activity and plasticity in the four areas. Aim 4 will evaluate neonatal temporal windows of vulnerability to structural and behavioral effects. Aim 5 will test whether the cerebellar effects are observed with gestational exposur or whether exposure that extends into the hypothesized critical period of vulnerability is required for cerebellar damage.

Website: http://crisp.cit.nih.gov/crisp/Crisp_Query.Generate_Screen

- **Project Title: ALCOHOL AND STRESS—INTERACTIVE EFFECTS**

  Principal Investigator & Institution: Weinberg, Joanne K.; Professor; University of British Columbia 2075 Wesbrook Pl Vancouver,

  Timing: Fiscal Year 2001; Project Start 01-AUG-1988; Project End 31-MAY-2003

  Summary: (Adapted from the Investigator's Abstract) The ability to respond to stress is an important basic adaptive mechanism; hypothalamic-pituitary-adrenal (HPA) activation is known to be a central feature of this response. Hyperresponsiveness and/or deficits in recovery of HPA activity following stress could have adverse behavioral and physiological consequences for the organism and thus hyperresponsiveness, as well as altered behavioral and immune responsiveness, particularly following exposure to stressors. The present proposal will investigate mechanisms mediating the effects of prenatal ethanol exposure on HPA regulation as well as the role of the HPA hormones in mediating the alterations in immune function seen in E offspring. The Specific Aims are 1) to explore further the mechanisms underlying the increased HPA activity observed in E animals. Experiments will test two possible and not incompatible hypotheses: a) that HPA hyper-responsiveness in E animals result, at least in part, from deficits in feedback regulation of the HPA axis. Experiments will examine effects of repeated exposure to restraint (increased HPA activity and feedback) and of adrenalectomy (adx, removal of the feedback signal) and corticosterone (CORT) replacement (restoration of the feedback signal) on plasma hormone levels, hypothalamic and pituitary gene expression, and hippocampal glucocorticoid receptor gene expression ND activation; b) that HPA hyper-responsiveness in E animals results, at least in part, from enhanced stimulatory input to the HPA axis. Experiments will examine effects of acute and repeated restraint stress and/or of adx and CORT replacement on hypothalamic and pituitary gene expression, corticotropin releasing fracture (CRF) and CRF1 receptor expression, and pituitary CRF binding protein expression. 2) to examine effects of prenatal ethanol exposure on immune function of offspring. Experiments will test the hypothesis that the HPA hyper-responsiveness induced by prenatal ethanol may mediate at least in part the adverse changes in immune competence of E animals. Experiments will examine the role of HPA hormones in mediating altered antibody responses, and the role of the transcription factor NF-kB in mediating possible CORT-induced immunosuppression. The proposed work will have relevance to our understanding of the adverse effects of prenatal ethanol on adaptive functioning in adulthood.

  Website: http://crisp.cit.nih.gov/crisp/Crisp_Query.Generate_Screen

- **Project Title: ALCOHOL SERVER EDUCATION AS A FAS PREVENTION METHOD**

  Principal Investigator & Institution: Dresser, Jack W.; Oregon Research Institute 1715 Franklin Blvd Eugene, or 97403

  Timing: Fiscal Year 2001; Project Start 24-SEP-1999; Project End 30-JUN-2004

  Summary: Fetal alcohol syndrome is by some estimates the leading cause of developmental disability in the Western world, and one which is entirely preventable. Efforts at prevention heretofore have been largely clinic-based, which fails to access many high-risk women in time to intervene effectively. This study will investigate the potential effectiveness of intervention in another venue perhaps more frequently visited by drinking gravidas than the prenatal clinic: the public drinking establishment. Much damage can be prevented by intervention in the second trimester, when pregnancy is ordinarily visible to others such as alcohol service personnel. This study has two principle goals. First, we will examine the effectiveness of alcohol server training legislation to prevent FAS, comparing two approaches and a control: state-mandated training in two states with varying degrees of formal emphasis on FAS, and one state with no formal server training system. Second, we will develop, provide, and evaluate the effectiveness of a supplementary server training program in FAS prevention under all three state systems. Dependent variables measuring implementation and effectiveness will include: FAS knowledge, attitudes, and establishment policies assessed by large sample mail surveys; knowledge, attitudes, and self-reported practices of servers assessed by interviews in subsamples of establishments; observed server adherence to responsible practices using pseudopatrons in subsamples of establishments; and records of self-referrals to community health resources by gravidas resulting from server interventions.

Website: http://crisp.cit.nih.gov/crisp/Crisp_Query.Generate_Screen

- **Project Title: AN ENHANCED BRIEF INTERVENTION FOR PRENATAL ALCOHOL USE**

Principal Investigator & Institution: Chang, Grace; Brigham and Women's Hospital 75 Francis Street Boston, Ma 02115

Timing: Fiscal Year 2001; Project Start 27-SEP-1999; Project End 31-AUG-2003

Summary: No universally safe level of prenatal alcohol consumption has been identified. The consequences of drinking while pregnant range from subtle developmental problems to **fetal alcohol syndrome.** Yet, the rate of frequent drinking by pregnant women has increased substantially in recent years. Brief interventions have been generally recommended as the first approach to treatment for mild to moderate alcohol problems, and their effectiveness documented in several well designed studies. Pregnant women at risk for antenatal consumption are an especially appropriate group to receive brief interventions, given the potential consequences of prenatal drinking and the relative infrequency of dependent alcohol use in this population. Our previous efforts to improve the identification and modification of alcohol use in pregnancy have demonstrated higher rates of abstinence among women randomized to a brief intervention. The purpose of this study is to test the effectiveness of an enhanced brief intervention involving an individual chosen by the pregnant woman. This support partner will assist in the maintenance and application of skills learned as a result of the brief intervention. Three hundred pregnant women initiating prenatal care, who are alcohol screen positive and currently drinking, or drank during a previous pregnancy, or drank at least one drink daily before pregnancy will be randomized to either the enhanced brief intervention with assessment or assessment only. The aim specific to this proposed randomized clinical trial is to test the hypothesis that 70 percent of the women will be abstinent after the enhanced brief intervention in contrast to 50 percent of the women after the assessment only. This proposed study seeks interventions to prevent drinking by pregnant women, and builds upon our previous research by incorporating advances in feminine psychology which recognize the importance of relationships in women's lives.

Website: http://crisp.cit.nih.gov/crisp/Crisp_Query.Generate_Screen

- **Project Title: ANALYZING FUNCTIONAL AND STRUCTURAL MRI IN FAS CHILDREN**

Principal Investigator & Institution: Sowell, Elizabeth R.; Assistant Professor; Neurology; University of California Los Angeles 10920 Wilshire Blvd., Suite 1200 Los Angeles, Ca 90024

Timing: Fiscal Year 2002; Project Start 27-SEP-2002; Project End 30-JUN-2005

Summary: (provided by applicant): The overarching goal of the proposed studies is to understand better the effects of severe prenatal alcohol exposure on the structure and function of the developing human brain by using advanced image analysis technology to combine functional and structural magnetic resonance imaging (MRI) data. While severe prenatal exposure to alcohol is known to cause mental retardation and generalized microcephaly, little is yet known about the subtler toxic effects of prenatal alcohol exposure on brain structure and function. Recent structural MRI studies have shown brain shape abnormalities in parietal and anterior frontal brain regions in alcohol-exposed individuals that exceed their generalized microcephaly. One might expect brain functional activity to be altered in regions of brain structural abnormality, but to date, no functional MRI studies have been reported in the **fetal alcohol syndrome** (FAS) literature. In these proposed studies, we will assess differences in brain activation between children and adolescents with FAS and those who were not exposed to alcohol prenatally. We expect that regional patterns of functional abnormality will parallel regional patterns of structural abnormality. Advanced image analysis technology is required to address this issue when the groups to be compared have different brain shapes. Traditional functional image analysis techniques require brain image data to be scaled into standard space, typically by using automated procedures. Unfortunately, brain anatomy is less likely to be well matched with the automated algorithms in regions where brain shape differs between groups, greatly reducing the likelihood that subtle differences in brain function can be measured in these regions. We will address this problem by refining existing and developing new high-dimensional continuum mechanical image warping algorithms to align functional images of FAS and control subjects based on gyral landmarks identified in each individual's structural image data. We will design functional MRI experimental paradigms which have been shown to recruit both structurally "normal" and structurally "abnormal" brain regions to assess the specificity of alteration in brain function, and we will compare results from the more traditional and the novel spatial normalization procedures. The results of these studies will help us in planning intervention strategies to optimize development in FAS children and provide more optimal image analysis techniques for other pediatric populations.

Website: http://crisp.cit.nih.gov/crisp/Crisp_Query.Generate_Screen

- **Project Title: ARND--IMPACT ON SYNAPTIC PLASTICITY MECHANISMS**

Principal Investigator & Institution: Perrone-Bizzozero, Nora I.; Professor of Neurosciences; Biochem and Molecular Biology; University of New Mexico Albuquerque Controller's Office Albuquerque, Nm 87131

Timing: Fiscal Year 2001; Project Start 01-FEB-1998; Project End 31-JAN-2003

Summary: (Adapted from the Investigator's Abstract) Learning disabilities are among the most subtle yet most pervasive deficits related to prenatal alcohol exposure in children. These learning deficits, which may not become apparent until a child is school-aged, can occur in the absence of other physical evidence of **alcohol-related birth defects.** Offspring of rats exposed to moderate levels of alcohol during gestation also show a significant impairment in learning when tested as young adults, validating the use of this animal model in studies of the effect of fetal alcohol exposure (FAE). Initial studies by our integrative research program suggested that these deficits are related to specific alterations in synaptic plasticity mechanisms which correlated with a failure in the establishment of long-term potentiation (LTP). The long-term objectives of this Integrated Research Program Grant (IRPG) are two-fold: 1)to delineate more clearly the molecular and neurochemical alterations of synaptic plasticity mechanisms caused by prenatal alcohol exposure and 2) to explore new treatment strategies to overcome these deficits. The overall hypothesis for the IRPG is that prenatal exposure to moderate levels of ethanol produces multiple defects in the mechanisms underlying glutamate levels of ethanol produces multiple defects in the mechanisms underlying glutamate receptor-dependent LTP in the hippocampus and medial frontal cortex. The specific goal of Project 3 in this IRPG is to define the impact of FAE on the levels and function of proteins involved in synaptic plasticity mechanisms. Based upon preliminary studies, our hypothesis is that protein kinase C (PKC) activity and the levels and phosphorylation of GAP-43 and other important plasticity-associated proteins is altered in specific brain regions of FAE rats. To test this idea, we propose the following Specific Aims: 1)to study PKC activity and the phosphorylation of GAP-43 and other PKC substrate proteins in the hippocampus and medial frontal cortex of FAE rats, both under basal conditions and after electrical stimulation 2)to examine the impact of FAE on activity-dependent changes in GAP-43 phosphorylation and gene expression during behavioral conditioning, 3) to characterize the causes for the deficit in PKC activity in FAE rats and to evaluate its significance in synaptic plasticity mechanisms and 4) to investigate the effects of different pharmacological treatments on PKC activity and GAP-43 phosphorylation in control and FAE rats and 5) to relate these to the behavioral and electrophysicological properties of the animals. The identification of the neurochemical basis for the alterations in synaptic plasticity in the hippocampus and medial frontal cortices of FAE rats will improve our understanding of the effects of prenatal alcohol exposure in the function of these important brain structures. Ultimately, this information will help design better therapeutic strategies to overcome behavioral and cognitive deficits in children affected with Alcohol Related Neurodevelopmental Disorders (ARND).

Website: http://crisp.cit.nih.gov/crisp/Crisp_Query.Generate_Screen

- **Project Title: AXONAL AND DENDRITIC DIFFERENTIATION IN GRANULE NEURONS**

Principal Investigator & Institution: Carr, Catherine E.; Professor; Zoology; University of Maryland College Pk Campus College Park, Md 20742

Timing: Fiscal Year 2001; Project Start 01-JUL-1997; Project End 31-MAY-2003

Summary: The objective of this proposal is to understand the mechanisms that control axonal and dendritic differentiation and morphology in granule neurons. To determine how cues intrinsic to the cell, or present in the extracellular environment, direct the differentiation and maturation of granule cell axons and dendrites, the following hypotheses will be tested: 1) The initial site of unipolar process extension is determined by the cytoplasmic location of the Golgi apparatus; after unipolar extension, the GA re-orients within the cytoplasm to support the growth of the second axonal process. To test this hypothesis, time-lapse confocal microscopy will be used to determine the dynamic behavior of the GA during the initial stages of granule clel axon outgrowth in. 2) After initial bipolar parallel fiber (PF) axon outgrowth is completed, diffusible or contact-mediated signals from developing Purkinje cells (PC) and/or granule cells within the molecular layer (ML) cause a down-regulation in expression of the axonal cell adhesion molecule, TAG-1, on granule cells located at the deep external granule layer (EGL)/ML border. To test this hypothesis, it will determined whether granule cell/PC contact in , or conditions that mimic the onset of synaptic activity between granule cells and Pcs, provide an "off-signal" for TAG-1 expression on initial granule cell axons. 3) Exposure of immature granule cells to depolarizing conditions inhibits axonogenesis and promotes dendritic differentiation. To test this hypothesis, immature granule cells will be exposed to depolarizing condition from the time of plating in. 4) Complete granule cell dendritic differentiation, which is characterized by the formation of characteristic claw-like dendrites, proceeds only after direct cell-cell contact with mossy fiber afferents. To test this hypothesis, granule cells will be co-cultured with pontine explants to provide a source of mossy fiber afferent input, to determine whether direct cell-cell contact with mossy fibers 'drives' further dendritic differentiation. Understanding the mechanisms that control the normal differentiation of granule neurons is critical in understanding the etiology of the various cerebellar ataxias and birth defects such as **fetal alcohol syndrome.**

Website: http://crisp.cit.nih.gov/crisp/Crisp_Query.Generate_Screen

- **Project Title: BEHAVIORAL, EEG, AND MRI EVALUATION OF PRENATAL ALCOHOL**

Principal Investigator & Institution: Riley, Edward P.; Professor; Psychology; San Diego State University 5250 Campanile Dr San Diego, Ca 92182

Timing: Fiscal Year 2001; Project Start 01-JAN-1995; Project End 31-DEC-2003

Summary: Fetal alcohol syndrome (FAS) encompasses a broad range of disabilities involving both structural and functional changes. Among the most devastating effects are those caused by alterations in the central nervous system (CNS). These CNS changes result in the cognitive and behavioral deficits reported in most studies of FAS. In addition, there is a growing body of literature that suggests that brain and behavioral changes can occur in the absence of the facial features required for an FAS diagnosis. In our study, children with heavy prenatal exposure to alcohol (PEA), who do not have the obvious physical features of FAS, show changes in both brain and behavior similar to those seen in FAS. Previous work has documented broad, fairly general, deficits in general intellectual ability. More recently, attention has been paid to specific aspects of neuropsychological functioning, documenting deficits as well as relative strengths across various cognitive domains. Needed is greater understanding of the details of these strengths and weaknesses. This level of examination, coupled with brain imaging, will provide the framework for intervention and remediation strategies for alcohol-exposed children. The proposed project is multidisciplinary in nature, including neuropsychological assessment, magnetic resonance imaging (MRI), and electrophysiological evaluation. This proposal represents a continuation of work that we have been conducting for the last three years. We plan to continue our general evaluation and are proposing to expand the investigation of our three research domains. In the neuropsychological domain, in addition to our general test battery, we are proposing specific measures of learning, memory, and emotional functioning. In the MRI component, along with continuing to evaluate brain structure in children with FAS and PEA, we are proposing a study of developmental brain changes and a pilot study in functional MRI. Finally, in the electrophysiological component, we are proposing to continue to collect EEG and ERP data on children with PEA as well as a new component addressing emotional responses in alcohol-exposed children. We believe that our approach has been successful thus far, and that this multidisciplinary project will expand our understanding of the devastating effects of prenatal alcohol exposure, perhaps leading to new treatment strategies.

Website: http://crisp.cit.nih.gov/crisp/Crisp_Query.Generate_Screen

- **Project Title: BRAIN DEVELOPMENT & ETHANOL: MICROGLIAL PATHOGENESIS**

  Principal Investigator & Institution: Kane, Cynthia Jm.; Associate Professor; Anatomy; University of Arkansas Med Scis Ltl Rock 4301 W Markham St Little Rock, Ar 72205

  Timing: Fiscal Year 2001; Project Start 01-JUL-2000; Project End 30-JUN-2003

  Summary: Intervention in the extensive CNS pathology that underlies **fetal alcohol syndrome** is a high priority for alcohol researchers and is the long-term goal of this laboratory. There is no treatment for the brain damage associated with fetal ethanol exposure since the cellular and molecular mechanisms by which ethanol causes developmental neuropathogenesis are not yet understood. Although many years of study have focused on the neuronal and macroglial pathology caused by ethanol, the impact of ethanol upon an important, major cell type in the brain - the microolial cell - has not been probed until these recent studies. This is surprising since ethanol damage to microglia may produce serious consequences within developing neuronal populations. Microglia communicate directly with neurons and the immune system to influence neuronal survival and function. They are the first line of defense against CNS insults, are the principal immune cells within the brain, and are active in cytokine secretion, reactive oxygen species secretion, antigen presentation and phagocytosis. Pilot studies reveal that damage to microglia occurs at ethanol concentrations far below that required to cause direct neuronal death. Parallel studies in the cerebellum and cultures of microglia have led to the HYPOTHESIS that ethanol pathogenesis in microglia occurs via specific cellular mechanisms: (1) ethanol inhibits microglial genesis and survival, (2) ethanol suppresses microglial maturation to further reduce the population of mature microglia, (3) the activity and functionality of microglia are impaired as a result, and (4) since there is no turnover of microglia, the impaired microglial functionality persists in the adult. This study will define the mechanisms of ethanol pathogenesis within the microglial population. A causal relationship between microglial pathology and neuronal toxicity will be defined. The critical period of microglial sensitivity to the teratogenic effects of ethanol will be determined. The acute, transient or persistent nature of ethanol pathogenesis within the microglial population will be distinguished. The molecular mechanisms of ethanol activity will be identified. The intracellular signaling pathways underlying ethanol activity will be manipulated in order to block ethanol pathogenesis in microglia. Block of ethanol-induced microglial pathology may provide a new opportunity to intervene in the brain damage caused by fetal ethanol exposure.

  Website: http://crisp.cit.nih.gov/crisp/Crisp_Query.Generate_Screen

- **Project Title: BRAIN GLUCOSE TRANSPORT AND UTILIZATION IN FAS**

  Principal Investigator & Institution: Snyder, Ann; Associate Professor, Research; Pharmacol & Molecular Biology; Finch Univ of Hlth Sci/Chicago Med Sch North Chicago, Il 60064

  Timing: Fiscal Year 2001; Project Start 01-FEB-1998; Project End 31-JAN-2002

  Summary: (Adapted from the Investigator's Abstract) Mechanisms of ethanol-induced damage of developing brain remain to be elucidated. In cultures of rat astrocytes or intact embryos, ethanol inhibits both glucose transport and glucose oxidation via the pentose phosphate pathway (PPP). Developmental changes in the expression of brain glucose transporters, GLUT 1 and GLUT 3, suggest that these genes are regulated to meet the changing metabolic requirements of immature brain. Glucose is not only the primary energy substrate of brain, but its oxidation via the PPP is essential for production of ribose-5-phosphate which is necessary for synthesis of nucleosides and polysaccharides. The PPP is also involved in the production of NADPH for removal of free radicals and synthesis of lipids and neurotransmitters. Brief exposure to ethanol during the brain growth spurt reduces glucose transport, as well as GLUT 1 and GLUT3 proteins of neurons and astrocytes. It is proposed that these reductions result from specific regulation of the GLUT1 and GLUT3 genes by ethanol. This regulation may differ for the two transporter isoforms, and is likely to involve post-transcriptional mechanisms. In vitro studies with astrocytes and rat embryos also show that ethanol specifically inhibits activity of the PPP. It is proposed that PPP is particularly vulnerable to reduced glucose transport and that reduced activity of this pathway has significant toxicological impact on cells with critical requirements for its products. Goals of the proposed research will be to identify and characterize the mechanism by which ethanol alters glucose transporter expression in neurons and glia of developing brain. Proposed studies will use immunocytochemistry and in situ hybridization histochemistry for detecting regional changes in transporter proteins and mRNAs and for quantitation of mRNAs by northern analysis and nuclear transcription assays in specific brain regions. Transporter proteins and mRNA stabilities and post-transcriptional mechanisms will be studied in cultured neurons, astrocytes and oligodendroglia. The second major aim will be to characterize alterations in glucose utilization, indicators of oxidative stress and parameters of cell function and viability under the same conditions and to define the toxicological significance of these effects, including those on intercellular relations which might affect growth or survival.

Website: http://crisp.cit.nih.gov/crisp/Crisp_Query.Generate_Screen

- **Project Title: BRIEF ALCOHOL INTERVENTION--HEALTHY MOMS PROJECT**

Principal Investigator & Institution: Fleming, Michael F.; Professor; Family Medicine; University of Wisconsin Madison 750 University Ave Madison, Wi 53706

Timing: Fiscal Year 2001; Project Start 01-JUL-2001; Project End 31-MAR-2006

Summary: Background: The prevention of **Fetal Alcohol Syndrome** and fetal alcohol exposure is an important national priority. A 1995 national survey conducted by the Centers for Disease Control estimates that as many as 140,000 children born in the US are exposed to. potentially harmful effects of alcohol. during fetal development (3.5% of 4 million live births). One prevention strategy is to establish screening and intervention procedures that can be administered in primary care settings to women who are drinking above recommended limits. Goal: This study is designed to test the efficacy of a primary care-based brief intervention for women who resume heavy drinking during the post partum period and who used alcohol during their last pregnancy. The ultimate goal is to reduce alcohol use, alcohol-related harm, and fetal alcohol exposure in subsequent pregnancies. Method: The trial will utilize methods successfully employed by the PI in three brief intervention trials (Project TrEAT, Project GOAL, and an ongoing trial in Poland). Women will be asked to complete an embedded alcohol questionnaire (Health Screening Survey) while seeing their obstetrician for a routine post partum visit. Women who screen positive for heavy drinking (>7 drinks/week in the past month, 4 or more drinks/occasion, or two or more positive responses on the T-ACE) will be invited by a researcher to participate in a health interview. Women who meet eligibility criteria for the trial will be randomized to a usual care control group or a physician/nurse brief intervention group. The intervention will consist of two 10-15 minute physician/nurse visits and two 2- minute follow-up phone calls. All subjects will be contacted at 6, 12, 18 and 24 months by telephone to assess outcomes of interest which include alcohol use, quality of life, mental health problems, accidents, and health care utilization. Power analysis suggests that 250 women in each arm of the trial will have sufficient power to detect a difference for the main outcome variables of interest. Significance: The proposed study would significantly increase our understanding of how to reduce alcohol use in post partum patients and how to limit FAS and fetal alcohol exposure.

Website: http://crisp.cit.nih.gov/crisp/Crisp_Query.Generate_Screen

- **Project Title: BRIEF INTERVENTION TO PREVENT PRENATAL ALCOHOL USE**

Principal Investigator & Institution: Kraemer, Kevin L.; Medicine; University of Pittsburgh at Pittsburgh 350 Thackeray Hall Pittsburgh, Pa 15260

Timing: Fiscal Year 2001; Project Start 23-SEP-1999; Project End 31-AUG-2003

Summary: Prenatal alcohol use by women is the most frequent and preventable known cause of mental retardation and birth defects in the United States. Although most women who drink abstain from alcohol after learning they are pregnant, 10 percent to 20 percent continue to drink during pregnancy and many will return to levels of alcohol intake after delivery that place their next pregnancy at risk. Brief motivational interventions to encourage women to change their prenatal alcohol use have the potential to prevent alcohol-related injury to the fetus in the current and subsequent pregnancies. The specific aims of this randomized, controlled, single-blinded, study are to: 1) assess the effect of brief motivational interventions on the alcohol intake of women during pregnancy and at 12 months postpartum, 2) assess how readiness to change and self-efficacy for change moderate or mediate the relationship between brief intervention and alcohol use, 3) identify maternal and intervention factors that predict drinking behaviors and mediate the effect of brief intervention, and 4) determine in what way the knowledge, attitudes, and beliefs of the significant other (male partner, family member, or friend) affect maternal alcohol use following intervention. The primary hypothesis of this study is that, compared to usual care, women randomized to the brief intervention group will be more likely to abstain or to significantly decrease alcohol intake during pregnancy and at 12 months postpartum. Pregnant women presenting for their first prenatal clinic visit will be screened for alcohol use. Four hundred twenty-eight protocol-eligible subjects will be enrolled over an 18-month period and randomized to usual care or to brief intervention. Subjects in the brief intervention arm will meet with a nurse therapist for motivational interviews at time of enrollment, 4 and 8 weeks later, and at 6 weeks postpartum. The significant others of study subjects in the intervention arm will be given brief telephone advice on supporting healthy prenatal drinking behaviors at baseline and at 6 weeks postpartum. Research assistants who are blinded to treatment assignment will perform telephone assessments at 6 and 12 months postpartum, and in-person assessments of the study subject and newborn infant at delivery. The primary study outcome measure will be alcohol use during pregnancy and at 12 months postpartum. If proven effective, this type of intervention could be broadly implemented as a method to decrease the incidence of **fetal alcohol syndrome, alcohol-related birth defects,** and alcohol-related neurodevelopmental defects. This study will also provide valuable data on maternal and social factors that influence the effect of brief interventions and on which components of a brief intervention are most crucial for producing behavioral change in this population.

Website: http://crisp.cit.nih.gov/crisp/Crisp_Query.Generate_Screen

- **Project Title: CAM TARGETING /SIGNALING--FETAL ALCOHOL SYNDROME MODEL?**

Principal Investigator & Institution: Benson, Deanna L.; Associate Professor; Neurobiology; Mount Sinai School of Medicine of Nyu of New York University New York, Ny 10029

Timing: Fiscal Year 2001; Project Start 01-JUN-2001; Project End 31-MAY-2004

Summary: The neuropathology observed in **fetal alcohol syndrome** (FAS) is strikingly similar to that observed in humans with mutations in the cell adhesion molecule L1. Since these L1 mutations are known to disrupt extracellular adhesion and some are presumed to block intracellular signaling, the effects of FAS may be due in part to disrupted LI adhesive signal transduction during development. During development cell adhesion molecules (CAMS) mediate many of the cell-cell interactions essential for appropriate axon pathfinding and synapse formation. In order for CAMS to do this, they are restricted to particular cell types, targeted to either axons or dendrites, and in many cases, to particular regions within axons and dendrites. Virtually nothing is known about how CAMS become targeted to particular cellular domains, how they are retained or for molecules of the Ig superfamily, how adhesive signals are transduced from the surface to the cytoskeleton. The overall goal of this proposal is to define intracellular sorting strategies and signaling pathways that are employed by the axonal CAM L1 and to determine whether these strategies are undermined by exposure to alcohol. To do this, we will identify the molecular domains required to mediate some of the functions of L1 so that ultimately we may identify signaling pathways that are disrupted by alcohol during critical developmental. periods.

Website: http://crisp.cit.nih.gov/crisp/Crisp_Query.Generate_Screen

- **Project Title: CHRONIC BRAIN IMAGING USING FLUORESCENCE ENDOSCOPY**

Principal Investigator & Institution: Schnitzer, Mark J.; Applied Physics; Stanford University Stanford, Ca 94305

Timing: Fiscal Year 2003; Project Start 30-SEP-2003; Project End 31-JUL-2005

Summary: (provided by applicant): Many forms of drug addiction lead to longstanding behavioral sensitization and to changes in neural circuits that persist well after administration of the addictive substance is terminated. Neuronal changes can involve drug-induced alterations in patterns of gene expression, increased levels of particular proteins, or morphological changes in specific neuron types. These changes likely contribute to the enduring behavioral effects of drug addiction. Understanding of such long-lasting cellular changes is important for medical efforts towards counteracting their contributions to addiction and to cognitive deficits. Unfortunately, current studies are severely hampered by the dearth of methods that can track long-term progression of cellular properties in live animals. This proposal explores an exciting new in vivo imaging technology that will enable longitudinal studies of how abused substances affect individual neurons and neuronal dendrites. The proposed research will rely on newly developed high-resolution fluorescence endoscopes that are 350-1000 um in diameter and that enable in vivo imaging of neurons and dendrites with micron-scale resolution. The first specific aim seeks to establish the ability to monitor chronically individual neurons deep in the mammalian brain over days to months. This would be powerful for studying cellular consequences of drug abuse, because specific fluorescence probes can reveal changes in neuronal morphology, gene expression, or protein distribution. The second aim seeks to demonstrate the broad utility of this methodology by using chronic endoscopic imaging to visualize long-term structural effects of fetal ethanol exposure on mouse CA1 hippocampal pyramidal cell dendrites.

Website: http://crisp.cit.nih.gov/crisp/Crisp_Query.Generate_Screen

- **Project Title: CRANIOFACIAL DEFECTS IN ETHANOL-EXPOSED ZEBRAFISH**

  Principal Investigator & Institution: Ahlgren, Sara C.; None; California Institute of Technology Mail Code 201-15 Pasadena, Ca 91125

  Timing: Fiscal Year 2002; Project Start 30-SEP-2002; Project End 31-AUG-2003

  Summary: (provided by applicant): Craniofacial abnormalities are characteristic of embryonic exposure to alcohol. In typical **fetal alcohol syndrome** poor development of a number of facial features, all of which are derived from the cranial neural crest, is observed. This grant seeks to establish a zebrafish model to study the craniofacial defects associated with embryonic alcohol exposure, and to establish that such environmental insults produce craniofacial defects by interfering with normal signals that control growth. We will first establish what the optimal dose and time schedule for alcohol application is, with respect to deficits in cranial neural crest cells, taking into consideration doses which would be relevant to **fetal alcohol syndrome.** The zebrafish is an excellent model for comparing teratogens, like alcohol, with genetic defects, to determine what candidate genes might be altered by environmental conditions. In addition, it is possible to overexpress genes of interest by directed injection or transgenesis. The defects in **fetal alcohol syndrome** partially overlap with some features of holoprosencephaly, which is typically a more dramatic malformation of the central nervous system with associated midline facial features, arising from both genetic and environmental factors. One such genetic cause is a heterozygous mutation in the human Sonic Hedgehog gene. Partial inhibition of Sonic hedgehog in the chick embryo using function-blocking antibodies results in a phenotype similar to a mild holoprosencephaly that is intriguingly similar to **fetal alcohol syndrome.** The morphological similarity between embryos exposed to alcohol and partial inhibition of Sonic hedgehog suggests a potential mechanistic link. Zebrafish have multiple hedgehog genes, so it is possible that alcohol interferes with a common signaling pathway. To test the hypothesis that ethanol leads to cranial neural crest cell death via a decrease in the availability of zebrafish hedgehog genes, the experiments described in this grant will examine the effect of ethanol on the message levels of genes in the hedgehog signaling pathway. We will also examine the fate of cranial neural crest cells, as well as the growth of the craniofacial structures. We will further attempt to rescue the cranial neural crest cells after ethanol treatment by application of exogenous Sonic hedgehog. These experiments will lay the groundwork to expand our understanding of the mechanisms of craniofacial defects following embryonic exposure to alcohol.

  Website: http://crisp.cit.nih.gov/crisp/Crisp_Query.Generate_Screen

- **Project Title: CRANIOFACIAL MORPHOGENESIS IN PRENATAL ALCOHOL EXPOSURE**

  Principal Investigator & Institution: Smith, Susan M.; Associate Professor; Nutritional Sciences; University of Wisconsin Madison 750 University Ave Madison, Wi 53706

  Timing: Fiscal Year 2001; Project Start 01-JUL-1996; Project End 30-APR-2006

  Summary: Prenatal alcohol exposure (PAE) is the leading known cause of mental retardation and birth defects. Its teratogenicity originates, in part, through its initiation of apoptosis in critical cell populations. Under previous NIAAA support, we developed a chick embryo model of PAE and showed that ethanol causes the selective apoptosis of the neural crest, an embryonic cell population containing craniofacial and neuronal precursors. Here, we hypothesize that ethanol induces neural crest apoptosis by activating the phospholipase C-dependent release of intracellular Ca2+. This hypothesis is tested using pharmacologic approaches, taking advantage that we can locally target agonists and antagonists of Ca2+ signaling pathways to the premigratory neural crest in ovo, and thus test their ability to attenuate ethanol's effects upon the embryo. Experiments in this proposal test three sub-hypotheses: 1) Acute ethanol induces neural crest apoptosis by stimulating the release of intracellular Ca2+. The requirement for Ca2+ release is tested through the use of fluorescent Ca2+ indicators, Ca2+ ionophores and chelators, and the direct assay of downstream, Ca2+-dependent signaling proteins (CaM kinase, calcineurin). 2) Ethanol mobilizes intracellular Ca2+ and induces apoptosis by activating inositol triphosphate (IP3) receptors. Pharmacologic agonists and antagonists test that the ethanol-released Ca2+ originates from IP3-mediated stores; this IP3 release will be quantified directly. Potential contributions of ryanodine receptors and extracellular Ca2+ also are tested. 3) Ethanol's activation of Phospholipase C (PLC) is responsible for the Ca2+ release and neural crest apoptosis. PLC activation is measured by direct assay and by targeted inhibitors. Contributions of diacylglycerol, receptor-mediated tyrosine kinases, and receptor-mediated G proteins are investigated. these results address the molecular mechanism underlying the neural crest's sensitivity to ethanol, and, thus, contribute to understanding the basis for ethanol's teratogenicity. Results also may provide possible explanations for genetic-based variations in fetal responses to prenatal ethanol exposure.

Website: http://crisp.cit.nih.gov/crisp/Crisp_Query.Generate_Screen

- **Project Title: DEVELOPMENT ALCOHOL AND CIRCADIAN CLOCK FUNCTION**

Principal Investigator & Institution: Earnest, David J.; Associate Professor; Human Anatomy and Medical Neurobiology; Texas A&M University Health Science Ctr College Station, Tx 778433578

Timing: Fiscal Year 2001; Project Start 01-JUL-2001; Project End 31-MAR-2006

Summary: (Provided by applicant): It is estimated that 2,000-12,000 babies are born each year with **fetal alcohol syndrome** (FAS) (Stratton et al., 1996). By far the most debilitating feature of FAS in CNS dysfunction that results from structure are known to persist into adulthood. However, information on the long-term neurobehavioral correlates of this alcohol-related brain damage is limited. The circadian regulation of most body processes by the clock in the suprachiasmatic nucleus (SCN) represents an area in which limited information is available on the consequences of developmental alcohol exposure in humans or animal models. Offspring exposed to heavy maternal alcohol consumption during pregnancy have been reported to show disturbances in their sleep-wake patterns (Rosett et al., 1979). Consistent with this finding, our PRELIMINARY STUDIES demonstrate that alcohol exposure during the third trimester equivalent in rats produces permanent changes in the circadian rhythm of activity. Therefore, experiments in this proposal will utilize multidisciplinary approaches to examine the long-term effects of three different alcohol doses on the circadian rhythm of activity on the anatomical, cellular and molecular organization of the SCN clock. The patterns of wheel- running behavior in adult rats will be assessed for alcohol-related changes in fundamental properties such as circadian period and rhythm amplitude. Subsequent to this behavioral analysis, the SCN will be evaluated for evidence of general cell loss and perturbations in its rhythmic expression of the putative clock genes, Perl, Per2 and Cry2, and the output signals, vasopressin (AVP), vasoactive intestinal polypeptide (VIP) and brain-derived neurotrophic factor (BDNF). Unlike CNS involvement in the neural regulation of most other behaviors, the discrete localization of circadian clock function to the SCN provides a unique opportunity to identify cellular and molecular correlates of alcohol-related neurobehavioral disturbances. By determining how the SCN and its circadian function are affected by developmental alcohol exposure, these studies are expected to yield important information on the basic mechanisms underlying alcohol-induced brain injury during development. Such information could lead to new strategies in the treatment of known behavioral correlates of FAS related to sleep problems and to mental and physical disorders associated with sleep-wake abnormalities.

Website: http://crisp.cit.nih.gov/crisp/Crisp_Query.Generate_Screen

- **Project Title: DEVELOPMENTAL BIOLOGY AND PATHOLOGY CENTER**

Principal Investigator & Institution: Kinney, Hannah C.; Associate Professor; Children's Hospital (Boston) Boston, Ma 021155737

Timing: Fiscal Year 2003; Project Start 26-SEP-2003; Project End 31-JUL-2006

Summary: (provided by applicant): This application is a response to the Request for Application (RFA) entitled: Prenatal Alcohol Exposure Among High-Risk Populations: Relationship to Sudden Infant Death Syndrome (SIDS) (RFA: HD-03-004). Our group is applying for the award of the Developmental Biology and Pathology Center. As requested in the RFA, we plan to conduct basic and applied research related to molecular and biological aspects of alcohol related injury to the brain, systemic organs, and placenta in the subject population. We hypothesize that prenatal exposure to alcohol adversely affects the development of the serotonergic (5-HT) system in the medulla oblongata of the brainstem, and thereby puts the vulnerable fetus/infant at risk for sudden death by compromising an array of homeostatic reflexes which are all influenced by the medullary 5-HT neurons, and which protect the fetus/infant from life-threatening stressors, e.g., hypoxia, hypercarbia, and hypotension. This hypothesis is a direct outgrowth of our brainstem analysis in two independent databases of SIDS and control cases, including in the Northern Plains Indians, a high-risk population. We propose 5 Specific Aims for the sample study to examine inter-relationships between brainstem 5-HT and vasoactive intestinal peptide (VIP), the latter shown to play a pivotal role in the pathogenesis of alcohol-induced injury in animal models. In Specific Aim 1 we will determine if abnormalities in the medullary 5-HT system correlate with VIP abnormalities in this system in fetuses and/or infants with sudden death who were exposed to prenatal alcohol. In Specific Aim 2, we will determine if markers of oxidative stress correlate with5-HT-related abnormalities in the medullary 5-HT system in such fetuses/infants. In Specific Aim 3, we address the question if the same brainstem abnormalities reported by us in SIDS infants are present in unexplained stillbirth, data which would substantiate the idea that there is a continuum of disease-effect from the fetal period through infancy. In Specific Aim 4, we seek to know if polymorphisms or mutations in 5-HT-related markers are associated with medullary 5-HT system abnormalities and an increased risk for sudden death in fetuses/infants exposed to prenatal alcohol. In Specific Aim 5, we address issues related to VIP expression in the placenta, the key organ of maternal-fetal homeostasis, based upon reports of alcohol-induced reductions in placental VIP in animal models. These human studies should help provide the necessary critical steps to translate basic science findings into therapeutic strategies for the prevention or amelioration of prenatal alcohol-induced injury to the developing human brain.

Website: http://crisp.cit.nih.gov/crisp/Crisp_Query.Generate_Screen

- **Project Title: DEVELOPMENTAL NEUROTOXICITY OF ETHANOL**

Principal Investigator & Institution: Costa, Lucio G.; Professor; Environmental Health; University of Washington Seattle, Wa 98195

Timing: Fiscal Year 2003; Project Start 27-SEP-1991; Project End 30-APR-2006

Summary: This abstract is not available.

Website: http://crisp.cit.nih.gov/crisp/Crisp_Query.Generate_Screen

- **Project Title: DOPAMINE FUNCTION AFTER PRENATAL ETHANOL EXPOSURE**

Principal Investigator & Institution: Shen, Roh-Yu; Senior Research Scientist; None; State University of New York at Buffalo Suite 211 Ub Commons Amherst, Ny 14228

Timing: Fiscal Year 2001; Project Start 01-APR-1999; Project End 31-MAR-2004

Summary: Our previous studies demonstrate that prenatal ethanol exposure produces a persistent reduction in the electrical activity of midbrain dopamine neurons and alters dopamine receptor sensitivity. These changes are normalized by DA agonist administration. Midbrain DA neurotransmission is involved in many important CNS functions including reward, motor control attention, and locomotor activity. Therefore, prenatal ethanol exposure-induced dopamine hypofunction may contribute to the attention/hyperactivity problems commonly observed in children with fetal alcohol effects, **fetal alcohol syndrome** (FAE/FAS). In the proposed studies, we will use extracellular and intracellular electrophysiological recording techniques to further characterize the postnatal developmental process of dopamine systems that prenatal ethanol exposure. We will study how these changes may be normalized by dopamine agonists. We will also initiate behavioral experiments to correlate dopamine hypofunction and attention problems. In addition, the cellular leading to a reduction in the electrical activity of dopamine neurons after prenatal ethanol exposure will be examined. The results of these studies will better our understanding in the etiology of behavioral symptoms in FAE/FAS and help us to develop more appropriate animal models to advance the pharmacological treatment of FAE/FAS.

Website: http://crisp.cit.nih.gov/crisp/Crisp_Query.Generate_Screen

- **Project Title: DYSMORPHOLOGY CORE (U24 CORE)**

Principal Investigator & Institution: Jones, Kenneth L.; Pediatrics; University of California San Diego 9500 Gilman Dr, Dept. 0934 La Jolla, Ca 92093

Timing: Fiscal Year 2003; Project Start 30-SEP-2003; Project End 31-AUG-2006

Summary: (provided by applicant): Diagnosis of the Fetal Alcohol Spectrum Disorder (FASD) is dependent on the identification of a pattern of malformation including alterations in growth and neurobehavioral development as well as a constellation of specific minor craniofacial anomalies. In that a neurobehavioral phenotype specific for prenatal alcohol exposure has not yet been identified, it is presently not possible to diagnose FASD in the absence of the clinical phenotype. It will be the responsibility of the Dysmorphology Core to assure accurate and consistent diagnosis of FASD in children at all consortium sites through implementation of a standard protocol based on documentation of the clinical phenotype which will be used at all sites. In that this consortium will integrate investigators from different sites throughout the world, it is imperative to have a small core of individuals with extensive experience in evaluation of children prenatally exposed to alcohol responsible for diagnosis of FASD at all sites. Identification of large numbers of children with FASD at various ages, each of whom has received a standardized clinical evaluation will provide the opportunity to gain new insight into a variety of issues relating to the clinical phenotype including the full range of structural defects in the disorder, physical features that are predictive of alterations in neurobehavioral development, the extent to which degrees of growth deficiency should be used to enhance specificity of diagnosis without loss of sensitivity, and will provide the opportunity to develop strategies to diagnose this disorder in the newborn period.

Website: http://crisp.cit.nih.gov/crisp/Crisp_Query.Generate_Screen

- **Project Title: ECONOMIC ANALYSIS OF FAS PREVENTIVE INTERVENTION**

Principal Investigator & Institution: Kenkel, Donald S.; Interim Director and Associate Professor; Policy Analysis & Management; Cornell University Ithaca Office of Sponsored Programs Ithaca, Ny 14853

Timing: Fiscal Year 2001; Project Start 19-SEP-2000; Project End 31-JUL-2004

Summary: (Adapted from applicant's abstract): The proposed study will conduct econometric investigations of four types of naturally occurring interventions that have the potential to prevent **fetal alcohol syndrome** and fetal alcohol effects. First, the project will extend economics research on the effectiveness of alcohol tax and availability policies to examine their role in reducing alcohol consumption and abuse by pregnant women. Second, the project will examine the extent to which alcohol consumption by pregnant women is reduced by state and local legislation, requiring point of sale alcohol health warning signs. Third, the project will employ econometric methodology to estimate the treatment effect of the receipt of physician advice on alcohol consumption by pregnant women. Fourth, the project will re-visit the impact of the 1989 federal requirement of warning labels on alcohol beverage containers. To accomplish these aims, the project will analyze data from the 1988 National Maternal and Infant Health Survey (NMIHS) conducted by the National Center for Health Statistics. The public use national files provide a sample of almost 19,000 pregnant women. The data contain measures of the women's alcohol consumption, prenatal care, and receipt of advice from a health care professional about drinking while pregnant. Information on state alcoholic beverage tax rates and legal requirements for point-of-sale alcohol health warning signs will be merged with the individual-level data in the NMIHS. The project will also use the 1991 Longitudinal Follow-up Survey to the 1988 NMIHS to investigate the impact of alcohol beverage warning labels. By fortunate timing, the 1988 NMIHS and its 1991 Follow-up Survey provide information on pregnant women's alcohol consumption before and after the implementation of required alcohol beverage warning labels. The results of the study will provide estimates of the effectiveness of current interventions, to provide information for policymakers on the relative benefits and costs of alternative approaches.

Website: http://crisp.cit.nih.gov/crisp/Crisp_Query.Generate_Screen

- **Project Title: EFFECTS OF ALCOHOL ON NEURONAL CELL MIGRATION**

Principal Investigator & Institution: Komuro, Hitoshi; Cleveland Clinic Foundation 9500 Euclid Ave Cleveland, Oh 44195

Timing: Fiscal Year 2002; Project Start 01-MAY-2002; Project End 30-APR-2006

Summary: (provided by applicant): Maternal alcohol consumption during pregnancy can cause serious birth defects, of which **fetal alcohol syndrome** (FAS) is the most devastating. Recognized by characteristic craniofacial abnormalities and growth deficiency, this condition includes severe alcohol-induced damage to the developing brain. FAS children experience deficits in intellectual functioning; difficulties in learning, memory, problem solving, and attention; difficulties with mental health and social interactions. The long-term goal of present proposal is to elucidate the cellular and molecular mechanisms underlying alcohol-induced malformation of brain. Specially, we will focus on the effects of alcohol on neuronal cell migration in the developing brain, since many ectopic neurons are found in the brain of FAS patients, suggesting that alcohol exposure causes abnormal migration of immature neurons. To this end, we use cerebellum as a model system, because the effect of alcohol on brain growth is especially marked in the cerebellum. We will determine the effects of alcohol on the cerebellar granule cell migration. First, we will determine when, where and how alcohol alters the migration of cerebellar granule cells in a real-time manner with the use of acute cerebellar slice preparations and microexplant cultures. In particularly, we will examine a relationship between mounts and durations of alcohol administration and inhibition of cell movement. Second, we will determine whether changes in intracellular Ca2+ fluctuations and membrane potential of migrating granule cells are involved in alcohol-induced alteration of neuronal migration. Third, we will determine whether manipulations of intracellular Ca2+ fluctuations and membrane potentials by activating NMDA receptor or inhibiting K+ channel activity can overcome the alcohol-induced changes in cell migration. The fundamental mechanisms whereby ethanol administration leads to the disturbances of brain development have not been delineated definitively. Answers to the questions raised in this project will provide a new insight for understanding how prenatal and early postnatal exposure to alcohol causes malformation of brain.

Website: http://crisp.cit.nih.gov/crisp/Crisp_Query.Generate_Screen

- **Project Title: EFFECTS/PRENATAL ALCOHOL EXPOSURE/DERMATOGLYPHIC TRAITS**

Principal Investigator & Institution: Holman, Darryl J.; Ctr/Studs/Demography & Ecology; University of Washington Seattle, Wa 98195

Timing: Fiscal Year 2003; Project Start 29-SEP-2003; Project End 31-AUG-2006

Summary: (provided by applicant): This research will examine the relationship between prenatal alcohol exposure and asymmetry in dermatoglyphic traits (the system of ridges on the hand). The primary aim is to develop new methods for studying developmental perturbations resulting from prenatal alcohol exposure. The dermatoglyphic system is a sensitive indicator of prenatal alcohol exposure; thus, these traits may prove useful in early diagnosis of fetal alcohol effects (FAE). Quantitative and qualitative dermatoglyphic traits will be read from finger and palm prints from two samples. The first sample consists of 282 individuals diagnosed with **fetal alcohol syndrome** (FAS) or fetal alcohol effects (FAE) and 175 unexposed controls. The second sample consists of 410 individuals whose mother's were recruited during prenatal care visits by the 5th month of pregnancy from two Seattle hospitals, and who provided detailed information on the use of alcohol throughout pregnancy. A new statistical method is proposed that quantifies both the ordinary asymmetry found in all bilateral traits and the additional asymmetry associated with prenatal alcohol exposure. Methods will be developed for using dermatoglyphic traits to predict the expression of FAE in exposed individuals. Additionally, we will develop a statistical method to map the effects of alcohol exposure across a spatial gradient of the developing dermal ridge system by estimating spatial correlations in asymmetry among traits. Using an approach based on the gradient of development in the hand, the possibility that the relative timing of alcohol exposure can be detected in the dermatoglyphic system will be explored. This would enable mapping of the periods of development most sensitive to prenatal alcohol exposure.

Website: http://crisp.cit.nih.gov/crisp/Crisp_Query.Generate_Screen

- **Project Title: ETHANOL AND BCL-2 GENE INTERACTIONS IN DEVELOPING CNS**

Principal Investigator & Institution: Heaton, Marieta B.; Professor; Neuroscience; University of Florida Gainesville, Fl 32611

Timing: Fiscal Year 2001; Project Start 01-AUG-2001; Project End 30-APR-2006

Summary: The proposed research will investigate the relationship between developmental ethanol neurotoxicity and the expression of apoptosis effector and repressor molecules of the Bcl-2 family. Members of this family can inhibit apoptosis (e.g., Bcl-2, Bcl- xl) or promote it (e.g., Bax, Bad, Bcl-xs). These relationships will be explored in the developing cerebellum, which exhibits a differential temporal susceptibility to ethanol during the early postnatal period, with a brief period of sensitivity on postnatal days 45 (P45), which results in loss of Purkinje and granule cells, followed by a period during which this region is relatively refractory to ethanol effects (P7-8). We hypothesize that alterations in the expression of Bcl-2-related molecules contribute significantly to this population's relative temporal vulnerability to ethanol. Neonatal rats will be exposed to ethanol via artificial rearing, which we have found to produce increases in bax and bcl-xs mRNA on P4, but not on P7. In specific experiments we will use quantitative Western blot procedures to characterize the dynamics of expression of Bcl-2- related proteins following ethanol exposure at P4 and P7. We will also examine the influence of ethanol on certain post- translational modifications of Bcl-2-related proteins (e.g., dimerization, phosphorylation, and altered molecular integrity). Such processes affect the capacity of these molecules to implement or inhibit cell death. We will determine the regional distribution of Bcl-2-related proteins within the developing cerebellum following ethanol exposure at a vulnerable time (P4) and at a "protected" time (P7), using immunohistochemical procedures. Finally, we will establish whether a causal relationship exists between expression of Bcl-2-related proteins and ethanol-induced neurotoxicity. For this study we will use genetically engineered animals lacking the pro-apoptotic bax gene. Homozygous, heterozygous and wild-type animals will be exposed to ethanol on P45 and Purkinje and granule cell counts subsequently made. We hypothesize that loss of this apoptosis promoter will eliminate or significantly mitigate ethanol-induced cerebellar neuronal death. These studies will be important in producing the first characterization of the role of cell death effector and repressor molecules in developmental ethanol neurotoxicity, and will provide new information concerning a critical mechanism underlying the devastating central nervous system damage seen in the **Fetal Alcohol Syndrome.**

Website: http://crisp.cit.nih.gov/crisp/Crisp_Query.Generate_Screen

- **Project Title: ETHANOL AND L1 MEDIATED NEURITE OUTGROWTH**

Principal Investigator & Institution: Bearer, Cynthia F.; Associate Professor; Pediatrics; Case Western Reserve University 10900 Euclid Ave Cleveland, Oh 44106

Timing: Fiscal Year 2001; Project Start 01-JAN-1999; Project End 31-DEC-2003

Summary: The ultimate goal of this work is to identify the role of L1, a neural adhesion molecule, in alcohol related neurodevelopmental disorder. Patients with the most severe form of this disorder, **fetal alcohol syndrome,** possess neuroanatomic features which are strikingly familiar to those with genetic defects in L1. These observations suggest that L1 plays a role in the pathogenesis of alcohol related neurodevelopmental disorder. Our preliminary results show that ethanol inhibits L1 mediated neurite outgrowth at concentrations comparable to social drinking in rat postnatal day 6 cerebellar granule neurons. L1 is a developmentally regulated cell surface glycoprotein which is critical for proper neural migration, axon guidance and axon-fascicle formation through binding to itself or other molecules at the cell surface. Binding of L1 to itself is followed by cascades of signaling events critical for neurite outgrowth. These cascades can be divided into two pathways: A pathway common to several cell adhesion molecules involving activation of the fibroblast growth factor receptor and subsequent release of arachidonic acid, and pathways unique to L1 with phosphorylation of L1 on the cytoplasmic domain. Our hypothesis is that ethanol disrupts central nervous system development by altering those L1 mediated signaling cascades which lead to neurite outgrowth. This hypothesis will be tested in rat cerebellar granule cells and in a rat model of ARND. Using assays of neurite outgrowth, immunoprecipitation and Western blot, the ethanol sensitivity of the common pathway will be tested by determining the effect of ethanol on: 1) neurite outgrowth stimulated by other cell adhesion molecules, 2) levels of phosphotyrosine modified proteins, and 3) phosphorylation of the fibroblast growth factor receptor. For the L1 unique pathways, in vitro kinase assays, metabolic labeling, and immunocytochemistry will be used to determine the effects of ethanol on: 1) serine kinases associated with L1, 2) the serine and tyrosine phosphorylation of LI, 3) the binding of L1 to ankyrin, and 4) the cellular distribution of L1. In vitro experiments will be correlated to in vivo experiments. These experiments will provide important information on the underlying mechanism of ethanol's inhibitory effect on L1 mediated neurite outgrowth.

Website: http://crisp.cit.nih.gov/crisp/Crisp_Query.Generate_Screen

- **Project Title: ETHANOL AND NEURONAL DEVELOPMENT**

Principal Investigator & Institution: Lindsley, Tara A.; Professor; Ctr/Neuropharmacology/Neurosci; Albany Medical College of Union Univ Union University Albany, Ny 12208

Timing: Fiscal Year 2001; Project Start 01-APR-1998; Project End 31-MAR-2003

Summary: (Adapted from the Investigator's Abstract) The long term objectives of this research are to identify and characterize the cellular mechanisms underlying ethanol induced changes in neuronal development, and to assess the role of these changes in the etiology of CNS abnormalities associated with **Fetal Alcohol Syndrome** (FAS). Key neuropathologic features of FAS include altered neuronal morphogenesis and synapse formation in the hippocampus. Recent studies have elucidated some of the molecules and processes responsible for the distinct growth characteristics of axons and dendrites, thus providing the basis for novel experiments to determine the mechanisms underlying ethanol's disruption of neuronal development. The use of primary cultures of embryonic rat hippocampal pyramidal neurons is integral to the objectives of the project. Neurons in these cultures develop axons, dendrites, and synapses in a sequence of events that mimics their development in vivo. Experiments in this proposal are designed to use immunofluorescent cytochemistry coupled with quantitative morphometric analysis, time lapse videomicroscopy, and Fura-2 intracellular free calcium measurements in the following specific aims: (1) Compare the sensitivity of cultured hippocampal neurons exposed to ethanol at different times relative to development of axons, dendrites and synapses, (2) Distinguish whether ethanol induced changes in neuronal development result from direct effects of ethanol on neurons, or indirect effects on neurons mediated by astrocytes, (3) Determine whether ethanol's effects on process outgrowth involve altered regulation of intracellular calcium levels. The results of these studies will establish whether a disruption of process outgrowth and molecular compartmentalization is a key aspect of ethanol's neurodevelopmental toxicity and will provide important insight into the mechanism(s) underlying these actions. This fundamental knowledge can be expected to provide a basis for improving the identification and treatment of affected individuals.

Website: http://crisp.cit.nih.gov/crisp/Crisp_Query.Generate_Screen

- **Project Title: ETHANOL EFFECTS ON GLUTAMATE RECEPTORS**

  Principal Investigator & Institution: Yasuda, Robert P.; Pharmacology; Georgetown University Washington, Dc 20057

  Timing: Fiscal Year 2001; Project Start 01-AUG-1997; Project End 31-JUL-2003

  Summary: (Adapted from the Investigator's Abstract) The excitatory amino acid pathways in the brain are widespread and are involved in synaptic plastic events such as long-term potentiation in the hippocampus. Long-term potentiation is thought to be part of the process of learning and memory. Excitatory amino acids are thought to also play a role in excitotoxicity as related to seizures and may be involved in ethanol withdrawal induced seizures. At least two glutamatergic receptor systems are thought to regulate long-term potentiation in the hippocampus. These receptor systems are the metabotropic receptors and the NMDA receptor complex. The metabotropic receptors are G-protein linked receptors that are coupled to several intracellular enzymes such as phospholipase C. The NMDA receptor is a complex of several protein subunits that form a glutamate gated ion channel that has high permeability for calcium. Each subunit imparts a different character to the NMDA receptor function. Acute and chronic treatment with ethanol alters the function of these receptors. Prenatal exposure to ethanol can affect the offspring even when they are quite old. Alteration of these receptors in the hippocampus by ethanol can influence the process of learning and memory. We now know that chronic ethanol treatment increases the function of NMDA receptor in the hippocampus and that an increase in the protein for NR1 NMDA subunit is observed as well as an increase in binding sites for NMDA. Prenatal exposure to ethanol causes a decrease in both NMDA receptor function and metabotropic receptor function. The specific aims of these investigations are to examine what metabotropic receptor subtypes and/or what NMDA receptor subunits change after chronic ethanol exposure or prenatal ethanol exposure and how these changes in protein expression correllate with functional chages. We will be using receptor subtype and subunit specific antibodies to identify and quantify metabotropic receptor subtypes and NMDA receptor NR1 splice variants and NR2 subunits that may change after such an insult. My long-term goal is to understand how differences in the expression of metabotropic receptors and NMDA receptor subunits occur during chronic and prenatal ethanol treatments. These studies will help us to understand some of the underlying mechanism in **fetal alcohol syndrome** as well as the effects of chronic alcoholism.

  Website: http://crisp.cit.nih.gov/crisp/Crisp_Query.Generate_Screen

- **Project Title: ETHANOL EFFECTS ON GLYCINE RECEPTOR/CHANNEL FUNCTION**

  Principal Investigator & Institution: Ye, Jiang-Hong; Associate Professor of Anesthesiology; Anesthesiology; Univ of Med/Dent Nj Newark Newark, Nj 07103

  Timing: Fiscal Year 2001; Project Start 01-APR-1999; Project End 31-MAR-2004

  Summary: Ethanol (EtOH) is an effective brain depressant and an additive drug. Emerging evidence suggests that glycine receptor/channels (GlyRs) are sensitive to pharmacologically relevant concentrations of EtOH. Since glycine inhibits neuronal activity, potentiation of GlyR function would be expected to enhance neuronal inhibition and perhaps contribute to the neuronal depressant effects of EtOH. Therefore, we propose to examine the effects of EtOH on glycine-induced responses of dopaminergic neurons from the ventral tegmental area (VTA) of the brain, the reward center for drug abuse. The overall objective of this study is to investigate the mechanisms by which EtOH alteration of GlyR function contributes to the central nervous system (CNS) consequences of alcohol in vivo. To achieve this objective the following three hypotheses will be tested. HYPOTHESIS I is that EtOH interacts with the GlyR. EtOH regulates the excitability of dopaminergic neurons by altering functions of GlyRs. HYPOTHESIS II is that EtOH interactions with the GlyR are modulated by the protein phosphorylation status of the GlyR, the intracellular activity of PKA, PKC and G-proteins. HYPOTHESIS III is that GlyR structure, intracellular C1-concentration of dopaminergic neurons and, consequently, glycine-induced responses and their response to EtOH change with development. These hypotheses will be tested on VTA neurons freshly isolated from both neonatal and mature rats. Whole-cell patch- clamp technique (especially gramicidin perforated patch technique) will be used to record glycine-induced responses, including membrane current, potential and the alteration of spontaneous firing in the absence and presence of EtOH. Specific activators and inhibitors of protein kinases A and C and of Gproteins will be used to identify the enzyme pathways involved in any effects, of EtOH on GlyRs. These studies will significantly advance our understanding of the effects of EtOH on CNS GlyRs at the molecular and cellular levels. A better knowledge of the actions of EtOH in the brain will improve our understanding of related reinforcement mechanisms, which will, in turn, facilitate the identification of strategies which might be of value in the treatment of alcohol abuse and **fetal alcohol syndrome.**

Website: http://crisp.cit.nih.gov/crisp/Crisp_Query.Generate_Screen

- **Project Title: ETHANOL, RETINOIDS, AND CONGENITAL HEART MALFORMATIONS**

Principal Investigator & Institution: Gelineau-Van Waes, Janee; Munroe-Meyer Institute; University of Nebraska Medical Center Omaha, Ne 681987835

Timing: Fiscal Year 2002; Project Start 01-JUL-2002; Project End 30-JUN-2004

Summary: (provided by applicant): Congenital malformations of the heart have been reported following maternal exposure to various environmental toxins, but the precise mechanism(s) by which these teratogenic exposures disrupt normal morphogenesis remains unknown. Prenatal exposure to ethanol (Fetal Alcohol Syndrome) or maternal vitamin A (retinoic acid) deficiency or excess during gestation have been shown to cause conotruncal heart defects. In the proposed research program, the complex processes underlying embryological development of the mammalian heart and the impact of prenatal exposure to ethanol and perturbed retinoic acid levels leading to cardiac dysmorphogenesis will be studied using molecular-genetic approaches. The proposed studies will focus on a critical gestational timepoint during murine heart development when the cardiac neural crest cells are migrating from the dorsal neural tube to the heart. Alterations in the network of developmentally regulated genes in this cell population will be analyzed following teratogen exposure through the use of genetic microarrays. Potential mechanisms suggested by altered gene expression profiles will be further evaluated relative to the observed cellular dysmorphology by examining protein expression of critical candidate genes identified in the cDNA arrays, as well as proteins associated with changes in cell proliferation and apoptosis. The goal will be to identify significant gene/protein interactions that take place during normal heart development, and the mechanism(s) by which in utero ethanol exposure disrupts this process. We will also further investigate the possibility that malformations of the heart subsequent to prenatal alcohol exposure are a result of decreased endogenous retinoic acid synthesis due to competition between alcohol and retinol for alcohol dehydrogenase enzymatic pathways. The proposed research program will therefore test the hypothesis that prenatal ethanol exposure leads to congenital heart malformations by disrupting normal retinoid signaling pathways critical for cell fate determination in the migrating cardiac neural crest cells/conotruncus.

Website: http://crisp.cit.nih.gov/crisp/Crisp_Query.Generate_Screen

- **Project Title: ETHANOL-INDUCED PURKINJE CELL APOPTOSIS**

  Principal Investigator & Institution: Light, Kim E.; Pharmaceutical Sciences; University of Arkansas Med Scis Ltl Rock 4301 W Markham St Little Rock, Ar 72205

  Timing: Fiscal Year 2001; Project Start 01-JUL-2000; Project End 30-JUN-2002

  Summary: One of the most extensively studied aspects of ethanol-induced neural toxicity is the specific loss of Purkinje ce s the cerebellum The consequences of Purkinje cell loss are thought to be involved in the deficiencies of motor coordination and gait exhibited by children diagnosed with **fetal alcohol syndrome.** Although loss of Purkinje cells has been repeatedly demonstrated to be a consistent and reliable consequence of early postnatal ethanol exposure in the rat, the manner and time course of this cell loss has not been clearly identified. We hypothesize that Purkinje cell loss in the cerebellum results from the induction of apaptosis in a manner similar to an acute toxic response (time course related to peak blood ethanol concentration). Thus, a linear relationship will exist between ethanol concentrations and the extent of apoptosis. Evaluation of this hypothesis will include in vivo exposures to ethanol using the intra gastric intubation technique and in vitro experiments using the organotypic slice culture model. Throughout these studies we will use ethanol exposures on PN4 (or the in vitro equivalent) in the rat, since the strongest relationship between peak BEC and percent reduction of Purkinje cells has been demonstrated to occur on this day. This exposure paradigm is a model of third trimester ethanol exposure in the human. Two specific aims will guide this research: (1) The first aim involves the identification of the relationship between peak blood ethanol concentration (BEC) and Purkinje cell death following in vivo ethanol administration. These experiments will identify the timing and manner of Purkinje cell death as well as the linear relationship between the magnitude of cell death to peak BEC. Apoptotic cell death will be identified by the presence of fragmented DNA, apoptotic cell morphology, increased expression of pro-apoptotic associated antigens (Bax, caspase-3) and decreased expression of anti-apoptotic associated antigens (p53). (2) The second specific aim will use the in vitro organotypic slice culture technique to further explore the nature and mechanisms of ethanol-induced Purkinje cell apoptosis. Initially, these studies will parallel those described under the first specific aim in order to confirm the ability of ethanol to produce Purkinie cell apoptosis. These studies will also establish the direct linear relationship between ethanol concentration and the magnitude of Purkinje cell death. This second specific aim provides the foundation for the use of this technique as an experimental paradigm to determine the mechanism and specific pathway(s) involved in ethanol-induced apoptosis as well as to dissect the regulation of these pathway(s) with standard biochemical and pharmacological techniques.

  Website: http://crisp.cit.nih.gov/crisp/Crisp_Query.Generate_Screen

- **Project Title: ETHANOL-RETINOID INTERACTION IN INNER EAR MALFORMATIONS**

  Principal Investigator & Institution: Van Waes, Janee; University of Nebraska Medical Center Omaha, Ne 681987835

  Timing: Fiscal Year 2003; Project Start 30-SEP-2003; Project End 30-JUN-2008

  Summary: Using a molecular genetic approach, this project will focus mechanistically on alterations in developmental events that result in congenital malformations of the inner ear following prenatal alcohol exposure (Fetal Alcohol Syndrome). The ovedying hypothesis is that malformations of the inner ear subsequent to prenatal alcohol exposure are a result of decreased endogenous retinoic acid synthesis due to competition between alcohol and retinol for alcohol dehydrogenase enzyme pathways. Specific Aim 1 will examine the severity and range of malformations in the inner ear subsequent to prenatal ethanol exposure, or as a result of maternal vitamin A deficiency or excess. Additionally, alterations in gene pathways likely to result in dysmorphogenesis and/or cellular dysfunction will be analyzed using cDNA microarrays. The analysis will focus primarily on those genes known to be relevant for inner ear morphogenesis (e.g. FGF, EYA, GATA, BMP) and cell fate determination (e.g. Ngn1, Math1, Hes1, Hes5). Alternations in the spatio-temporal pattern of these genes will be analyzed using such methods as hierarchical and kmeans clustering, self-organizing maps, and principal components analysis. Results will be verified using quantitative PCR (Q-PCR). Specific Aim 2 will confirm and extend the data from Specific Aim 1 by localizing expression of "critical genes" during inner ear development through the use of in situ hybridization and immunohistochemical techniques. Specific Aim 3 will directly test the suggested molecular interaction of ethanol and retinoic acid competition for common enzymatic pathways by using two different techniques (HPLC and a bioassay using retinoic acid responsive reporter cell lines). In a future RO1 submission, the identified candidate genes will be further analyzed in the teratogenic context using existing mutant and transgenic mouse strains (e.g. FGF10 null, ngn1 BAC) to probe for enhanced susceptibility.

  Website: http://crisp.cit.nih.gov/crisp/Crisp_Query.Generate_Screen

- **Project Title: ETHNIC FACTORS IN ALCOHOL ABUSE AMONG AFRICAN AMERICANS**

  Principal Investigator & Institution: Taylor, Robert E.; Scientific Advisor; Pharmacology; Howard University 2400 6Th St Nw Washington, Dc 20059

  Timing: Fiscal Year 2001; Project Start 30-SEP-1997; Project End 31-AUG-2003

  Summary: This application proposes the establishment of a Collaborative Minority Alcohol Research Development (CMIARD) Program at Howard University. The goal is to stimulate, strengthen, and facilitate multi-disciplinary research and collaborations which will lead to the reduction of alcohol morbidity/mortality among minority populations with emphasis on African Americans. Under the theme of Ethnic Factors in Alcohol Abuse Among African Americans, Howard University will create a strong and effective infrastructure of facilities, staff, and an optimum research environment to (1) support new exploratory and ongoing research; (2) motivate and cultivate interest by well trained research investigatory in the area of alcohol research; (3) train students in the area of alcohol research; and (4) create and implement mechanisms for the transfer of pertinent information gleaned from the research to health professionals and the local and world community. The CMIARD will be housed within the Department of Pharmacology, Howard University College of Medicine and Hospital which will serve as the hub for the management of all administrative and scientific functions. Under the direction and leadership of the PI, an Administrative Core will be established with the following components: (1) a Project Advisory Committee (PAC) to provide overall direction and guidance, (2) an Executive Committee to serve as an adjunct to the PAC, assisting with general decision making and very timely input into the Centers operation, (3) Working Groups to include experienced scientists and new investigators to help stimulate interest in alcohol research, and (4) the Scientific Research Project component. The research component of the Administrative core have five initial research projects for inclusion in this application representing a broad spectrum of promising research. These projects are designed to further research in **fetal alcohol syndrome,** ethnogenetic determinants of alcohol abuse, and basic science experimental models of alcohols effects. Ten additional projects offer strong consideration for future research projects, a five year research plan is proposed which focuses on a well integrated, multi disciplinary approach to expand current and develop new research capabilities.

Website: http://crisp.cit.nih.gov/crisp/Crisp_Query.Generate_Screen

- **Project Title: EXPERIMENTAL FETAL ALCOHOL SYNDROMEN**

Principal Investigator & Institution: Miller, Michael W.; Professor and Chair; Neuroscience and Physiology; Upstate Medical University Research Administration Syracuse, Ny 13210

Timing: Fiscal Year 2001; Project Start 01-DEC-1993; Project End 31-MAR-2004

Summary: Studies of humans with **fetal alcohol syndrome** (FAS) and rats with experimental FAS show that brain structure and function are profoundly affected by early exposure to ethanol. Ethanol-induced defects include microencephaly, a thinner cerebral cortex, and reductions in the number of cortical neurons. These findings may result from a single cause- the toxic effects of ethanol to cause neuronal death. We will test the hypotheses that ethanol-induced neuronal death results from interference with the survival-promoting activities of nerve growth factor (NGF) and that this interference results in the altered expression of genes coding for known and/or novel proteins. In vivo studies will examine the effect of prenatal exposure to ethanol on the expression of NGF and on the expression of death- associated proteins, specifically p75 and bcl proteins. p75 serves as the low affinity receptor for NGF and is affected by ethanol treatment, and bcl proteins can repress (e.g., bcl-2) or facilitate (e.g., bax) neuronal death. These studies will focus on three components of the trigeminal/somatosensory system: the somatosensory cortex, the ventrobasal thalamus, and the principal sensory nucleus of the trigeminal nerve. A series of in vitro studies will test the above hypotheses and the corollary that NGF and ethanol treatments are mutually antagonistic. Two types of cells will be examined: purified cultures of cortical neurons and conditionally immortalized neuroblasts. Cells will be raised in a serum-free medium alone, a medium supplemented with NGF or ethanol, or a medium with NGF and ethanol. This design will be used to determine the effects of NGF and ethanol (a) on neuronal survival (cell counts, thymidine nick-end labeling procedure (TUNEL) and electron microscopy) and (b) on the expression of bcl gene products. Subsequently, the effects of NGF and ethanol on the gene expression will be determined using a technique relying on the differential display of induced mRNAs. The expression of these novel proteins in living and dying neurons will be determined using double-labeling techniques in which the dying cells are positively identified (e.g., with TUNEL). The spatiotemporal expression of the newly developed probes in the trigeminal/somatosensory system will be examined in vivo. Animals will be exposed to ethanol prenatally and their offspring will be assayed for the expression of the differentially displayed mRNAs. The proposed experiments explore a mechanism of FAS and test the hypothesis that CNS defects associated with FAS result from alterations in NGF-mediated protein expression.

Website: http://crisp.cit.nih.gov/crisp/Crisp_Query.Generate_Screen

- **Project Title: FAS: NEUROPSYCHOLOGICAL ASSESSMENT OF CHILDREN**

Principal Investigator & Institution: Mattson, Sarah N.; Assistant Professor; Psychology; San Diego State University 5250 Campanile Dr San Diego, Ca 92182

Timing: Fiscal Year 2003; Project Start 01-APR-1997; Project End 31-MAR-2008

Summary: (provided by applicant): The effects of heavy prenatal alcohol exposure reach beyond the diagnosis of **Fetal Alcohol Syndrome** and can result in a complex pattern of neurodevelopmental disorders. Although the precise nature of this pattern is not well defined, current research is progressing toward this end. Similarly, brain imaging studies point to a pattern of effects in the brain structure of children with heavy prenatal alcohol exposure with some structures affected to a greater degree than others. The current application proposes studies based on recent neuropsychological and neuroanatomical studies of children with heavy prenatal alcohol exposure. The proposed studies are aimed at clarifying three important functional comparisons: "what" vs. "where" visuospatial processing, "global" vs. "local" hierarchical visuospatial processing, and "disengaging" vs. "shifting" of visual attention. These areas have been linked to the parietal lobe, an area of the brain affected by prenatal alcohol exposure. Although previous studies of individuals with brain damage have assessed these three areas separately, the research proposed herein aims to assess the three domains in one population. First, assessment of "what-where" visuospatial functioning will be conducted using computerized and traditional tests. Based on preliminary data, relative weaknesses in "where" processing are predicted. Second, assessment of global-local processing will be conducted using tests of both recall and potential biasing effects of hierarchical figures. Based on previous research, a relative weakness in local processing is predicted. Finally, assessment of disengaging-shifting of visual attention will be conducted using a classic measure of spatial orienting of attention. Based on both brain imaging studies and previous studies of attentional shifting, a relative weakness in disengagement is predicted. Thus, the proposed series of studies targets three important functional dissociations that are anatomically linked. The underlying rationale and hypotheses for these studies are based on previous neuropsychological and imaging studies. Clarification of these dissociations will help define the profile of weaknesses and strengths in children with heavy prenatal alcohol exposure and help identify core deficits in this population.

Website: http://crisp.cit.nih.gov/crisp/Crisp_Query.Generate_Screen

- **Project Title: FETAL ALCOHOL EFFECTS AND IMMUNE DEVELOPMENT**

Principal Investigator & Institution: Wolcott, Robert M.; Microbiology and Immunology; Louisiana State Univ Hsc Shreveport P. O. Box 33932 Shreveport, La 71103

Timing: Fiscal Year 2001; Project Start 01-JAN-1994; Project End 31-DEC-2002

Summary: (Adapted from the Investigator's Abstract) The teratogenic potential of alcohol is well known and the offspring of mothers who abuse alcohol have been shown to have a broad spectrum of anomalies that have been termed alcohol related birth defects (ARBD). The manifestation of ARB span from reduced birth weight to the unique constellation of features termed **fetal alcohol syndrome** (FAS). FAS children are the offspring of chronic alcoholic women. However, clinical studies have shown that even moderate drinking during pregnancy can affect fetal development suggesting that alcohol abuse may be one of the leading causes of birth defects. Most studies of the teratogenic effects of alcohol have focused on the morphological and neurological features of the affected infants. However, recent studies have shown ARBD children to be at high risk of having some degree of immune deficiency and consequent increased incidence and severity of infection. Since the immune system is not fully developed at birth the infant's ability to cope with infection is fragile. Therefore, it is important to identify environmental factors that might delay normal immune development and put infants at risk. Recent studies from this laboratory using a murine model of ARBD have shown that in utero exposure to alcohol caused a retarded development of B lymphocytes in fetal liver and neonatal bone marrow and spleen. Phenotypic analysis of developmental intermediates in the B lineage showed several to be affected by in utero alcohol exposure. In particular, the investigator's observed that a previously unreported B cell precursor was decreased in neonatal marrow and spleens of animals exposed in utero to alcohol. In this proposal the applicants will use a model consisting of fetal alcohol exposed and pair-fed and chow-fed control animals to assess he effects of alcohol on B lymphopoiesis during fetal and neonatal life. They will use multiparameter flow cytometry to ascertain the absolute number of B cell intermediates and the phenotype of these cells within the fetal liver and neonatal bone marrow and spleen. The developmental potential of the B cell intermediates will be determined by sorting B-lineage cells and other hematopoietic precursors and stem cells and using clonal analysis to determine if alcohol exposure alters the frequency of cells that are capable of differentiation. They will also follow fetal alcohol exposed animals in to adulthood to determine if the exposure affected the function of the humoral immune system and the longevity of the effect.

Website: http://crisp.cit.nih.gov/crisp/Crisp_Query.Generate_Screen

- **Project Title: FETAL ALCOHOL EFFECTS IN MONKEYS: DOPAMINE AND BEHAVIOR**

Principal Investigator & Institution: Schneider, Mary L.; Professor; Kinesiology; University of Wisconsin Madison 750 University Ave Madison, Wi 53706

Timing: Fiscal Year 2001; Project Start 01-AUG-2001; Project End 31-MAY-2006

Summary: Fetal alcohol syndrome, (FAS) is the leading known cause of mental retardation today and currently represents an enormous problem for our society. The central question addressed by this proposal is whether moderate alcohol exposure constitutes a danger to the developing offspring. To address this issue, we propose to assess the behavior and physiology in 50 monkeys from four conditions: 1) mothers consumed moderate level alcohol daily throughout pregnancy 2) mothers experienced psychological stress; 3) mothers consumed moderate level alcohol and experienced psychological stress; and 4) mothers consumed sucrose (controls) (Schneider et al., 1997). The specific aims are as follows: 1) to characterize dopamine D2 receptor densities in striata of offspring using in vivo PET imaging techniques 2) to characterize dopamine synthesis in these same cohorts, also using PET imaging, and to uncouple presynaptic synthesis of dopamine from postsynaptic receptor binding availability; 3) to evaluate these monkeys with a standard battery of widely accepted tests and measurements, which index cognitive functioning and behavior; and 4) to determine the effects of a dopamine agonist, methylphenidate, on behavior and cognitive performance in this cohort of monkeys. Our primate model has allowed control of the exact timing and level of alcohol exposure to the fetus and the separation of the effects of alcohol from other life-style factors, such as psychological stress The proposed studies provide a unique and unprecedented opportunity not only to better understand the underlying neurobiology of fetal alcohol effects, but also to discover potential in vivo diagnostic markers for detecting fetal alcohol- induced brain damage. Increasing our understanding of the association between behavior, cognition, and molecular mechanisms of neuronal function in fetal alcohol-exposed primates could aid in early identification and appropriate treatment of children with prenatal alcohol exposure.

Website: http://crisp.cit.nih.gov/crisp/Crisp_Query.Generate_Screen

- **Project Title: FETAL ALCOHOL EXPOSURE AND NMDA RECEPTOR INTERACTION**

Principal Investigator & Institution: Elberger, Andrea J.; Professor of Anatomy & Neurobiology; Anatomy and Neurobiology; University of Tennessee Health Sci Ctr Health Science Center Memphis, Tn 38163

Timing: Fiscal Year 2001; Project Start 01-JUL-2000; Project End 30-JUN-2003

Summary: The corpus callosum (CC) can be absent or reduced in children with **fetal alcohol syndrome** (FAS) or alcohol related birth defect (ARBD). Histological studies have shown that the CC in the rat is also negatively affected by prenatal alcohol exposure that produces a wide range of blood alcohol concentrations (BACS) during the first, second, or first + second trimester equivalent. The abnormalities consist of temporally altered CC development, disorganization of laminar distribution of CC projection neurons (CCpn), misoriented CCpn, misshapen CCpn, and abnormal growth of apical and basilar dendrites of CCpn. Using the same histological techniques, a transgenic strain of mouse with total (-/-) deletion of the NMDA-R1 receptor has also been shown to have altered CC development which is opposite to that of rats with prenatal ethanol exposure. For NR1-/-, the alteration consists exclusively of accelerated CC development without the abnormal CCpn morphology or spatial disorganization. The goal of this project is to test the hypothesis that a significant in vivo mechanism in the negative effects of prenatal alcohol exposure on CC development is the action of ethanol on the NMDA-R1 receptor. This proposal will be used to obtain pilot data to support this hypothesis by giving prenatal alcohol exposure to pregnant NRl transgenic mice. Doses of alcohol that produce a High (>250 mg/dl) or Moderate (<200 mg/dl) BAC will be applied daily to NRl transgenic mice in a binge model during the first + second trimester equivalent. Controls will consist of NR1 transgenic mice that are ad-lib chow fed, or weight-matched pairfed mice that undergo the same handling and testing. A superficial morphological analysis of CC development will be carried out on offspring sacrificed at gestational day 15 and 17, and postnatal day 0 to tentatively pair the morphological phenotype with a presumed genotype. Following this initial analysis, tissue samples taken at the time of sacrifice will be analyzed by PCR amplification to determine the genotype of each pup. Only the NR1-/- and NR1+/+ offspring (the latter are controls) will undergo detailed histological analysis to evaluate the location, orientation, shape, and dendritic arbor of CCpn in all groups. There are three possible outcomes for the NR1-/- mice prenatally exposed to alcohol. 1) The CCpn will display the abnormalities typical of prenatal ethanol exposure, indicating that activation of the NMDA-R1 receptor is not a significant in vivo mechanism for prenatal ethanol neurotoxicity. 2) The CCpn will display the alteration typical of NR1-/-, indicating that activation of the NMDA-R1 receptor is a highly significant in vivo mechanism for prenatal ethanol neurotoxicity. 3) The CCpn will have intermediate effects in terms of temporal development, types of CCpn morphological abnormalities, or number of CCpn showing abnormalities. The results will be interpreted in comparison to existing data on the effects of ethanol on NMDA receptors in mature cells in vitro. The results of this proposal will serve as pilot data for a subsequent grant application to study possible mechanisms for neurotoxicity induced by fetal alcohol exposure, specifically the in vivo interaction of ethanol with receptors such as NMDA-R1 in terms of effects on CCpn and cortical cells at different stages of development.

Website: http://crisp.cit.nih.gov/crisp/Crisp_Query.Generate_Screen

- **Project Title: FETAL ALCOHOL EXPOSURE AND SCHOOL AGE COGNITION**

Principal Investigator & Institution: Jacobson, Sandra W.; Professor; Psychiatry & Behav Neuroscis; Wayne State University 656 W. Kirby Detroit, Mi 48202

Timing: Fiscal Year 2001; Project Start 01-MAR-1993; Project End 31-MAR-2004

Summary: Recent studies have identified specific patterns of intellectual impairment in **fetal alcohol syndrome** (FAS) patients, but only limited data are available on the specific deficits associated with lower level prenatal exposure to alcohol. In our recent 7.5-year follow-up evaluation of 340 Detroit children recruited to overrepresent moderate-to-heavy prenatal alcohol exposure, we have begun to identify a distinct "neurobehavioral profile" associated with this exposure. This profile differs from FAS in that IQ and verbal learning appear to be spared but resembles FAS and the effects reported in the Seattle study in that deficits in focused attention, arithmetic, and working memory are particularly salient. Preliminary 7.5-year follow-up data also indicate an alcohol-related increased incidence in clinically-significant levels of childhood aggression and social problems, after control for confounders and current caregiver alcohol use. Because these effects are only partially mediated by the attentional deficits, these data suggest that, in addition to its effects on attention, prenatal alcohol may directly disrupt CNS pathways that mediate affective response and emotional regulation. We now propose to reevaluate our Detroit cohort at 12 years of age. The principal aims of this study are (1) to confirm and further refine the distinctive pattern of alcohol-related attentional deficits seen at 7.5 years and (2) to examine the relation between prenatal alcohol and socioemotional function using a new test battery focusing on social judgment, social competence, and emotionality; a clinical assessment of psychopathology; and adolescent alcohol and drug use. We will also focus on dose-response relations, threshold, pattern of pregnancy drinking associated with developmental deficit, and the importance of the observed deficits for the day-to-day function of the individual child. The data to be generated from this study have the potential to help refine the diagnosis of alcohol- related neurodevelopmental disorder (ARND) and to contribute to the design of interventions specifically targeted to alcohol-exposed children.

Website: http://crisp.cit.nih.gov/crisp/Crisp_Query.Generate_Screen

- **Project Title: FETAL ALCOHOL EXPOSURE--NEUROIMMUNE INTERACTIONS**

Principal Investigator & Institution: Taylor, Anna N.; Professor; Neurobiology; University of California Los Angeles 10920 Wilshire Blvd., Suite 1200 Los Angeles, Ca 90024

Timing: Fiscal Year 2001; Project Start 01-JUL-1994; Project End 31-MAR-2003

Summary: Fetal alcohol exposure (FAE) impairs the functioning of the immune system and decreases resistance to various infectious diseases. FAE also alters the development of neural and neuroendocrine systems, and thus may interfere with the bidirectional communications between the immune and the nervous system of offspring. Data indicate that FAE impairs the interactions between the immune and nervous systems. For example, we have shown that FAE blunts the febrile response induced by a pathogen product, lipopolysaccharide (LPS), and one of the cytokines, interleukin-1 beta

(IL1), induced by LPS. Moreover, maternal adrenalectomy was found to prevent the blunted febrile response. The effects of FAE are probably mediated by developmentally-induced alterations in brain mechanisms, since FAE also blunts the febrile response following intracerebroventricular (icv) administration of IL1. Given the essential role of fever in the host defense response to infection, we hypothesize that the attenuated febrile response following FAE reflects a general impairment in neuroimmune interactions which may contribute to the predisposition to infection resulting from FAE. One corollary hypothesis states that FAE affects the adult expression of neural mediators of the febrile component of the acute phase response to infection. A second corollary hypothesis states that prevention of FAE-induced alterations in neuroimmune interactions mediating the febrile response to LPS can be achieved by hormonal manipulations pre-or postnatally. Specifically, we aim to: 1) Characterize the effects of LPS administered ip on certain mediators of the febrile response in adult male fetal alcohol-exposed and control rats, i.e., a) prostaglandin E2 (PGE), b) norepinephrine (NE), c) nitric oxide (NO), d) arginine vasopressin (AVP), e) alpha-melanocyte stimulating hormone (MSH), f) ACTH and corticosterone and g) IL1; 2) Investigate a possible role for neonatal or adult testosterone levels in mediating the effects of FAE on the LPS-induced febrile response and on its neurochemical mediators, as identified in Aim 1; and 3) Determine whether the prevention of the blunted LPS-induced febrile response by maternal adrenalectomy is (a) mediated by adreno-medullary or -cortical products, (b) is accompanied by changes in any of the neurochemical mediators of the febrile response identified as being affected by FAE in Aim 1, and (c) is accompanied by a reversal of the FAE-induced reduction in testosterone levels in neonatal and/or adult rats.

Website: http://crisp.cit.nih.gov/crisp/Crisp_Query.Generate_Screen

- **Project Title: FETAL ALCOHOL SYNDROME BIOMARKERS BY ANTIBODY MICROARRAY**

Principal Investigator & Institution: Kim, Hyesook S.; Detroit R & D, Inc. Metro Center for High Tech. Bldg. Detroit, Mi 48201

Timing: Fiscal Year 2003; Project Start 15-SEP-2003; Project End 31-AUG-2005

Summary: (provided by applicant): **Fetal Alcohol Syndrome** (FAS) is defined as a pattern of growth retardation, characteristic facial anomalies and mental retardation in children born to alcoholic women. It is essential to begin remedial treatment of FAS children as early as possible. Therefore biomarkers linked to infants destined to develop FAS are being sought. The discovery of biomarkers for FAS could also help to identify potential physiological mechanisms that mediate alcohol teratogenesis. Our long-term goal is to produce antibody microarrays for rat, mouse and human and screen various biological fluids and tissues to identify chemical, gene and pathway biomarkers for FAS and other fetal alcohol effects. We will produce hypothesis-driven targeted antibody arrays for selected (a) proteins and chemicals primarily involved with oxidative stress, (b) phosphorylated/non-phosphorylated protein pairs involved in cellular signaling through protein phosphorylation and (c) biologically active fatty acids and their ethyl esters. We will also produce protein chips to screen autoantibodies and protein-protein interactions. Durin.q Phase I, we will produce rat oxidative stress chips and phosphorylated/non-phosphorylated protein pair chips and biomarkers of FAS will be searched by screening proteins obtained from fetal liver tissues and rat placentas. In addition, we will produce antibodies for biologically active fatty acids.

Website: http://crisp.cit.nih.gov/crisp/Crisp_Query.Generate_Screen

- **Project Title: FETAL ALCOHOL SYNDROME: GENETIC STUDIES IN ZEBRAFISH**

  Principal Investigator & Institution: Carvan, Michael J.; Assistant Professor; None; University of Wisconsin Milwaukee Box 413, 2200 Kenwood Blvd Milwaukee, Wi 53201

  Timing: Fiscal Year 2001; Project Start 01-JUN-2001; Project End 31-MAY-2003

  Summary: This application is being submitted for consideration as a small grant (R03). I am a new investigator planning to expand my research focus to include the area of ethanol-induced birth defects. The long-range goal of this project is to elucidate the molecular mechanisms by which ethanol perturbs embryonic and fetal development and to identify genes that play a role in the sensitivity to ethanol-induced teratogenesis. **Fetal Alcohol Syndrome** (FAS) is a constellation of congenital anomalies seen in some newborns exposed to alcohol through maternal consumption and is characterized by prenatal and postnatal failure to thrive, central nervous system disorders, and a distinctive set of patterning defects that affect the cardiovascular system, facial structures and limbs. Data from twin studies and animal models argue strongly for a robust genetic component to FAS. Our hypothesis is that mutations in single genes influence one's resistance to ethanol-induced teratogenesis. The zebrafish vertebrate model system has proven to be very powerful for the purpose of identifying genes that play a role in specific physiological events. The specific aims of this proposal are to: [1] Analyze the non-lethal teratogenic effects of ethanol in selected zebrafish strains, and [2] Map and isolate the genomic region(s) containing the gene(s) responsible for the differential sensitivity of zebrafish strains to the embryolethal effects of ethanol exposure. Comparing sensitive and resistant zebrafish strains will elucidate the genetic and molecular mechanisms behind the sensitivity of vertebrate embryos to alcohol toxicity, and may apply directly to alcohol sensitivity in humans. The final products of the project described herein will be a thorough characterization of the nonlethal teratogenic effects of ethanol exposure in zebrafish that are characteristic of FAS, and the identification of several large genomic clones containing candidate genes that influence the sensitivity of zebrafish to the effects of ethanol exposure.

  Website: http://crisp.cit.nih.gov/crisp/Crisp_Query.Generate_Screen

- **Project Title: FETAL ETHANOL EFFECTS ON THE PERIPHERAL NERVOUS SYSTEM**

  Principal Investigator & Institution: Johnson, Mary I.; Neurology; University of New Mexico Albuquerque Controller's Office Albuquerque, Nm 87131

  Timing: Fiscal Year 2003; Project Start 01-AUG-2003; Project End 31-JUL-2005

  Summary: (provided by applicant): Fetal ethanol exposure results in life-long and devastating effects on the nervous system. The most recognizable child with **fetal alcohol syndrome** (FAS) has growth retardation, craniofacial abnormalities and central nervous system (CNS) dysfunction, but represents only a portion of those children exposed to alcohol. For the affected individuals and their families the impact is immeasurable; the economic costs are difficult to estimate but significant. Central nervous system abnormalities may not be the entire basis for the motor deficits of the children including weakness and low muscle tone. Alcohol affects many systems in the developing nervous system and, understandably, most research on the effects of prenatal ethanol exposure is focused on the CNS. We know far less about fetal ethanol exposure and its effect on the peripheral nervous system (PNS), despite its importance in the maintenance of the body's internal milieu as well as in the function of the peripheral sensorimotor system. This system includes motor and sensory neurons, their glia (Schwann cells), peripheral nerves, neuromuscular junctions, and muscle cells. In an in vitro model of neuronal-glial interaction, we know that ethanol dramatically decreases Schwann cell numbers. Our hypothesis is that prenatal ethanol exposure alters the development and long term function of the PNS. While the Schwann cell may be a vulnerable target, the other PNS components may also be affected. The consequence is an abnormal neuromuscular system that contributes both to the motor deficits manifest by children with FAS and the persistent growth retardation. We have preliminary data that exposure of pregnant rats to ethanol results in reduced grip strength in female offspring. We specifically propose to develop and characterize an in vivo rat model that demonstrates an effect of fetal ethanol exposure on the PNS. Evidence of the effects of ethanol on the PNS will be monitored by testing grip strength in rats exposed to increasing concentrations of ethanol. Electrophysiological studies to record compound action potentials will test for abnormalities in the conduction properties of the sciatic nerve. We also propose preliminary experiments using immunocytochemical staining to investigate morphological correlates of the functional and physiological findings. We will focus on two components of the sciatic nerve, Schwann cells and axons. Our long term goal is to study the mechanism by which ethanol acts on the PNS, what components are adversely affected and what approaches may ameliorate these effects

Website: http://crisp.cit.nih.gov/crisp/Crisp_Query.Generate_Screen

- **Project Title: FETO-MATERNAL PHARMACOKINETICS OF ABUSED INHALANTS**

Principal Investigator & Institution: Gatley, Samuel J.; Scientist; Brookhaven Science Assoc-Brookhaven Lab Brookhaven National Lab Upton, Ny 11973

Timing: Fiscal Year 2002; Project Start 30-SEP-2002; Project End 30-JUN-2005

Summary: (provided by applicant): Striking phenotypic similarities have been noted between infants exposed to toluene in utero and infants diagnosed with **fetal alcohol syndrome.** However, data are lacking to relate the degree of maternal exposure to toluene and other inhalant drugs of abuse to their effects on the fetus. This is an important issue because a majority of persons who abuse inhalants are females in their prime childbearing years, and the National Pregnancy and Health Survey has indicated that 12,000 pregnant women each year abuse inhalants. There are no quantitative data on transplacental transfer of toluene or any other inhalants in humans, although rodent studies indicate that 10% of an inhaled dose of toluene reaches the fetus whereas this fraction is 2% -4% for chlorinated hydrocarbons or for more highly substituted aromatics such as xylene and styrene. The proposed work builds on our previous extensive neuroimaging studies of drugs of abuse using positron emission tomography (PET) and high-field magnetic resonance spectroscopic imaging, and our recent preliminary preclinical studies with the abused inhalant, toluene, labeled with the PET radioisotope carbon-11. The objective is to develop methodologies for quantifying exposure of fetal macaques after administration of the positron labeled inhalants [11C] toluene and [11C] butane to the macaque mother. This work with two inhalants with somewhat different physical properties and reported subjective effects will set the stage for hypothesis driven PET studies with these and other inhalants in pregnant non-human primates. Ultimately, the hope is to relate the mother's exposure to inhalants to the dose received by the fetus and to post-natal behavioral deficits.

Website: http://crisp.cit.nih.gov/crisp/Crisp_Query.Generate_Screen

- **Project Title: GENE THERAPY VECTORS FOR PEDIATRIC BRAIN DISEASE**

Principal Investigator & Institution: Messer, Anne; Director/Research Scientist; Wadsworth Center Empire State Plaza Albany, Ny 12237

Timing: Fiscal Year 2001; Project Start 20-APR-2001; Project End 31-MAR-2004

Summary: (application abstract): Since the cerebellum develops over a considerable period of time, it is vulnerable to a wide range of genetic, environmental and pharmaceutical perturbants. It is also increasingly clear that the cerebellum participates in both motor and cognitive learning; therefore cerebellar defects can underlie or participate in a wide range of developmental brain disorders including **fetal alcohol syndrome,** seizures due to brain malformations, hereditary cerebellar degenerations, infantile autism, ataxia telangiactasia, and possibly dyslexia. Because of the extended developmental and plastic time-period, it may also be feasible to treat such disorders by enhancing cell outgrowth during infancy and early childhood. However, more knowledge of both the cellular factors that influence cerebellar development, and optimal methods for altering these will be required, The long-term goal of this project is to establish methods to manipulate the cerebellum genetically. This will require both knowledge of the hierarchy of gene expression, and a capacity to deliver and control gene therapies. Experiments in this proposal will encompass both the underlying developmental neurobiology and vector technology to manipulate the genes. initial experiments will test a feline lentivirus as a transfer vector, under circumstances where quantitative parameters of success are available. The mouse mutant staggerer (sg) will be used as a model system, since it shows a well-characterized defective cerebellar development, the gene has been cloned, and many of its morphological, genetic and biochemical effects are already known. The system can then be used to optimize cellspecific promoters and vector targeting strategies. Once this assay system is in place for one vector, it can also be used to test modifications of vector specificity and expression, as well as additional vectors such as AAV complexes.

Website: http://crisp.cit.nih.gov/crisp/Crisp_Query.Generate_Screen

- **Project Title: GENETIC ANALYSIS OF ETHANOL SENSITIVITY IN MICE**

Principal Investigator & Institution: Muglia, Louis J.; Associate Professor; Pediatrics; Washington University Lindell and Skinker Blvd St. Louis, Mo 63130

Timing: Fiscal Year 2001; Project Start 30-SEP-2001; Project End 31-AUG-2006

Summary: (provided by applicant): The long-term goals of our laboratory are to understand the molecular mechanisms for the neurotoxic effects of ethanol on the developing brain. Alcohol consumption by pregnant women can result in intrauterine fetal neurotoxicity, i.e. **fetal alcohol syndrome** (FAS), with sequelae in affected children including hyperactivity, learning disorders, mental retardation, depression, and psychosis. Previous pharmacological evidence has implicated N-methyl-D-aspartate (NMDA) receptor inhibition as an important direct effect of ethanol, and increased sensitivity to the sedative effect of ethanol occurs with mutations in the cAMP second messenger pathway in drosophila. We will utilize mice genetically deficient in the calcium-stimulated adenylyl cyclases type I (AC1) and VIII (AC8), important mediators of N-methyl-D-aspartate (NMDA) receptor signaling, to determine if alteration in mammalian AC function modulates ethanol sensitivity in vivo. The specific aims of this proposal will test the hypotheses that AC1 and/or AC8 deficiency results in 1) increased sensitivity to the apoptotic actions of ethanol during the synaptogenesis period of brain development; increase in sensitivity to the NMDA receptor antagonist component of ethanol action; and 3) greater long-term behavioral deficits for similar degrees of ethanol-mediated neuronal death in the perinatal period.] The results of these genetic, pharmacological, and molecular biological studies will further elucidate the molecular mechanisms by which ethanol alters neuronal physiology and survival and provide the basis for considering isoform-specific modulation of AC function as a therapeutic target for **fetal alcohol syndrome.**

Website: http://crisp.cit.nih.gov/crisp/Crisp_Query.Generate_Screen

- **Project Title: GENETIC DISSECTION OF ALCOHOL/RETINOL METABOLIC PATHWAYS**

Principal Investigator & Institution: Duester, Gregg L.; Burnham Institute 10901 N Torrey Pines Rd San Diego, Ca 92037

Timing: Fiscal Year 2001; Project Start 01-APR-1995; Project End 31-MAR-2003

Summary: (Adapted from the Investigator's Abstract) Vitamin A (retinol) must be metabolized to an active retinoid ligand in order to fulfill all of its roles in vertebrate development. During retinoid signaling retinol is first converted to retinal followed by conversion of retinal to the active ligand retinoic acid which modulates nuclear retinoic acid receptors. The alcohol dehydrogenase (ADH) enzyme family may function in the metabolism of retinol, the alcohol form of vitamin A, as well as ethanol metabolism. Some members of the ADH family prefer retinol as a substrate over ethanol, and the ability to oxidize retinol is competitively inhibited by intoxicating levels of ethanol. Likewise, there exists an aldehyde dehydrogenase (ALDH) family containing members preferring retinal, the aldehyde form of vitamin A, as a substrate over acetaldehyde. The spatiotemporal expression patterns of mouse ADHs and ALDHs overlap, suggesting that these enzymes may cooperate to upregulate retinoic acid synthesis during development. Retinoic acid synthesis may be decreased by excess ethanol consumption due to the ability of ethanol to act as a competitive inhibitor of ADH-catalyzed retinol oxidation. This suggests a mechanism whereby ethanol damage may occur during alcohol abuse. Treatment of mouse embryos at the neurulation stage with an intoxicating amount of ethanol leads to a reduction in retinoic acid levels, thus suggesting ADH participates in the retinoic acid synthetic pathway. This may be a contributing factor in **fetal alcohol syndrome,** characterized by malformations of neural and craniofacial tissues known to require retinoic acid for proper development. The in vitro properties and gene expression profiles of the ADH and ALDH enzyme families suggest a role in both alcohol and retinol metabolism, but there is a need for genetic loss-of-function studies in mice to address their true physiological roles. The mouse ADH gene family consists of three classes (ADH-I, ADH-III, and ADH-IV), with only ADH-I and ADH-IV known to oxidize retinol in vitro. The extent of the mouse ALDH gene family is unknown, but ALDH-I has been shown to oxidize retinal in vitro and has an expression pattern overlapping that of ADH-I and ADH-IV. Mutational analysis of all three mouse ADHs and ALDH-I is proposed here. Goals: (1) Complete the genetic analysis of ADH now in progress by preparing mice carrying knockout mutations of ADH-I, ADH-III, and ADH-IV, as well as mice carrying mutations of multiple ADHs since redundancy of function is suspected. (2) Analyze the phenotype of mice carrying mutations in single or multiple ADH genes for morphological defects during development and adulthood, for the ability to metabolize ethanol and retinol, and for the ability to survive and reproduce during vitamin A deficiency. (3) Prepare and ALDH-I knockout mouse plus mice mutated for one or more ADHs and ALDH-I, then analyze their phenotype as above.

Website: http://crisp.cit.nih.gov/crisp/Crisp_Query.Generate_Screen

- **Project Title: HOW MUCH DOES SHE REALLY DRINK? AN HMO INTERVENTION**

Principal Investigator & Institution: Armstrong, Mary Anne; Kaiser Foundation Research Institute 1800 Harrison St, 16Th Fl Oakland, Ca 94612

Timing: Fiscal Year 2003; Project Start 30-SEP-1999; Project End 30-JUN-2004

Summary: Alcohol abuse during pregnancy is a serious problem. Research suggests that 1) abstinence is the optimum strategy, but any decrease in alcohol consumption during pregnancy is beneficial; 2) drinkers underestimate their ethanol consumption; 3) supportive counseling is better than impersonal or purely medical approaches; and 4) in the context of a supportive environment, desire for a healthy baby is a powerful motivator. We propose to test a simple intervention in a mature managed care organization. The Kaiser Permanente Medical Care Program has implemented a substance abuse harm reduction program known as Early Start in 15 obstetrics clinics in California. We propose to enhance Early Start by helping women recognize how much alcohol they consume. We will use sample vessels, photographs of similar containers, and a simple software application that permits a counselor to show a pregnant woman what the Quantity and Frequency of her ethanol consumption actually is. Our Specific Aims are to test two hypotheses. HYPOTHESIS 1: Eligible women who abuse alcohol and who are provided with intensive education and careful quantification of their ethanol consumption (Group 1, Early Start Plus, or intervention arm) will have better perinatal outcomes (e.g., lower rates of neonatal assisted ventilation) than eligible women who simply receive confidential counseling (Group 2, Early Start, or "usual care" arm). Women in these two groups will have significantly better perinatal outcomes than those who receive no counseling at all (Group 3, comparison arm). HYPOTHESIS 2: Substance abusing women in Group 1 (Early Start Plus) will have higher rates of abstinence or cutting down on their drinking than those in Group 2 (Early Start). Women in these two groups will have significantly higher rates of abstinence or cutting down on their drinking than those who receive no counseling at all (Group 3, comparison arm). These hypotheses will be tested by randomizing 15 Early Start clinics to either the intervention or usual care arms. Each arm will consist of 7-8 obstetrics clinics. In addition, 2 KPMCP clinics where Early Start is not implemented will serve as comparison sites. We anticipate retaining 600 women in each of the 3 treatment arms during a 36 month period. We will then compare rates of a combined perinatal outcome measure (which includes mortality and morbidity) as well as decreases in maternal alcohol intake in the intervention, "usual care," and comparison arms. Our long term goals are to increase patient, provider, and policymaker awareness of the importance of alcohol abuse in pregnancy and to demonstrate the applicability of a simple, targeted intervention in a managed care organization.

Website: http://crisp.cit.nih.gov/crisp/Crisp_Query.Generate_Screen

- **Project Title: IN VITRO MECHANISMS OF ETHANOL INDUCED NEURONAL DEATH**

Principal Investigator & Institution: Mennerick, Steven J.; Assistant Professor; Psychiatry; Washington University Lindell and Skinker Blvd St. Louis, Mo 63130

Timing: Fiscal Year 2001; Project Start 30-SEP-2001; Project End 31-AUG-2006

Summary: Fetal alcohol effects and **fetal alcohol syndrome** account for a large percentage of metal retardation and behavioral disorders in the United States and impose a tremendous personal and social burden. Understanding how the immature nervous system responds to ethanol is critical to rational intervention strategies.

Electrical activity promotes survival of central nervous system (CNS) neurons in vitro and in vivo and prevents natural cell death (NCD) in neurons from many CNS regions. Ethanol depresses CNS electrical activity through interactions with both N-methyl-D-aspartate (NMDA) and gamma-aminobutyric acid (GABA) postsynaptic receptors. Thus it is possible that ethanol enhances developmental NCD. Recent evidence suggests that ethanol exposure is indeed toxic to immature neurons of the forebrain in vivo. The pattern of cell loss is similar to that produced by a combination of glutamate receptor blockade and GABA receptor potentiation. Our evidence suggests that immature hippocampal neurons in vitro are also susceptible to ethanol- induced cell loss, suggesting that susceptibility is intrinsic to neuronal populations affected and that ethanol itself, rather than associated metabolic or nutritional variables, induces the neuronal loss. Hippocampal neurons in culture also die when chronically exposed to GABAmimetics or NMDA receptor blockade. Cell death elicited by all three treatments is prevented by chronically depolarizing neurons. Thus, we have an in vitro model of ethanol-induced neuronal death that will allow us to explore mechanistic questions. We will examine the ultrastructural and biochemical profile of ethanol-induced hippocampal neuronal death in vitro. We will determine whether the interaction of ethanol with NMDA receptors and/or GABA receptors is sufficient to explain the neuronal loss observed in vitro. We will also address whether permanent or acute decreases in calcium signaling are important in cell loss and will determine the time course over which increases in intracellular calcium provide neuroprotection against ethanol-induced cell loss. The proposed experiments should lead to a better fundamental understanding of the mechanisms by which forebrain neurons are susceptible to ethanol-induced death.

Website: http://crisp.cit.nih.gov/crisp/Crisp_Query.Generate_Screen

- **Project Title: INFORMATICS CORE ON FETAL ALCOHOL SPECTRUM DISORDER**

Principal Investigator & Institution: Stewart, Craig A.; Instructional Systems Technol; Indiana University Bloomington P.O. Box 1847 Bloomington, in 47402

Timing: Fiscal Year 2003; Project Start 30-SEP-2003; Project End 31-AUG-2006

Summary: (provided by applicant): The Informatics Core is part of the Consortium for the "Collaborative Initiative on Fetal Alcohol Spectrum Disorders" (CIFASD). The theme of this collaborative initiative is a cross-cultural assessment of "fetal alcohol spectrum disorder" (FASD). The CIFASD will coordinate basic, behavioral, and clinical investigators in a multidisciplinary research project to better inform approaches aimed at developing effective intervention and treatment approaches for FASD. It will involve the input and contributions from basic researchers, behavioral scientists, and clinical investigators with the willingness to utilize novel and cutting-edge techniques so as not to simply replicate previous or ongoing work, but rather to try and move it forward in a rigorous fashion. The Informatics Core will develop and maintain the CIFASD Data Repository, which will be used to collect, maintain and distribute data generated by the various participants in the consortium. The Informatics Core will be responsible for working with the other consortium participants to define a Data Dictionary to be used in standardizing data collection, enabling the transfer of data to and from the CIFASD Data Repository, consulting on how to establish local data management systems, providing both software tools and consulting to consortium participants, and producing status reports about the progress of the various projects within the consortium. The Informatics Core draws on a wealth of resources, experience, and expertise at Indiana University in information technology infrastructure and data management, The CIFASD

Data Repository will be developed on Indiana University's state-of-the-art central supercomputing facilities, taking advantage of Indiana University's strong commitment to institutional computational resources. Resources that will be used to implement the CIFASD Data Repository include multiple supercomputers, an array of readily available database and statistical software, and a highspeed, secure, robust data archiving system capable of storing duplicate copies in multiple physical locations separated by more than fifty miles. The Informatics Core will use these extraordinary computational resources to provide a single, highly secure location for consortium participants to obtain the cross-cultural data that will enable the CIFASD to meet its goals of developing novel techniques for intervention and treatment of FASD.

Website: http://crisp.cit.nih.gov/crisp/Crisp_Query.Generate_Screen

- **Project Title: INTERNATIONAL NEUROPSYCHOLOGICAL STUDY OF FASD--U01**

Principal Investigator & Institution: May, Philip A.; Professor of Sociology; None; University of New Mexico Albuquerque Controller's Office Albuquerque, Nm 87131

Timing: Fiscal Year 2003; Project Start 30-SEP-2003; Project End 31-AUG-2006

Summary: The long-term objective of this proposal is to determine if there is a unique neurobehavioral profile in children exposed to alcohol prenatally. Even though a large body literature exists on cognitive-emotional functioning in alcohol-exposed children, it is unknown if there is a signature neurobehavioral profile in children with **fetal alcohol syndrome** (FAS) or other fetal alcohol spectrum disorder (FASD). Specific aims of the current investigation are: 1.) to assess cognitive-emotional functioning in children diagnosed with FASD from a community in South Africa and a number of American Indian reservations in the Northern Plains States. A core test battery designed by the NiAAA-supported Consortium of International Collaborative Research on FASD will be utilized in this international study; 2.) to test a specific statistical model of neurocognitive functioning (radex model) with the aim of further elucidating cognitive dysfunction in alcohol-affected children. The identification of a neurobehavioral profile in children with prenatal alcohol exposure will help clinicians diagnose children with FASD, specifically those alcohol-exposed children without evidence of dysmorphia. Identification of a profile of strengths and weaknesses of cognitive-emotional functioning is also essential for developing evidence-based interventions for children with FASD. Specifically, clinicians will be able to design programs that capitalize on strengths to address weaknesses in cognitive emotional functioning. The proposed research design involves a comparison of test performance of FASD children with that of typically developing children matched for age, sex, SES, and ethnicity. Potential participants in South Africa will be 150 children previously diagnosed as having FAS by our epidemiologic studies utilizing an international team of dysmorphologists. Case controls (n=150) will also be studied. The American Indian sample volunteers are from a large group of children diagnosed with FASD (n-100) through the University of New Mexico FAS Epidemiology Research and Prevention Project. Case controls will be selected from the same communities. The test battery will be comprised of tests designed to measure general cognitive ability, attention, executive functioning, language, visual perception, memory, motor skills and emotional functioning. Data gathered through the core test battery will be combined with those collected elsewhere in the international collaborative project (e.g. Russia, Finland, Italy, and the US) to create a large data base. This international collaborative project will provide a rare opportunity to researchers to answer many questions pertaining to cognitive-emotional functioning of FASD children to define a behavioral phenotype and to design evidence-based.

Website: http://crisp.cit.nih.gov/crisp/Crisp_Query.Generate_Screen

- **Project Title: MATERNAL ALCOHOL AND FETAL THYMIC GENE EXPRESSION**

Principal Investigator & Institution: Aird, Fraser; Psychiatry and Behavioral Scis; Northwestern University Office of Sponsored Programs Chicago, Il 60611

Timing: Fiscal Year 2001; Project Start 01-SEP-1997; Project End 31-AUG-2002

Summary: (Adapted from the Investigator's Abstract): Maternal alcohol consumption during pregnancy can adversely affect T-cell function in the offspring. This has been demonstrated in both man and animals. T-cell differentiation occurs in the thymus and involves interactions with regulatory factors produced by thymic stromal cells. It is proposed that prenatal exposure to alcohol and/or alcohol induced changes in maternal hormones induce a permanent change in expression of one or more of the stromal factors required for normal T-cell maturation, resulting in an immunosuppressive "imprinting" of the fetus. Thus, the overall goal of the proposal is to identify the genes encoding these factors, and determine their role in prenatal alcohol-induced immunosuppression. The strategy for identifying these genes is based upon previously described observations that maternal adrenalectomy reverses the T-cell dysfunction observed in fetal alcohol-exposed male rats. Therefore, this proposal will examine the developing fetal thymus for changes in gene expression brought about by FAE and maternal adrenalectomy. The specific aims are: 1) to analyze expression of known candidate genes in the fetal thymic stromal and lymphoid compartments that may contribute to FAE-induced T-cell dysfunction. 2) Identify new genes with altered expression of fetal thymic stromal cells due to FAE. 3) Establish a fetal thymic cell culture model of FAE. 4) Manipulate expression of specific genes in the fetal thymic cell culture model. Expression of genes identified in experiments 1 and 2 will be manipulated using antisense oligonucleotides to inhibit their expression, or expression vectors to overexpress these genes. Thus, a causal relationship may be established between altered expression of these genes and the observed changes in thymocyte differentiation in response to FAE.

Website: http://crisp.cit.nih.gov/crisp/Crisp_Query.Generate_Screen

- **Project Title: MATERNAL ALCOHOLISM AND CNS DEVELOPMENT OF OFFSPRING**

Principal Investigator & Institution: Druse-Manteuffel, Mary J.; Professor; Molecular & Cellular Biochem; Loyola University Medical Center Lewis Towers, 13Th Fl Chicago, Il 60611

Timing: Fiscal Year 2001; Project Start 01-JAN-1980; Project End 31-AUG-2003

Summary: Many studies of **fetal alcohol syndrome** (FAS) emphasize the relationship between the severity of abnormalities and the timing of ethanol administration relative to vulnerable periods in brain development. Chronic in utero ethanol exposure markedly impairs the early development of the serotonin (5-HT) system by encompassing a critical vulnerable period. During this period, 5-HT neurons are generated, differentiate, and extend projections to target areas; also during this period 5-HT normally exerts neurotrophic effects by stimulating astrocyte 5HT/1A receptors to increase production of S100beta, a neurotrophic factor (NTF) that is essential for the normal development of 5-HT neurons. Despite the frequency of FAS and the tremendous public health costs associated with FAS, there is no therapeutic treatment that prevents the CNS damage. This grant will investigate a mechanism by which ethanol may impair the development of the 5-HT system and a therapeutic intervention that may prevent this damage. A potential mechanism underlying the aberrant development of the 5-HT system is an ethanol-induced reduction of S100beta. This grant will investigate the use of a 5-HT/1A agonist because research suggests that this agonist prevents ethanol-associated damage to the developing 5-HT system in rats, and because this agonist increases production of S100beta. This grant proposal will investigate the following questions: Does ethanol impair the astrocyte-mediated neurotrophic stimulation of the development of serotonergic neurons? Can the damaging effects of ethanol be prevented by stimulation with a 5-HT/1A agonist? These questions will be examined using both an in vivo and in vitro experiments. In vivo experiments use a rat model to assess the effects of in utero ethanol exposure on the development of 5-HT neurons and astrocyte production of S100beta; Separate in vitro studies will use astrocytes, neurons, and astrocyte-neuron co-cultures to identify the cellular level at which these effects are mediated. Analyses will include in situ hybridization, northern and western blots, immunohistochemistry, [3H]5-HT reuptake, HPLC, and cell culture.

Website: http://crisp.cit.nih.gov/crisp/Crisp_Query.Generate_Screen

- **Project Title: MECHANISMS OF ARND RELATED SYNAPTIC PLASTICITY DEFICITS**

Principal Investigator & Institution: Savage, Daniel D.; Professor & Chair; Neurosciences; University of New Mexico Albuquerque Controller's Office Albuquerque, Nm 87131

Timing: Fiscal Year 2001; Project Start 21-SEP-2000; Project End 30-JUN-2003

Summary: (Adapted from the Investigator's Abstract) Learning disabilities are among the more subtle, yet most pervasive, of fetal alcohol exposure-related defects in children. These learning deficits may not manifest until a child is school-aged and can occur in the absence of other physical evidence of **alcohol-related birth defects.** Deficits in hippocampal glutamatergic neurotransmission and synaptic plasticity have been observed in rats whose mothers consumed moderate quantities of ethanol during gestation. As glutamate receptor-dependent synaptic plasticity is important in learning, these defects are one candidate mechanism for the learning disabilities observed in offspring whose mothers drank moderate quantities of ethanol during pregnancy. The long-term objectives of our research program are two-fold: First, to more clearly delineate the neurobiological and behavioral mechanisms of activity-dependent synaptic plasticity deficits caused by prenatal ethanol exposure. Then, once these teratologic effects are better characterized, develop and explore rational treatment strategies for overcoming fetal ethanol exposure-induced learning deficits. The working hypothesis for this project states that: Prenatal ethanol exposure decreases metabotropic glutamate receptor (mGluR5)-mediated potentiation of amino acid transmitter release in dentate gyrus slices. In this proposal, we will focus on the initial steps in the process, the coupling of the mGluR5, the G-proteins Galphaq/11 and phospholipase C-beta1 (PLC-beta1) in the production of inositol 1, 4, 5 trisphosphate (IP3). The proposed deficit may be a function of: 1) Decreased mGluR5-coupled, phospholipase C (PLC)-stimulated IP3 production, which in turn, may result from 2) decreased levels of mGluR5, Galphaq/11 or PLC-beta1 proteins or 3) alterations in agonist-mediated desensitization of mGluR5-stimulated IP3 production. These studies will provide important new information about the effects of prenatal ethanol exposure on mGluR5 regulation of transmitter release, a critical component of synaptic plasticity in the hippocampal formation. Further, these results could provide insights into whether agents that affect mGluR function could be used to treat synaptic plasticity deficits and, ultimately, learning deficits in prenatal ethanol-exposed offspring.

Website: http://crisp.cit.nih.gov/crisp/Crisp_Query.Generate_Screen

- **Project Title: MODERATE ETHANOL PRENATALLY ON NMDA PHOSPHORYLATION**

Principal Investigator & Institution: Leslie, Steven W.; Professor; Institute for Neuroscience; University of Texas Austin 101 E. 27Th/Po Box 7726 Austin, Tx 78712

Timing: Fiscal Year 2001; Project Start 01-AUG-1999; Project End 30-APR-2004

Summary: Studies in our laboratory and by others indicate that prenatal and early postnatal ethanol exposure results in a significant reduction of NMDA receptor function and number. NMDA receptors are linked with important aspects of brain development and learning and memory. Ethanol-related deficits in NMDA function, therefore, may be of key importance not only in the severe cognitive and behavioral deficiencies of **fetal alcohol syndrome** (FAS) but also in alcohol-related neurodevelopmental disorders (ARND) typically expressed as behavioral symptoms associated with fetal alcohol effects (FAE). We have recently found that decreases in NMDA receptor function resulting from prenatal ethanol exposure in rats are accompanied by reductions in some, but not all, of the subunits comprising the NMDA receptor complex. NMDAR2A and NMDAR2B subunits are significantly reduced, while the NMDAR1 subunit is unaffected. Studies conducted thus far have examined the effects of high doses of ethanol prenatally and postnatally on NMDA receptor function and subunit levels. Studies proposed in specific aims 1 through 4 are designed to determine the dose-response relationships of prenatal ethanol treatment on 1) functional measures of NMDA receptor activation using fura-2 loaded dissociated neurons and H-MK801 binding, 2) NMDAR1 and NMDAR2 subunit protein (Western blot analysis) and messenger RNA levels (RNase protection assay), and 3) changes in NMDA receptor subunit composition as measured by immunoprecipitation studies. Specific aim 4 will examine the relationship(s) of NMDA receptor subunit changes with changes in subunit phosphorylation. The overall hypothesis of this proposal is that prenatal ethanol exposure, even at modest concentrations, will result in demonstrable deficits in the function of NMDA receptors. We expect the magnitude of the deficits to be dose-related. It is hypothesized further that ethanol's actions in this regard may be linked with abnormalities of NMDA receptor phosphorylation.

Website: http://crisp.cit.nih.gov/crisp/Crisp_Query.Generate_Screen

- **Project Title: MOLECULAR TOXICOLOGY OF PLACENTAL CARBOXYLESTRASE**

Principal Investigator & Institution: Yan, Bingfang; Pharmacology and Toxicology; University of Rhode Island 70 Lower College Road, Suite 2 Kingston, Ri 028810811

Timing: Fiscal Year 2001; Project Start 01-FEB-1997; Project End 31-JAN-2003

Summary: APPLICANT'S ABSTRACT: Carboxylesterases are known to play an important role in xenobiotic metabolism and detoxication of pesticides The long-term objective of the proposed studies is to determine the molecular basis for the existence of multiple forms of human carboxylesterases, and to determine the structure, function and regulation of these enzymes. The central hypothesis of the proposed project is that the multiple forms of carboxylesterases expressed in human placenta are distinct gene products that have different substrate specificities, and are independently regulated. The specific aims of the project are (1) to isolate from a human placental library full-length cDNAs encoding two carboxylesterases (HP-1 and HP-2), and (2) to characterize by biochemical, immunochemical and molecular techniques the structure, function and regulation of these enzymes. As part of enzymatic and immunochemical studies, recombinant enzymes and antibodies against the recombinant proteins will be produced. To test the hypothesis that HP-1 and HP-2 have different substrate specificities, the recombinant enzymes will be examined for their ability to hydrolyze selected esters and amides, and their ability to catalyze the transesterification of cocaine and the synthesis of fatty acid ethyl esters. Immunoprecipitation from placental samples will be conducted to compare enzymatic characteristics between the natural and recombinant enzymes. To test the hypothesis that HP-1 and HP-2 are independently regulated, the MRNA and protein levels will be determined with samples from individual placenta and cultured placental slices treated with xenobiotics. Samples for these studies will cover a broad range of genetic (i.e., ethnic) and environmental (i.e., smoking) factors. Some progress has been made toward the goals of the project. The enzymatic activity of placental microsomes to hydrolyze several esters has been determined. Two partial cDNAs (348 bp each) that apparently encode two distinct carboxylesterases have been isolated from human placentas. In addition to hydrolyzing numerous xenobiotics such as drugs and pesticides, carboxylesterases are known to catalyze a transesterification reaction and fatty acid ethyl ester synthesis. Ethylcocaine, a more potent metabolite of cocaine in mediating lethality and cardiac toxicity than the parent compound, is formed through the transesterification reaction. The accumulation of ethyl esters due to alcohol abuse during pregnancy has been shown to contribute significantly to the development of **fetal alcohol syndrome.** Therefore, the experiments outlined in this project will contribute significantly to our basic understanding of carboxylesterases as a family of enzymes involved in the detoxication and bioactivation of xenobiotics.

Website: http://crisp.cit.nih.gov/crisp/Crisp_Query.Generate_Screen

- **Project Title: MOTIVATING PREGNANT PROBLEM DRINKERS TO CHANGE**

Principal Investigator & Institution: Handmaker, Nancy S.; Visiting Assistant Professor; Psychology; University of New Mexico Albuquerque Controller's Office Albuquerque, Nm 87131

Timing: Fiscal Year 2001; Project Start 27-SEP-1999; Project End 30-JUN-2004

Summary: Prenatal alcohol exposure is known to cause brain damage. Persons with brain damage resulting from drinking during pregnancy have developmental disabilities and related lifetime problems in school, employment, and independent functioning. Alcohol counseling offered as part of prenatal care has been shown to decrease drinking among pregnant women and the adverse consequences to their babies. Few prenatal care clinics are prepared to offer specialized alcohol treatment. An alternative strategy is to improve the efficacy of minimal counseling and referrals offered within obstetric care settings. In two decades of clinical trials, brief interventions have been shown to reduce drinking, improve health, and increase the rate of successful referrals to alcohol treatment. Motivational Interviewing has been shown in a pilot study to reduce drinking among high-risk pregnant women. The proposed project aims to replicate these findings with a larger sample to develop motivational strategies that can be implemented during early prenatal care in primary health care settings to decrease maternal and fetal risks due to drinking. A brief counseling approach will be tested in a randomized clinical trial. A sample of 300 at-risk drinkers receiving prenatal care will be assigned to one of three conditions prior to their referral for alcohol treatment: (1) Motivational Enhancement Therapy (MET); (2) a comparison group who will also receive MET, but 6 weeks later; or (3) Treatment- As-Usual, screening and advice to abstain. Maternal outcomes to be assessed include drinking and other drug use during subsequent pregnancy and postpartum, risk perception and motivation for change, alcohol treatment adherence, and psychological status. Infant psychomotor, physical, and cognitive development will also be assessed at 6 and 14 months. It is predicted that motivational counseling as a prelude to alcohol treatment, will significantly increase adherence to alcohol change programs and suppress maternal drinking. Project data will also be used to develop predictors of alcohol-related effects among infants, and of maternal response to intervention. Finally, the larger screened sample of 6,000 pregnancies will provide valuable epidemiological data on alcohol use and its relationship to pregnancy health complications.

Website: http://crisp.cit.nih.gov/crisp/Crisp_Query.Generate_Screen

- **Project Title: NEURAL BASIS OF THE ONTOGENY OF EYEBLINK CONDITIONING**

Principal Investigator & Institution: Freeman, John Henry.; Assistant Professor; Psychology; University of Iowa Iowa City, Ia 52242

Timing: Fiscal Year 2001; Project Start 10-APR-2000; Project End 31-MAR-2004

Summary: (Adapted from the Investigator's Abstract) Associative learning plays a key role in early development by providing a means for learning predictive relationships between events. The ontogeny of associative learning is thought to depend on developmental processes within the central nervous system. However, little information exists concerning the cellular mechanisms of associative learning during development. The proposed research project is designed to examine developmental changes in neuronal function that underlie the ontogeny of classically conditioned eyeblink responses in rats. The cerebellum is an essential component of the neural circuitry that mediates eyeblink conditioning in adult organisms and exhibits extensive morphological development during the first four postnatal weeks in rats. Preliminary studies showed that the eyeblink conditioned response (CR) also developed during the first four postnatal weeks in rats. Moreover, disrupting cerebellar maturation experimentally impaired the ontogeny of eyeblink conditioning. These data provided compelling evidence for a link between cerebellar maturation and the development of eyeblink conditioning. However, the ability to determine the specific changes in neural processes that underlie the development of the eyeblink CR requires a physiological analysis of learning-related neural plasticity within the cerebellum and brainstem. Three experimental approaches will be used for examining the relationship between neural maturation and the ontogeny of eyeblink conditioning. First, the experiments of Specific Aims 1 and 2 will use extracellular recording methods to examine ontogenetic changes in neuronal activity within various components of the eyeblink conditioning neural circuitry. Second, the experiments of Specific Aim 3 will determine whether electrical stimulation of either the conditioned or unconditioned stimulus neural pathways could be used to alter the time-course of the ontogeny of eyeblink conditioning. Third, the experiments of Specific Aim4 will evaluate developmental changes in the induction of neuronal plasticity in the cerebellum. This research will yield unique data concerning the specific changes in neuronal function that could underlie associative eyeblink conditioning. This work may also lead to the discovery of general principles concerning the relationship between neural and behavioral development, which could be applied to the analysis of other types of behavioral responses. In addition to the basic research goals of this project, the results of these studies may lead to a better understanding of the functional pathology associated with various developmental disorders that affect the nervous system including **fetal alcohol syndrome,** exposure to environmental neurotoxins, infantile autism, and Down's syndrome.

Website: http://crisp.cit.nih.gov/crisp/Crisp_Query.Generate_Screen

- **Project Title: NEUROANATOMIC/PSYCHOLOGIC ANALYSES OF FAS/FAE DEFICITS**

Principal Investigator & Institution: Streissguth, Ann P.; Psychiatry and Behavioral Scis; University of Washington Seattle, Wa 98195

Timing: Fiscal Year 2003; Project Start 01-AUG-1996; Project End 30-APR-2006

Summary: (provided by applicant): This research proposes to extend the successful work already completed in quantifying the neuroanatomic abnormalities underlying neuropsychological deficits among people with brain damage caused by prenatal alcohol exposure. Although **Fetal Alcohol Syndrome** (FAS) is a distinct diagnostic entity, it conceals substantial variability of deficits. Many individuals with substantial prenatal alcohol exposure exhibit dysfunctional behaviors that appear to be CNS-based, but do not have facial manifestations of FAS. These features are sometimes referred to as possible fetal alcohol effects (FAE). In prior work, we developed and demonstrated a new method of shape analysis targeting the corpus callosum (CC) that was above 80% accurate in separating FAS/FAE from controls, using a symmetrical four-quadrant data set of male and female adolescents and adults across three diagnostic groups: FAS, FAE, and age/sex matched non-exposed controls. Using newly developed methods, we now propose to reanalyze these magnetic resonance images for additional brain structures, targeting the cerebellum, and to compare these images with the full battery of neuropsychological tests obtained on our 180 subjects. We hypothesize that these new image analyses will reveal significant differences in mean or variance of brain form between FAS/FAE and controls, that FAS and FAE will not differ from each other, and that distinct profiles of association will be observed between neuroanatomy and neuropsychology. Over three years, we will pursue four aims: (1.) To quantify new morphological data from existing magnetic resonance images, to examine additional curves and shapes on and near the cerebellum that will be combined with CC and gray/white matter volumes in detecting FAS/FAE; (2.) To examine the behavioral phenotype of FAS/FAE, using already collected data augmented with new scores from existing data, to study the other three quadrants of subjects for profiles of Executive Function and Motor Function deficits that were related to different CC shape anomalies in adult males; (3.) To conclude the full four-quadrant neuroanatomic/neuropsychologic analysis, using the new data on cerebellar shape and size combined with the augmented behavioral phenotype data; (4.) To develop a data-driven diagnostic protocol based on the principles already demonstrated and utilizing entire data sets from both imaging and behavior. This will be the first systematic study to move directly from state-of-the-art image analysis techniques and neuropsychological testing, to a diagnostic protocol with practical utility, filling a compelling need for diagnosing fetal alcohol brain damage in adolescents and adults and in the absence of the typical facial characteristics.

Website: http://crisp.cit.nih.gov/crisp/Crisp_Query.Generate_Screen

- **Project Title: NORTHERN PLAINS PRENATAL AND INFANT HEALTH CONSORTIUM**

Principal Investigator & Institution: Elliott, Amy J.; Pediatrics; University of South Dakota 414 E Clark St Vermillion, Sd 57069

Timing: Fiscal Year 2003; Project Start 26-SEP-2003; Project End 31-JUL-2006

Summary: (provided by applicant): The 'Northern Plains Prenatal and Infant Health Consortium' is comprised of three institutions that each have existing links to communities across South and North Dakota and an Advisory Board with representatives from numerous community agencies and disciplines. The primary purpose behind the formation of this consortium is to provide a structure in which collaborative research projects can be conducted to clarify the role prenatal alcohol exposure plays in fetal death, stillbirth, and sudden infant death syndrome. Deciphering the impact of prenatal alcohol exposure on fetal/infant mortality and development will require the input of individuals from a variety of disciplines, in addition to input regarding community needs and concerns. The Northern Plains Consortium is committed to participating in the multidisciplinary steering committee that will result from this RFA and will work in a cooperative manner with the other Comprehensive Clinical Sites, the Developmental Biology and Pathology Center, the Data Coordinating and Analysis Center, and the NIH to design protocols that can be implemented across numerous clinical sites. It is hoped that this collaborative effort will result in answers that will decrease fetal and infant mortality rates, thereby improving child health in the communities we serve. The primary goal for Phase I of this project will be to formalize the collaborative relationships, with both the Steering Committee and the Northern Plains Advisory Board, which will serve as the basis for conducting multi-site research projects. These relationships will be formed through meetings which will occur 4 times in the first year for the Steering Committee and twice with the Advisory Board. We will meet with our advisory board twice each year, coincident with the bi-annual meetings of the Aberdeen Area Perinatal Infant Mortality Review Committee (PIMR). These meetings will lead to the creation of the collaborative structure and processes through which research projects suitable for multi-site implementation will be designed. Furthermore, the Advisory Board, which contains many community leaders, will help develop ways to strengthen the functional community partnerships that will be necessary to successfully carry out this research agenda. A final goal will be to refine the design of a potential pilot study that draws upon our expertise in the areas of exposure assessment and measurement of physiologic function during the fetal and early newborn period.

Website: http://crisp.cit.nih.gov/crisp/Crisp_Query.Generate_Screen

- **Project Title: OVINE MODEL SYSTEM FOR ALCOHOL RELATED BIRTH DEFECTS**

Principal Investigator & Institution: Cudd, Timothy A.; Veterinary Physiology & Pharmacology; Texas A&M University System College Station, Tx 778433578

Timing: Fiscal Year 2003; Project Start 01-SEP-1997; Project End 31-MAR-2007

Summary: This abstract is not available.

Website: http://crisp.cit.nih.gov/crisp/Crisp_Query.Generate_Screen

- **Project Title: PILOT--MATERNAL ALCOHOL ABUSE AND ITS EFFECTS ON PREMATURE INFANTS**

Principal Investigator & Institution: Gauthier, Theresa W.; Emory University 1784 North Decatur Road Atlanta, Ga 30322

Timing: Fiscal Year 2003; Project Start 01-FEB-2003; Project End 31-DEC-2007

Summary: Despite the well known neurological effects of alcohol on the developing fetus, its use during pregnancy remains a significant problem in our country. Even with modern neonatal intensive care units, chronic lung disease and bacterial sepsis continue to cause significant morbidity and mortality for the very low birth weight premature newborn. We have expanded the traditional focus of fetal alcohol exposure on the central nervous system to two other developing organ systems of the fetus, namely the lung and immune system. Recent prospective data implicates a history of alcohol abuse as the first reported co-morbid variable significantly increasing the incidence and severity of acute respiratory distress syndrome in adults. Additionally, alcohol exposure is associated with a decrease in lung antioxidant status, particularly glutathione. Glutathione is an essential antioxidant in the epithelial lining fluid of the lung. A reduction in alveolar glutathione, as seen in the premature infant, leaves the lung susceptible to increased pulmonary oxidative injury. We have novel experimental data describing reduced pulmonary glutathione, impairment of alveolar type II epithelial cell function and impaired cell function and impaired surfactant homeostasis in fetal guinea pig lungs exposed to alcohol in utero. Additionally, in a logistic regression analysis of 872 term newborns, we have demonstrated that maternal excessive alcohol use of 7 drinks/wk in either the 3 months prior to conception of the 2nd trimester significantly increased the risk of newborn infection by approximately 3 fold. Because of these data implicating adverse effects of fetal alcohol exposure on the developing fetus, we hypothesize the following: (1) alcohol exposure in (CLD), and (2) fetal alcohol exposure impairs fetal immune function thereby increasing the risk of infection, particularly late onset sepsis, in the premature newborn. We will address these hypotheses in the pilot clinical study by 1: Screening all women who deliver premature infants weighing <1500 gms for alcohol use during pregnancy with an extensive questionnaire. 2: Perform outcome analysis of these infants comparing alcohol-exposed to non-exposed premature infants, investigating the primary outcomes of chronic lung disease and late onset sepsis.

Website: http://crisp.cit.nih.gov/crisp/Crisp_Query.Generate_Screen

- **Project Title: POLYAMINES IN NEONATAL ALCOHOL NEUROTOXICITY**

Principal Investigator & Institution: Barron, Susan; Psychology; University of Kentucky 109 Kinkead Hall Lexington, Ky 40506

Timing: Fiscal Year 2003; Project Start 01-AUG-2003; Project End 31-JUL-2006

Summary: (provided by applicant): While it is well known that prenatal ethanol (ETOH) exposure has detrimental effects on the developing CNS, there are still numerous questions regarding the mechanisms underlying the CNS damage observed. The effects of ETOH on the glutamate/NMDA receptor (NMDAR) are well established. ETOH-induced alterations in NMDAR function during development causes hippocampal damage by at least two mechanisms; reduced NMDAR function during the presence of ETOH (via apoptosis) and enhanced NMDAR function during ETOH withdrawal (via excitotoxicity). Which of these mechanisms predominates may be age- dependent with suppression of NMDAR activity being more damaging at earlier developmental stages and overexcitation during ETOH WD being a more dominant component in older cultures. Polyamines are ubiquitous compounds that also play an important trophic role during CNS development and one of the mechanisms by which polyamines work is by potentiation of the NMDAR. Since hippocampal NMDAR subtypes and their response to polyamines change during the first neonatal weeks in rats, the timing when ETOH exposure occurs may have significant influences on response to polyamines, NMDAR and outcome. These hypotheses can be tested directly in vitro using the organotypic cell culture model and comparing cultures obtained from neonatal rats at PND 2 versus PND 8. The specific aims are 1) to examine how developmental age affects the response to ETOH as measured by cell damage in our in vitro organotyplc hippocampal model; 2) to examine how developmental age and ETOH exposure interact with polyamines as measured by cell damage in the in vitro hippocampal model and 3) To assess whether in vivo ETOH exposure correlates with the findings from in vitro exposure. The model proposed in this application will provide an innovative and novel approach for using hippocampal organotypic cell cultures to address specific developmental questions related to ETOH's effects and to assess the predictive validity of the model to predict in vivo results. With these findings, it may also be possible to gain a better understanding of some of the mechanisms underlying neonatal ETOH exposure and the role of polyamines that will provide grounds for pharmacological interventions that will reduce some of ETOH effects.

Website: http://crisp.cit.nih.gov/crisp/Crisp_Query.Generate_Screen

- **Project Title: PRENATAL ALCOHOL EXPOSURE: ADULT NEUROCOGNITION**

Principal Investigator & Institution: Coles, Claire D.; Professor; Psychiatry and Behavioral Scis; Emory University 1784 North Decatur Road Atlanta, Ga 30322

Timing: Fiscal Year 2003; Project Start 30-SEP-2003; Project End 31-AUG-2008

Summary: (provided by applicant): **Fetal Alcohol Syndrome** (FAS) and associated disorders are a major cause of lifelong developmental and behavioral disabilities. Maternal alcohol use during gestation produces dysmorphology, growth deficits and impacts the nervous system in ways that are not yet fully understood. Despite the need for accurate, databased information on the long-term effects of this teratogen, empirical research on adaptive functioning and neurocognition in alcohol-exposed and affected adults is still very limited. The proposed research will follow a well-characterized sample (N=275), part of a cohort identified prenatally between 1980 and 1986 based on maternal alcohol use during pregnancy, into early adulthood in order to describe their current functioning and to evaluate neurocognitive status. These outcomes will be correlated with the results of neuroimaging in a subsample (n=120) of individuals demonstrating behavioral effects of prenatal exposure. Previous research with this low socioeconomic status (SES), predominantly African-American cohort has demonstrated a pattern of neurodevelopmental deficits consistent with the hypothesis that alcohol exposure may have affected white matter tracts in the brain at both macrostructural and microstructural levels and that deficits related to such alterations may be associated with specific neurobehavioral outcomes. Using structural and functional MRI protocols and Diffusion Tensor Imaging (DTI), we will evaluate a series of hypotheses that prenatally exposed individuals demonstrating neuropsychological deficits relative to controls, matched for SES and disability status, will show measurable differences in brain structure and in indices of white matter integrity. A longitudinal follow-up portion of the study will examine social, adaptive and neuropsychological outcomes in alcohol-exposed and affected young adults and compare results to those of SES matched controls who have also been followed longitudinally and to members of a special education contrast group recruited during adolescence. A subsample of alcohol-affected individuals and controls will be selected for neuroimaging at 3T to evaluate effects of prenatal alcohol exposure on macrostructure, microstructure and function. We anticipate that these techniques will provide insight into the teratogenic effects of alcohol exposure on development as well as the relationship between white matter integrity and neuropsychological functioning in this disorder.

Website: http://crisp.cit.nih.gov/crisp/Crisp_Query.Generate_Screen

- **Project Title: RESPONSE SIGNATURES OF ALCOHOL RELATED BIRTH DEFECTS**

Principal Investigator & Institution: Knudsen, Thomas B.; Professor; Pathology, Anat/Cell Biology; Thomas Jefferson University Office of Research Administration Philadelphia, Pa 191075587

Timing: Fiscal Year 2001; Project Start 29-SEP-2001; Project End 31-AUG-2004

Summary: Fetal alcohol syndrome (FAS) refers to a recognized pattern of birth defects that occurs in a subset of children born to women who consume alcohol during pregnancy. Typical alcohol- related birth defects include microencephaly, microphthalmia, deficiencies of the facial prominences and visceral arches, as well as effects on the heart, great vessels, and thymus. Understanding disease mechanisms in prenatal alcohol exposure depends upon learning what metabolic and regulatory pathways mediate critical steps leading to dysmorphogenesis. The research proposed here uses gene expression arrays and bioinformatics to probe the origins of **alcohol-related birth defects** in an acute animal model. Many disease endpoints in human **alcohol-related birth defects** can be induced acutely in C57BL/6J mice during gastrulation-neurulation phases of development. Specific Aim 1 will survey the normal (developmental) gene expression for structures commonly malformed in **alcohol-related birth defects.** Parameterization will landmark key stages of ocular and hindbrain development across the window of vulnerability to ethanol-induced teratogenesis (days 8-10 of gestation) using C7BL/6J and CD-1 strains of mice that are differentially responsive to acute gestational exposure of ethanol. Conventional microdissection and laser capure microdissection will isolate specific precursor target cell populations from the test and reference samples. Specific Aim 2 will enumerate alcohol-related changes of gene expression within the exposure-disease continuum. Parameterization will entail dose-response, time after exposure, and strains differing in sensitivity. Emphasis will be the developing eye and hindbrain for exposure on day 9 of gestation. Specific Aim 3 is to initiate a functional genomics/computational biology pipeline for comprehensive pattern recognition, exploration, and validation of alcohol-related changes in developing target organs. Microarray data will be amalgamated into the first gene expression reference database for detecting alcohol-related effects on the developing embryo. This effort will enable computation of critical response signatures that represent core phenomena in disease mechanisms. By studying multigenic response signatures we hope to define the various metabolic and regulatory pathways set into disarray during critical periods of prenatal ethanol exposure. At ends, we expect this knowledge will enable researchers to identify mechanisms of **alcohol-related birth defects** and noninvasive strategies toward intervention. Project-generated resources will include the design and construction of specialized arrays focused on the genes emerging as responsive to ethanol intoxication, as well as a relational database made accessible to the scientific community through the world-wide web.

Website: http://crisp.cit.nih.gov/crisp/Crisp_Query.Generate_Screen

- **Project Title: RISK FACTORS AND THE VULNERABILITY OF THE DEVELOPING BRAIN**

  Principal Investigator & Institution: Edmond, John; University of California Los Angeles 10920 Wilshire Blvd., Suite 1200 Los Angeles, Ca 90024

  Timing: Fiscal Year 2001; Project Start 30-SEP-1983; Project End 30-NOV-2001

  Summary: This abstract is not available.

  Website: http://crisp.cit.nih.gov/crisp/Crisp_Query.Generate_Screen

- **Project Title: RISK FACTORS FOR FASD IN THE MOSCOW REGION**

  Principal Investigator & Institution: Chambers, Christina D.; Epidemiologist; Pediatrics; University of California San Diego 9500 Gilman Dr, Dept. 0934 La Jolla, Ca 92093

  Timing: Fiscal Year 2003; Project Start 30-SEP-2003; Project End 31-AUG-2006

Summary: (provided by applicant): Defining the range of expression, risk factors for, and incidence of FASD in children born to women who drink varying amounts of alcohol during pregnancy is of vital importance in terms of prevention, intervention and treatment. The proposed study entails a collaboration with the Moscow Region Ministry of Health to screen 26,000 pregnant women over two years. From these, 640 moderate to heavy drinkers and 640 controls will be selected for longitudinal follow-up including standardized physical exams and neurobehavioral testing of infants through twelve months of age. The specific aims of the project are: 1) To measure the birth prevalence and range of alcohol-related physical features and neurobehavioral impairment among children born to pregnant women in the Moscow Region who report consuming moderate to heavy amounts of alcohol by utilizing methods designed to permit earlier diagnosis of alcohol-related effects, and 2) To evaluate the contribution of maternal nutritional factors to increased risk for prenatal growth deficiency, neurobehavioral impairment, and alcohol-related physical features in infants prenatally exposed to moderate to heavy amounts of alcohol by conducting a randomized trial of a micronutrient supplementation intervention and measuring micronutrient levels in maternal blood. The proposed study will contribute to a better understanding of the incidence and range of FASD based on early diagnosis in a cross-cultural environment, and will for the first time specifically test a nutritional intervention that may have widespread applicability should undernutrition prove to be a modifiable risk factor for FASD.

Website: http://crisp.cit.nih.gov/crisp/Crisp_Query.Generate_Screen

- **Project Title: ROLE OF OPIATES IN ALCOHOL-INDUCED NEUROTOXICITY**

Principal Investigator & Institution: Sarkar, Dipak K.; Professor Ii and Director; None; Rutgers the St Univ of Nj New Brunswick Asb Iii New Brunswick, Nj 08901

Timing: Fiscal Year 2001; Project Start 01-AUG-1991; Project End 30-JUN-2005

Summary: (Adapted from the Investigator's Abstract) Exposure of a fetus to ethanol can lead to development of **fetal alcohol syndrome,** which is characterized by various morphological and behavioral deficits in fetal alcohol-exposed offspring. These offspring often show abnormalities in stress responses. Recent studies have revealed a possibility that the stress response anomalies seen in the FAE offspring are related to the functional abnormalities of hypothalamic beta-endorphin- (b-EP) producing neurons. However, there is not sufficient information available on the effect of ethanol on b-endorphin neuronal growth and differentiation. The present proposal will address this issue by studying the in vivo and in vitro effects of ethanol on beta-endorphin neuron growth and differentiation using rat as an animal model. The proposed research will test the hypotheses that ethanol exposure during the developmental period induces programmed cell death in b-EP neurons and that cAMP and transforming growth factor-beta1 (TGF-beta1) may be involved in controlling the ethanol-induced neurotoxicity. Specific objectives of this proposal are to: 1) determine the action of ethanol on b-EP neuronal growth and differentiation and the consequence on the development of the functional b-EP neurons, 2) identify the role of the cAMP system in ethanol neurotoxic action on b-EP neurons, 3) evaluate the role of TGF-beta in ethanol neurotoxic action on b-EP neurons, 4) study the signaling mechanisms of the ethanol neurotoxic action on b-EP neurons. Ethanol's action on programmed cell death in the b-EP neurons will be studied both in vivo and in vitro using biochemical and immunocytochemical techniques. The mechanism of ethanol's neurotoxic action on b-EP neurons will be determined using a rat fetal hypothalamic neuronal cell culture system. Two-pronged approaches will be applied to study the mechanisms of the ethanol neurotoxic action; one to pharmacologically manipulate the signal transduction systems, another to measure the intracellular level of these signal transducers by histological, biochemical and molecular techniques.

Website: http://crisp.cit.nih.gov/crisp/Crisp_Query.Generate_Screen

- **Project Title: SIDS DATA COORDINATING AND ANALYSIS CENTER**

Principal Investigator & Institution: Dukes, Kimberly A.; Dm-Stat, Inc. 407 Rear Mystic Ave, Unit 11A Medford, Ma 02155

Timing: Fiscal Year 2003; Project Start 30-SEP-2003; Project End 31-JUL-2006

Summary: (provided by applicant): In multi-center studies or collaborative projects, a centralized Data Coordinating and Analysis Center (DCAC) with strong leadership, organization and analytic skills is critical to the success of the project. DMSTAT, Inc. proposes to serve as the DCAC for the multi-disciplinary research network on prenatal alcohol exposure and sudden infant death syndrome (SIDS) that will be established through responses to RFA HD- 03-004. DM-STAT has a proven track record of success as the designated DCAC on NICHD and NIAAA sponsored multi-center trials and collaborations. Our goal is to make life easier for participating staff so that they can focus on their areas of expertise. To achieve that goal, DM-STAT will create and maintain a study-wide infrastructure to support the activities of and facilitate information sharing between members of the Network, including the NICHD, NIAAA, and governing boards. This infrastructure will revolve around a Network website containing administrative and data management components. The website will provide instant access to all project documentation and materials, data management reports, statistical analysis summaries, and will provide a forum (the Meeting Center) for sharing ideas and issues. The first phase (of two phases) calls for formalizing a collaborative structure between, Comprehensive Clinical Sites (CCS), Developmental Biology and Pathology Center(s) (DBPC) and the DCAC to investigate the relationship between prenatal alcohol exposure and the risk for sudden infant death syndrome (SIDS) and adverse pregnancy outcomes (e.g., stillbirth and **fetal alcohol syndrome (FAS)**). In addition, the Network will investigate social and behavioral factors that may be related to a woman's decision to drink alcohol during pregnancy and lactation. Phase I will require development of testable hypotheses, pilot testing of the core and site-specific protocols and producing an executive summary with recommendations based upon the results of these pilot studies in order to assess feasibility and justification for Phase II. DM-STAT will provide leadership and guidance to the network with respect to study design, protocol development, data management and statistical analysis. With a cohesive Network in place, DM-STAT will then be responsible for coordinating safe and consistent implementation of the core protocol, monitoring key indicators of quality, and performing analysis of pilot data. DM-STAT is committed to quality; it is the focal point of everything we do. We are proactive as opposed to reactive, innovative in streamlining and organizing processes and procedures, able to educate and communicate with study staff at all levels, and we are passionate and committed to getting the job done right the first time. We believe that DM-STAT is best positioned to serve the needs of this Network in an efficient and effective manner.

Website: http://crisp.cit.nih.gov/crisp/Crisp_Query.Generate_Screen

- **Project Title: THE MOLECULAR BASIS OF ALCOHOL'S ACTIONS.**

Principal Investigator & Institution: Jones, David N.; Assistant Professor; Pharmacology; University of Colorado Hlth Sciences Ctr P.O. Box 6508, Grants and Contracts Aurora, Co 800450508

Timing: Fiscal Year 2003; Project Start 01-FEB-2003; Project End 31-JAN-2008

Summary: (provided by applicant): Objectives and Health Related Issues. The intoxicating effects associated with exposure to ethanol have been linked to changes in the activities of several neurotransmitter receptors that are ligand-gated ion-channels. Acute exposure of the 7- amino-butyric acid (GABA) and N-methyl D-aspartate (NMDA) receptors to ethanol is directly implicated in the development of **fetal alcohol syndrome** and also in alcohol toxicity and alcohol dependency in the adult. There is increasing evidence that ethanol binds to specific sites on these receptors and induces a conformational change that modifies their activity. Characterization of alcohol-binding sites in ethanol sensitive proteins would provide potential targets for the development of pharmacological agents to control alcohol intoxication and alcohol dependency. At present there is no direct structural information available about the nature of potential binding sites of these important ethanol-sensitive proteins because of the inherent difficulties in studying integral membrane proteins. LUSH is a novel alcohol-binding protein from fruit flies that recognizes ethanol, n-propanol and n butanol. We have recently solved the structure of LUSH in the complex with ethanol. The long-term goal of this proposal is to characterize the molecular nature of this binding site in detail in order to define the molecular basis for alcohol-binding specificity. The structure of LUSH bound to a series of alcohols will be solved using X-ray crystallographic methods to reveal a molecular picture of alcohol specificity in a nonenzymatic protein. The effect of different alcohols on binding affinity and protein stability will be analyzed using biophysical and spectroscopic methods, and the differences correlated with changes to the protein structure in solution. The role of specific amino acids in alcohol binding and protein function will be tested using site directed mutagenesis to engineer proteins with modified ligand-binding properties. The ultimate goal is to develop a model for specific alcohol-binding sites in alcohol-sensitive proteins that will aid in an understanding of the molecular basis of alcohols actions in causing intoxication and toxicity.

Website: http://crisp.cit.nih.gov/crisp/Crisp_Query.Generate_Screen

- **Project Title: THE NEUROBIOLOGY OF ATTENTION IN FETAL ALCOHOL SYNDROMEN**

Principal Investigator & Institution: Lockhart, Paula J.; Kennedy Krieger Research Institute, Inc. Baltimore, Md 21205

Timing: Fiscal Year 2001; Project Start 01-JUL-2001; Project End 30-JUN-2006

Summary: This is a request for a NIAAA Mentored Patient Oriented Research Career Development Award (K23). This proposal describes a 5-year plan for the development of the candidate into an independent researcher in clinical child psychiatry and will include an investigation of attention problems in **Fetal Alcohol Syndrome** (FAS). This project will employ neurobehavioral paradigms and volumetric magnetic resonance imaging to evaluate the hypothesis that abnormalities of attention observed in individuals with FAS are due to disturbances in both an "anterior" frontostriatal network hypothesized to contribute to difficulties in motor impersistence and response inhibition, and a "posterior " parietal network, hypothesized to contribute to difficulties with orientation shifting attention. Through the mentorship of experts in the fields of developmental behavioral neurology, child psychiatry and neuropsychology, the candidate will embark on a course of study and mentored research that will characterize cortical networks of attention in FAS. The results of this study will lay the foundation for the future investigation of possible neurobiologic and neurobehavioral biomarkers of attention network impairment in this population of prenatally exposed individuals. Short term career goals are to become familiar with neurobehavioral paradigms used in the assessment of attention; to become proficient in the understanding and use of volumetric magnetic imaging; and to understand the basics of research design, ethics, epidemiology, and biostatistics as it applies to clinical child psychiatry. Additionally, the protected time will allow a more in depth evaluation of the FAS behavioral phenotype, with additional study in neuropharmacology, neurophysiology, neuroanatomy and psychopathology as it applies to brain-behavior relationships arising from teratogenic exposure. Long term career goals are to use the skills obtained in the didactic courses, tutorials and the mentored research project to perform independent clinical child psychiatry research in the pathogenesis of neuropsychiatric disorders associated with prenatal alcohol exposure will be investigated further in future projects, with the goal of helping design more focused mental health treatment and psychosocial remedies for the environmental disability present in many of these individuals.

Website: http://crisp.cit.nih.gov/crisp/Crisp_Query.Generate_Screen

- **Project Title: THERAPEUTIC MOTOR TRAINING AND FETAL ALCOHOL EFFECTS**

Principal Investigator & Institution: Greenough, William T.; Swanlund Professor of Psychology,; Psychology; University of Illinois Urbana-Champaign Henry Administration Bldg Champaign, Il 61820

Timing: Fiscal Year 2003; Project Start 01-AUG-1994; Project End 31-MAR-2007

Summary: (provided by applicant): Exposure to ethanol during brain development can permanently alter cerebellar and cerebral morphology and produce functional impairments in many aspects of behavior, including cognitive and motor performance. There currently is no known effective rehabilitation treatment for **fetal alcohol syndrome** (FAS). The long term objectives of this competing renewal are to identify methods to stimulate neuroplasticity that promotes rehabilitation of functional deficits resulting from brain damage induced by prenatal alcohol exposure. The general hypothesis is that complex motor learning, involving intensive training on an obstacle course, promotes structural neuroplasticity and ameliorates functional deficits in rats with brain damage induced by neonatal binge alcohol exposure. This period of brain development, comparable to that of the human 3rd trimester, is a time of heightened vulnerability to alcohol-induced cerebellar damage. Complex motor training in adulthood stimulated synaptic morphological plasticity of parallel fiber synapses in the cerebellar paramedian lobule (PML) and in motor cortex, and concurrently rehabilitated motor performance deficits. The three new aims build on this positive evidence of therapeutic rehabilitation, and now use early intervention initiated just after weaning. Aim 1 will identify other structural correlates of the rehabilitative effects in PML and motor cortex, including evaluation of plasticity of climbing fibers and effects on astrocytes and vasculature. Aim 2 will test whether the training can stimulate synaptogenesis in other regions of the cerebellum and in the hippocampus, and concurrently rehabilitate deficits in cerebellar-dependent and hippocampal dependent learning. Aim 3 will determine whether rats with alcohol- induced brain damage have the capacity for neurogenesis in the postweaning or adult brain, and whether stimulation of adult neurogenesis (or enhanced survival of newly-generated neurons) by behavioral experience, has merit as a potential mode of rehabilitation. These studies will provide important new data that can guide and inform efforts to develop a rational approach to rehabilitation for children with FAS

Website: http://crisp.cit.nih.gov/crisp/Crisp_Query.Generate_Screen

- **Project Title: TRAINING GRANT ON GENETICS ASPECTS OF ALCOHOLISM**

  Principal Investigator & Institution: Lumeng, Lawrence; Professor of Medicine and Biochemistry; Medicine; Indiana Univ-Purdue Univ at Indianapolis 620 Union Drive, Room 618 Indianapolis, in 462025167

  Timing: Fiscal Year 2001; Project Start 27-SEP-1985; Project End 30-JUN-2005

  Summary: This application is a competing renewal for an institutional research training program on the "Genetic Aspects of Alcoholism." Among the institutional training grants funded by NIAAA, our training program is one of five devoted to genetics of alcoholism. The main focus of research training is on the genetic, biological, and molecular basis of high alcohol-seeking behavior. Major topics of research include: neuronal mechanisms responsible for the reinforcing effects of ethanol; the genetics of alcohol metabolizing enzymes and receptors related to neurotransmission; the genetics (including QTL and finer mapping analyses) of alcohol preference and correlated phenotypes in selectively bred rat and mouse lines; studies of factors that regulate the expression of genes relevant to alcoholism; analysis of the extent hat genetically-influenced biobehavioral factors such as disinhibition/impulsivity and acute tolerance/insensitivity contribute to alcoholism risks in selectively bred rodents and in human populations; and the use of an alcohol clamp method to assess the effects of genetics (MZ twins and FHP vs FHN subjects) and recent drinking history on electrophysiologic, neuroendocrine, and subjective assessment of alcohol experience. Other topics of interest include; structure and function of mutated forms of alcohol and aldehyde dehydrogenases; the relationship of ethanol exposure to retinoid metabolism, the effect of ethanol on lipoprotein metabolism; and neurodevelopmental abnormalities of **fetal alcohol syndrome** in mouse and rat models. One major strength of our training program is the long history of collaboration with both M.D.S. and PhDs in research and research training and the involvement of multiple scientific disciplines. A number of important resources are available to foster research training; the selective bred P/NP, HAD/LAD, HARF/LARF rat lines and the HAP/LAP mouse lines that differ in alcohol preference, a large collection of DNA samples extracted from different human populations relevant for genetic studies of alcoholism and alcohol-related end-organ injuries, and NIAAA-funded Alcohol Research Center (Molecular Biology Core, Animal Production Core, Structural and Cellular Biology Core, Mouse Selective Breeding Component, and two Human Genetics Cores, a group of IRPG grants (they replaced a former Program Project grant) that focuses on identification of genes and neurobiological mechanisms underlying high alcohol seeking behavior through studies of the HAD/LAD and P/NP rats, and the participation as one of six sites for the "Collaborative Studies on the Genetics of Alcoholism (COGA)." The trainees for each year will include five predoctoral, five postdoctoral fellows (with one M.D. and four Ph.D. trainees), and six undergraduate students on short-term training during their summer or "off quarter". Training will be through an apprenticeship mode but seminars, research conferences and hands-on method courses are amply available.

  Website: http://crisp.cit.nih.gov/crisp/Crisp_Query.Generate_Screen

- **Project Title: TRAINING IN NEUROIMMUNOENDOCRINE EFFECTS OF ALCOHOL**

  Principal Investigator & Institution: Kovacs, Elizabeth J.; Professor; Cell Bio & Neurobio & Anatomy; Loyola University Medical Center Lewis Towers, 13Th Fl Chicago, Il 60611

  Timing: Fiscal Year 2002; Project Start 01-JUL-2002; Project End 30-JUN-2007

Summary: (provided by applicant): This is a new application for a Training Program in the Neuroimmunoendocrine Effects of Alcohol at Loyola University Stritch School of Medicine. An interdisciplinary group of nine well-funded basic scientists and clinicians with active research laboratories are studying the neurobiological, immune and endocrine responses to alcohol exposure. The training faculty hold primary appointments in the Departments of Cell Biology, Neurobiology & Anatomy, Medicine (primarily Divisions of Endocrinology and Gastroenterology), and Surgery, are all active members of the Alcohol Research Program and hold graduate appointments in Ph.D. granting programs: 1) Department of Cell Biology, Neurobiology, & Anatomy, 2) Molecular & Cellular Biochemistry Program, and 3) Neuroscience Program. The Director of the Training grant will be Elizabeth J. Kovacs, Ph.D., Professor of Cell Biology, Neurobiology, & Anatomy, a cellular immunologist with an international reputation for her work on endocrine effects on immunity after alcohol exposure. She will be assisted by Associate Director, Mary Druse-Manteuffel, Ph.D., Professor of Cell Biology, Neurobiology, & Anatomy, who works on neuronal consequences of **fetal alcohol syndrome,** and an internal Advisory Committee. The Advisory Committee, will be composed of senior faculty in the fields of cell biology, immunology, and neuroscience, who have extensive experience ill the administration training programs for pre-doctoral and post-doctoral fellows, but do not conduct alcohol research. This group, in conjunction with an Executive Committee, consisting of senior alcohol researchers, will oversee the Training Program. Pre-doctoral trainees will be selected from the pool of applicants applying to the Ph.D. programs in Cell Biology, Neurobiology, & Anatomy, Molecular & Cellular Biochemistry, and Neuroscience. These trainees will take courses in their respective graduate programs, including biochemistry, cell and molecular biology, immunology, neuroscience, etc., and will be instructed in oral and written communication through formal class work, seminars, and journal clubs. Post-doctoral trainees will spend a majority of their time in the laboratory of one of the members of the Training Program. All trainees will take a course in Ethics in Biomedical Sciences and, along with the Training Faculty, will attend Alcohol Research Program meetings. A plan to recruit trainees from under-represented minority backgrounds is included within the proposal. The commitment of the Training Faculty to excellence in research and teaching will insure the successful preparation of trainees for careers as academic scientists in the field of alcohol research.

Website: http://crisp.cit.nih.gov/crisp/Crisp_Query.Generate_Screen

- **Project Title: VIRTUAL REALITY AND WEB TOOLS FOR CHILDREN WITH FAS/FAE**

  Principal Investigator & Institution: Strickland, Dorothy C.; President; Virtual Reality Aids, Inc. 421 Orchis Rd Saint Augustine, Fl 32086

  Timing: Fiscal Year 2001; Project Start 30-SEP-2001; Project End 31-MAR-2003

  Summary: The broad long-term objectives of this project are to design, build, and evaluate the efficacy of a virtual reality instructional fire safety sequence for children with **Fetal Alcohol Syndrome** and Fetal Alcohol Effects. Specific aims are: 1) Analyze how virtual reality fire safety instructional learning programs developed by the company for children with autism could be modified to address the different learning needs of children with FAS and FAE; 2) Design and code one level of a fire safety program using virtual reality technology for home and school use; 3) Demonstrate the efficacy of the instructional software through use of applied behavior analysis and single subjects design. The learning environment afforded by virtual reality may improve skills training for individuals with mental, developmental, and attention disorders if virtual worlds can match their specialized needs. The research design and methods for achieving these goals are: 1) Choose children who have been diagnosed with FAS or FAE; 2) Design and program a PC based virtual reality critical environment to teach proper response to a home fire and be engaging to children with these disorders; 3) Conduct trials to evaluate the results using n, multiple baselines across subjects design. PROPOSED COMMERCIAL APPLICATIONS: Virtual reality learning environments would have a broad market appeal for children, parents, teachers, and health practitioners for treatment of FAS and FAE. A present company web site provides similar products for children with autism, allowing an in-place cost effective delivery and support system for this new product.

Website: http://crisp.cit.nih.gov/crisp/Crisp_Query.Generate_Screen

- **Project Title: ZEBRAFISH AS A MODEL FOR IDENTIFYING BIOMARKERS OF FAS**

Principal Investigator & Institution: Willett, Catherine E.; Senior Scientist; Phylonix Pharmaceuticals, Inc. 100 Inman St, Ste 300 Cambridge, Ma 02139

Timing: Fiscal Year 2001; Project Start 24-SEP-2001; Project End 31-MAR-2002

Summary: Using the zebrafish (danio rerio) embryo, this Phase I SBIR proposal aims to analyze the effects of ethanol on embryonic development and to identify biomarkers of **Fetal Alcohol Syndrome** (FAS). Using subtractive library technology, Phase I research will isolate genes involved in ethanol induced toxicity. Advantages of the zebrafish include transparency which facilitates visual analysis, rapid embryogenesis, a morphological and molecular basis of tissue and organ development that are either identical or similar to other vertebrates including man, and the low cost of maintaining and breeding large numbers of zebrafish. Embryo drug exposure and RNA isolation for gene expression testing are also simple procedures. In addition, high throughput, automated drug screening is possible C using the zebrafish. An eventual application of our model is to develop an assay to identify potential pharmacological interventions for fetuses at risk for FAS. The zebrafish could be used to screen therapeutic compounds that either protect fetal tissue from alcohol-related damage or aid in the restoration of damaged tissue. I PROPOSED COMMERCIAL APPLICATIONS: By providing a rapid method for identifying potential pharmacological interventions for fetuses at risk for FAS, the zebrafish assay will help to streamline the development of drugs and treatment protocols for FAS.

Website: http://crisp.cit.nih.gov/crisp/Crisp_Query.Generate_Screen

- **Project Title: ZEBRAFISH--A MODEL FOR FETAL ETHANOL INJURY**

Principal Investigator & Institution: Tanguay, Robert L.; Associate Professor; Pharmaceutical Sciences; University of Colorado Hlth Sciences Ctr P.O. Box 6508, Grants and Contracts Aurora, Co 800450508

Timing: Fiscal Year 2001; Project Start 01-JUN-2001; Project End 31-MAY-2004

Summary: One of the major causes of birth defects in North America is maternal ethanol consumption. Maternal alcohol consumption during critical windows of embryonic development can result in offspring with a number of predictable defects known as **Fetal Alcohol Syndrome** (FAS) and Fetal Alcohol Effects (FAE). The effects of ethanol on normal development is very costly to society since FAS and FAE children suffer from impaired development, cognitive deficits and behavior problems. In order to reduce the cost of the devastating effects of ethanol on human health, we must understand the mechanism of ethanol action. It is also essential that we determine the genetic factors involved. A greater understanding of underlying mechanisms) of ethanol action on developing embryos should lead to new ideas about prevention and intervention of FAS and FAE. Although several hypotheses have been proposed to explain the molecular mechanism of ethanol-mediated fetal injury, the cause remains uncertain. The long-range goal of this project is to establish zebrafish as a vertebrate model to understand the molecular mechanisms) of ethanol-induced fetal injury. Zebrafish embryos share many cellular, anatomical, and physiological characteristics with higher vertebrates including humans and they offer many practical advantages making them an excellent research model for teratogenic studies. We specifically propose to: (I) Investigate the potential involvement of ethanol metabolism by completely characterizing the metabolizing pathways in developing embryos. (II) Determine the critical developmental window for embryonic CNS injury. (III) Identify the impact of ethanol exposure on zebrafish nervous system development and test the hypothesis that cell death contributes significantly to the teratogenic actions of ethanol. Completion of this project will result in a powerful model system that will allow for a greater understanding of the molecular mechanisms underlying ethanol-mediated fetal injury.

Website: http://crisp.cit.nih.gov/crisp/Crisp_Query.Generate_Screen

The National Library of Medicine: PubMed

One of the quickest and most comprehensive ways to find academic studies in both English and other languages is to use PubMed, maintained by the National Library of Medicine.[3] The advantage of PubMed over previously mentioned sources is that it covers a greater number of domestic and foreign references. It is also free to use. If the publisher has a Web site that offers full text of its journals, PubMed will provide links to that site, as well as to sites offering other related data. User registration, a subscription fee, or some other type of fee may be required to access the full text of articles in some journals.

To generate your own bibliography of studies dealing with fetal alcohol syndrome, simply go to the PubMed Web site at **http://www.ncbi.nlm.nih.gov/pubmed**. Type "fetal alcohol syndrome" (or synonyms) into the search box, and click "Go." The following is the type of output you can expect from PubMed for fetal alcohol syndrome (hyperlinks lead to article summaries):

- **A case definition and photographic screening tool for the facial phenotype of fetal alcohol syndrome.**
  Author(s): Astley SJ, Clarren SK.
  Source: The Journal of Pediatrics. 1996 July; 129(1): 33-41.
  http://www.ncbi.nlm.nih.gov:80/entrez/query.fcgi?cmd=Retrieve&db=PubMed&list_uids=8757560&dopt=Abstract

---

[3] PubMed was developed by the National Center for Biotechnology Information (NCBI) at the National Library of Medicine (NLM) at the National Institutes of Health (NIH). The PubMed database was developed in conjunction with publishers of biomedical literature as a search tool for accessing literature citations and linking to full-text journal articles at Web sites of participating publishers. Publishers that participate in PubMed supply NLM with their citations electronically prior to or at the time of publication.

- **A cephalometric assessment of children with fetal alcohol syndrome.**
  Author(s): Gir AV, Aksharanugraha K, Harris EF.
  Source: American Journal of Orthodontics and Dentofacial Orthopedics : Official Publication of the American Association of Orthodontists, Its Constituent Societies, and the American Board of Orthodontics. 1989 April; 95(4): 319-26.
  http://www.ncbi.nlm.nih.gov:80/entrez/query.fcgi?cmd=Retrieve&db=PubMed&list_uids=2705412&dopt=Abstract

- **A challenge in managing a family with the fetal alcohol syndrome.**
  Author(s): Davis A, Lipson A.
  Source: Clinical Pediatrics. 1984 May; 23(5): 304.
  http://www.ncbi.nlm.nih.gov:80/entrez/query.fcgi?cmd=Retrieve&db=PubMed&list_uids=6538471&dopt=Abstract

- **A clinical neuropathological study of the fetal alcohol syndrome.**
  Author(s): Wisniewski K, Dambska M, Sher JH, Qazi Q.
  Source: Neuropediatrics. 1983 November; 14(4): 197-201.
  http://www.ncbi.nlm.nih.gov:80/entrez/query.fcgi?cmd=Retrieve&db=PubMed&list_uids=6686290&dopt=Abstract

- **A comprehensive local program for the prevention of fetal alcohol syndrome.**
  Author(s): Masis KB, May PA.
  Source: Public Health Reports (Washington, D.C. : 1974). 1991 September-October; 106(5): 484-9.
  http://www.ncbi.nlm.nih.gov:80/entrez/query.fcgi?cmd=Retrieve&db=PubMed&list_uids=1910181&dopt=Abstract

- **A decrease in the size of the basal ganglia in children with fetal alcohol syndrome.**
  Author(s): Mattson SN, Riley EP, Sowell ER, Jernigan TL, Sobel DF, Jones KL.
  Source: Alcoholism, Clinical and Experimental Research. 1996 September; 20(6): 1088-93.
  http://www.ncbi.nlm.nih.gov:80/entrez/query.fcgi?cmd=Retrieve&db=PubMed&list_uids=8892532&dopt=Abstract

- **A fetal alcohol syndrome screening tool.**
  Author(s): Astley SJ, Clarren SK.
  Source: Alcoholism, Clinical and Experimental Research. 1995 December; 19(6): 1565-71.
  http://www.ncbi.nlm.nih.gov:80/entrez/query.fcgi?cmd=Retrieve&db=PubMed&list_uids=8749828&dopt=Abstract

- **A fetal alcohol syndrome surveillance pilot project in American Indian communities in the Northern Plains.**
  Author(s): Duimstra C, Johnson D, Kutsch C, Wang B, Zentner M, Kellerman S, Welty T.
  Source: Public Health Reports (Washington, D.C. : 1974). 1993 March-April; 108(2): 225-9.
  http://www.ncbi.nlm.nih.gov:80/entrez/query.fcgi?cmd=Retrieve&db=PubMed&list_uids=8464980&dopt=Abstract

- **A hypothetical mechanism for fetal alcohol syndrome involving ethanol inhibition of retinoic acid synthesis at the alcohol dehydrogenase step.**
  Author(s): Duester G.
  Source: Alcoholism, Clinical and Experimental Research. 1991 June; 15(3): 568-72. Review.
  http://www.ncbi.nlm.nih.gov:80/entrez/query.fcgi?cmd=Retrieve&db=PubMed&list_ uids=1877746&dopt=Abstract

- **A macro-level fetal alcohol syndrome prevention program for Native Americans and Alaska Natives: description and evaluation.**
  Author(s): May PA, Hymbaugh KJ.
  Source: J Stud Alcohol. 1989 November; 50(6): 508-18.
  http://www.ncbi.nlm.nih.gov:80/entrez/query.fcgi?cmd=Retrieve&db=PubMed&list_ uids=2586104&dopt=Abstract

- **A multiple source methodology for the surveillance of fetal alcohol syndrome—The Fetal Alcohol Syndrome Surveillance Network (FASSNet).**
  Author(s): Hymbaugh K, Miller LA, Druschel CM, Podvin DW, Meaney FJ, Boyle CA; FASSNet Team.
  Source: Teratology. 2002; 66 Suppl 1: S41-9.
  http://www.ncbi.nlm.nih.gov:80/entrez/query.fcgi?cmd=Retrieve&db=PubMed&list_ uids=12239744&dopt=Abstract

- **A multiple-level, comprehensive approach to the prevention of fetal alcohol syndrome (FAS) and other alcohol-related birth defects (ARBD).**
  Author(s): May PA.
  Source: Int J Addict. 1995; 30(12): 1549-602. Review.
  http://www.ncbi.nlm.nih.gov:80/entrez/query.fcgi?cmd=Retrieve&db=PubMed&list_ uids=8557409&dopt=Abstract

- **A national survey of state-sponsored programs to prevent fetal alcohol syndrome.**
  Author(s): Baumeister AA, Hamlett CL.
  Source: Mental Retardation. 1986 June; 24(3): 169-73.
  http://www.ncbi.nlm.nih.gov:80/entrez/query.fcgi?cmd=Retrieve&db=PubMed&list_ uids=3736407&dopt=Abstract

- **A review of the neuroanatomical findings in children with fetal alcohol syndrome or prenatal exposure to alcohol.**
  Author(s): Roebuck TM, Mattson SN, Riley EP.
  Source: Alcoholism, Clinical and Experimental Research. 1998 April; 22(2): 339-44. Review.
  http://www.ncbi.nlm.nih.gov:80/entrez/query.fcgi?cmd=Retrieve&db=PubMed&list_ uids=9581638&dopt=Abstract

- **A review of the neurobehavioral deficits in children with fetal alcohol syndrome or prenatal exposure to alcohol.**
  Author(s): Mattson SN, Riley EP.
  Source: Alcoholism, Clinical and Experimental Research. 1998 April; 22(2): 279-94. Review.
  http://www.ncbi.nlm.nih.gov:80/entrez/query.fcgi?cmd=Retrieve&db=PubMed&list_uids=9581631&dopt=Abstract

- **A revised estimate of the economic impact of fetal alcohol syndrome.**
  Author(s): Abel EL, Sokol RJ.
  Source: Recent Dev Alcohol. 1991; 9: 117-25. Review.
  http://www.ncbi.nlm.nih.gov:80/entrez/query.fcgi?cmd=Retrieve&db=PubMed&list_uids=1758979&dopt=Abstract

- **A semiquantitative score system for epidemiologic studies of fetal alcohol syndrome.**
  Author(s): Vitez M, Koranyi G, Gonczy E, Rudas T, Czeizel A.
  Source: American Journal of Epidemiology. 1984 March; 119(3): 301-8.
  http://www.ncbi.nlm.nih.gov:80/entrez/query.fcgi?cmd=Retrieve&db=PubMed&list_uids=6702808&dopt=Abstract

- **A stereo-photogrammetric method to measure the facial dysmorphology of children in the diagnosis of fetal alcohol syndrome.**
  Author(s): Meintjes EM, Douglas TS, Martinez F, Vaughan CL, Adams LP, Stekhoven A, Viljoen D.
  Source: Medical Engineering & Physics. 2002 December; 24(10): 683-9.
  http://www.ncbi.nlm.nih.gov:80/entrez/query.fcgi?cmd=Retrieve&db=PubMed&list_uids=12460727&dopt=Abstract

- **A test-retest study of intelligence in patients with fetal alcohol syndrome: implications for care.**
  Author(s): Streissguth AP, Randels SP, Smith DF.
  Source: Journal of the American Academy of Child and Adolescent Psychiatry. 1991 July; 30(4): 584-7.
  http://www.ncbi.nlm.nih.gov:80/entrez/query.fcgi?cmd=Retrieve&db=PubMed&list_uids=1823538&dopt=Abstract

- **Acetaldehyde and the fetal alcohol syndrome.**
  Author(s): Ryle PR, Thomson AD.
  Source: Lancet. 1983 July 23; 2(8343): 219-20.
  http://www.ncbi.nlm.nih.gov:80/entrez/query.fcgi?cmd=Retrieve&db=PubMed&list_uids=6135053&dopt=Abstract

- **Alaska Fetal Alcohol Syndrome Prevention Project.**
  Author(s): Jones L, Nakamura P.
  Source: Alaska Med. 1993 April-June; 35(2): 179. No Abstract Available.
  http://www.ncbi.nlm.nih.gov:80/entrez/query.fcgi?cmd=Retrieve&db=PubMed&list_uids=8238775&dopt=Abstract

- **Alcohol dehydrogenase-2*2 allele is associated with decreased prevalence of fetal alcohol syndrome in the mixed-ancestry population of the Western Cape Province, South Africa.**
  Author(s): Viljoen DL, Carr LG, Foroud TM, Brooke L, Ramsay M, Li TK.
  Source: Alcoholism, Clinical and Experimental Research. 2001 December; 25(12): 1719-22.
  http://www.ncbi.nlm.nih.gov:80/entrez/query.fcgi?cmd=Retrieve&db=PubMed&list_uids=11781503&dopt=Abstract

- **Alpha-fetoprotein, human placental lactogen, and pregnancy-specific beta 1-glycoprotein in pregnant women who drink: relation to fetal alcohol syndrome.**
  Author(s): Halmesmaki E, Autti I, Granstrom ML, Heikinheimo M, Raivio KO, Ylikorkala O.
  Source: American Journal of Obstetrics and Gynecology. 1986 September; 155(3): 598-602.
  http://www.ncbi.nlm.nih.gov:80/entrez/query.fcgi?cmd=Retrieve&db=PubMed&list_uids=2428250&dopt=Abstract

- **Anterior segment anomalies associated with the fetal alcohol syndrome.**
  Author(s): Miller MT, Epstein RJ, Sugar J, Pinchoff BS, Sugar A, Gammon JA, Mittelman D, Dennis RF, Israel J.
  Source: Journal of Pediatric Ophthalmology and Strabismus. 1984 January-February; 21(1): 8-18.
  http://www.ncbi.nlm.nih.gov:80/entrez/query.fcgi?cmd=Retrieve&db=PubMed&list_uids=6707858&dopt=Abstract

- **Application of the fetal alcohol syndrome facial photographic screening tool in a foster care population.**
  Author(s): Astley SJ, Stachowiak J, Clarren SK, Clausen C.
  Source: The Journal of Pediatrics. 2002 November; 141(5): 712-7.
  http://www.ncbi.nlm.nih.gov:80/entrez/query.fcgi?cmd=Retrieve&db=PubMed&list_uids=12410204&dopt=Abstract

- **Appraisal of the epidemiology of fetal alcohol syndrome among Canadian native peoples.**
  Author(s): Robinson GC.
  Source: Canadian Journal of Public Health. Revue Canadienne De Sante Publique. 1989 September-October; 80(5): 382.
  http://www.ncbi.nlm.nih.gov:80/entrez/query.fcgi?cmd=Retrieve&db=PubMed&list_uids=2804872&dopt=Abstract

- **Appraisal of the epidemiology of fetal alcohol syndrome among Canadian native peoples.**
  Author(s): Bray DL, Anderson PD.
  Source: Canadian Journal of Public Health. Revue Canadienne De Sante Publique. 1989 January-February; 80(1): 42-5.
  http://www.ncbi.nlm.nih.gov:80/entrez/query.fcgi?cmd=Retrieve&db=PubMed&list_uids=2702544&dopt=Abstract

- **Audiologic manifestations in fetal alcohol syndrome assessed by brainstem auditory-evoked potentials.**
  Author(s): Rossig C, Wasser S, Oppermann P.
  Source: Neuropediatrics. 1994 October; 25(5): 245-9.
  http://www.ncbi.nlm.nih.gov:80/entrez/query.fcgi?cmd=Retrieve&db=PubMed&list_uids=7885533&dopt=Abstract

- **Auditory event-related potentials in fetal alcohol syndrome and Down's syndrome children.**
  Author(s): Kaneko WM, Ehlers CL, Philips EL, Riley EP.
  Source: Alcoholism, Clinical and Experimental Research. 1996 February; 20(1): 35-42.
  http://www.ncbi.nlm.nih.gov:80/entrez/query.fcgi?cmd=Retrieve&db=PubMed&list_uids=8651459&dopt=Abstract

- **Autism in fetal alcohol syndrome: a report of six cases.**
  Author(s): Nanson JL.
  Source: Alcoholism, Clinical and Experimental Research. 1992 June; 16(3): 558-65.
  http://www.ncbi.nlm.nih.gov:80/entrez/query.fcgi?cmd=Retrieve&db=PubMed&list_uids=1626656&dopt=Abstract

- **Behavioral phenotypes in four mental retardation syndromes: fetal alcohol syndrome, Prader-Willi syndrome, fragile X syndrome, and tuberosis sclerosis.**
  Author(s): Steinhausen HC, Von Gontard A, Spohr HL, Hauffa BP, Eiholzer U, Backes M, Willms J, Malin Z.
  Source: American Journal of Medical Genetics. 2002 September 1; 111(4): 381-7.
  http://www.ncbi.nlm.nih.gov:80/entrez/query.fcgi?cmd=Retrieve&db=PubMed&list_uids=12210296&dopt=Abstract

- **Bone age and growth in fetal alcohol syndrome.**
  Author(s): Habbick BF, Blakley PM, Houston CS, Snyder RE, Senthilselvan A, Nanson JL.
  Source: Alcoholism, Clinical and Experimental Research. 1998 September; 22(6): 1312-6.
  http://www.ncbi.nlm.nih.gov:80/entrez/query.fcgi?cmd=Retrieve&db=PubMed&list_uids=9756047&dopt=Abstract

- **Brain function in fetal alcohol syndrome assessed by single photon emission computed tomography.**
  Author(s): Bhatara VS, Lovrein F, Kirkeby J, Swayze V 2nd, Unruh E, Johnson V.
  Source: S D J Med. 2002 February; 55(2): 59-62.
  http://www.ncbi.nlm.nih.gov:80/entrez/query.fcgi?cmd=Retrieve&db=PubMed&list_uids=11865707&dopt=Abstract

- **Cardiac malformations in the fetal alcohol syndrome.**
  Author(s): Sardor GG, Smith DF, MacLeod PM.
  Source: The Journal of Pediatrics. 1981 May; 98(5): 771-3.
  http://www.ncbi.nlm.nih.gov:80/entrez/query.fcgi?cmd=Retrieve&db=PubMed&list_uids=7229757&dopt=Abstract

- **Cardiovascular malformations in the fetal alcohol syndrome.**
  Author(s): Steeg CN, Woolf P.
  Source: American Heart Journal. 1979 November; 98(5): 635-7.
  http://www.ncbi.nlm.nih.gov:80/entrez/query.fcgi?cmd=Retrieve&db=PubMed&list_uids=158960&dopt=Abstract

- **Caring for the child with fetal alcohol syndrome.**
  Author(s): Green HL, Diaz-Gonzalez de Ferris ME, Vasquez E, Lau EM, Yusim J.
  Source: Jaapa. 2002 June; 15(6): 31-4, 37-40. Review.
  http://www.ncbi.nlm.nih.gov:80/entrez/query.fcgi?cmd=Retrieve&db=PubMed&list_uids=12141072&dopt=Abstract

- **Cervical spine anomalies in fetal alcohol syndrome.**
  Author(s): Tredwell SJ, Smith DF, Macleod PJ, Wood BJ.
  Source: Spine. 1982 July-August; 7(4): 331-4.
  http://www.ncbi.nlm.nih.gov:80/entrez/query.fcgi?cmd=Retrieve&db=PubMed&list_uids=6890236&dopt=Abstract

- **Characteristics of mothers of children with fetal alcohol syndrome in the Western Cape Province of South Africa: a case control study.**
  Author(s): Viljoen D, Croxford J, Gossage JP, Kodituwakku PW, May PA.
  Source: J Stud Alcohol. 2002 January; 63(1): 6-17.
  http://www.ncbi.nlm.nih.gov:80/entrez/query.fcgi?cmd=Retrieve&db=PubMed&list_uids=11925060&dopt=Abstract

- **Characteristics of mothers of fetal alcohol syndrome children.**
  Author(s): Abel EL.
  Source: Neurobehav Toxicol Teratol. 1982 January-February; 4(1): 3-4. No Abstract Available.
  http://www.ncbi.nlm.nih.gov:80/entrez/query.fcgi?cmd=Retrieve&db=PubMed&list_uids=7070567&dopt=Abstract

- **Characteristics of parental response to fetal alcohol syndrome.**
  Author(s): Wilson PJ, Scott RV, Briggs FH, Ince SE, Quinton BA, Headings VE.
  Source: Birth Defects Orig Artic Ser. 1984; 20(6): 187-91. No Abstract Available.
  http://www.ncbi.nlm.nih.gov:80/entrez/query.fcgi?cmd=Retrieve&db=PubMed&list_uids=6543548&dopt=Abstract

- **Children with Fetal Alcohol Syndrome are impaired at place learning but not cued-navigation in a virtual Morris water task.**
  Author(s): Hamilton DA, Kodituwakku P, Sutherland RJ, Savage DD.
  Source: Behavioural Brain Research. 2003 July 14; 143(1): 85-94.
  http://www.ncbi.nlm.nih.gov:80/entrez/query.fcgi?cmd=Retrieve&db=PubMed&list_uids=12842299&dopt=Abstract

- **Chromosome abnormality in a patient with fetal alcohol syndrome.**
  Author(s): Qazi QH, Madahar C, Masakawa A, McGann B.
  Source: Curr Alcohol. 1979; 5: 155-61. No Abstract Available.
  http://www.ncbi.nlm.nih.gov:80/entrez/query.fcgi?cmd=Retrieve&db=PubMed&list_uids=755618&dopt=Abstract

- **Chronic intestinal pseudoobstruction associated with fetal alcohol syndrome.**
  Author(s): Uc A, Vasiliauskas E, Piccoli DA, Flores AF, Di Lorenzo C, Hyman PE.
  Source: Digestive Diseases and Sciences. 1997 June; 42(6): 1163-7.
  http://www.ncbi.nlm.nih.gov:80/entrez/query.fcgi?cmd=Retrieve&db=PubMed&list_
  uids=9201078&dopt=Abstract

- **Clinical and electroretinographic findings in fetal alcohol syndrome.**
  Author(s): Hug TE, Fitzgerald KM, Cibis GW.
  Source: J Aapos. 2000 August; 4(4): 200-4.
  http://www.ncbi.nlm.nih.gov:80/entrez/query.fcgi?cmd=Retrieve&db=PubMed&list_
  uids=10951294&dopt=Abstract

- **Clinical correlations between ethanol intake and fetal alcohol syndrome.**
  Author(s): Ernhart CB.
  Source: Recent Dev Alcohol. 1991; 9: 127-50. Review.
  http://www.ncbi.nlm.nih.gov:80/entrez/query.fcgi?cmd=Retrieve&db=PubMed&list_
  uids=1758980&dopt=Abstract

- **Clinical implications of recent research on the fetal alcohol syndrome.**
  Author(s): Russell M.
  Source: Bull N Y Acad Med. 1991 May-June; 67(3): 207-22. Review. No Abstract
  Available.
  http://www.ncbi.nlm.nih.gov:80/entrez/query.fcgi?cmd=Retrieve&db=PubMed&list_
  uids=1868274&dopt=Abstract

- **Clinical profile and prevalence of fetal alcohol syndrome in an isolated community in British Columbia.**
  Author(s): Robinson GC, Conry JL, Conry RF.
  Source: Cmaj : Canadian Medical Association Journal = Journal De L'association
  Medicale Canadienne. 1987 August 1; 137(3): 203-7.
  http://www.ncbi.nlm.nih.gov:80/entrez/query.fcgi?cmd=Retrieve&db=PubMed&list_
  uids=3607663&dopt=Abstract

- **Clinical, psychopathological and developmental aspects in children with the fetal alcohol syndrome: a four-year follow-up study.**
  Author(s): Spohr HL, Steinhausen HC.
  Source: Ciba Found Symp. 1984; 105: 197-217.
  http://www.ncbi.nlm.nih.gov:80/entrez/query.fcgi?cmd=Retrieve&db=PubMed&list_
  uids=6563987&dopt=Abstract

- **Closeup of fetal alcohol syndrome.**
  Author(s): Bock J.
  Source: Can Nurse. 1979 November; 75(10): 35. No Abstract Available.
  http://www.ncbi.nlm.nih.gov:80/entrez/query.fcgi?cmd=Retrieve&db=PubMed&list_
  uids=259024&dopt=Abstract

- **Coeliac disease coexistent with fetal alcohol syndrome.**
  Author(s): Hogh B, Stenhammar L.
  Source: European Journal of Pediatrics. 1984 November; 143(1): 74-5.
  http://www.ncbi.nlm.nih.gov:80/entrez/query.fcgi?cmd=Retrieve&db=PubMed&list_uids=6542523&dopt=Abstract

- **Cognitive deficits in nonretarded adults with fetal alcohol syndrome.**
  Author(s): Kerns KA, Don A, Mateer CA, Streissguth AP.
  Source: Journal of Learning Disabilities. 1997 November-December; 30(6): 685-93.
  http://www.ncbi.nlm.nih.gov:80/entrez/query.fcgi?cmd=Retrieve&db=PubMed&list_uids=9364906&dopt=Abstract

- **Comparison of social abilities of children with fetal alcohol syndrome to those of children with similar IQ scores and normal controls.**
  Author(s): Thomas SE, Kelly SJ, Mattson SN, Riley EP.
  Source: Alcoholism, Clinical and Experimental Research. 1998 April; 22(2): 528-33.
  http://www.ncbi.nlm.nih.gov:80/entrez/query.fcgi?cmd=Retrieve&db=PubMed&list_uids=9581664&dopt=Abstract

- **Computational modeling of a putative fetal alcohol syndrome mechanism.**
  Author(s): Whitmire D, Bowen JP, Shim JY, Whitmire PS.
  Source: Alcoholism, Clinical and Experimental Research. 1995 December; 19(6): 1587-93.
  http://www.ncbi.nlm.nih.gov:80/entrez/query.fcgi?cmd=Retrieve&db=PubMed&list_uids=8749832&dopt=Abstract

- **Conference on Fetal Alcohol Syndrome.**
  Author(s): Hearle JM.
  Source: Qrb Qual Rev Bull. 1980 August; 6(8): 24-9. No Abstract Available.
  http://www.ncbi.nlm.nih.gov:80/entrez/query.fcgi?cmd=Retrieve&db=PubMed&list_uids=6776470&dopt=Abstract

- **Consequences of prenatal maternal alcohol exposure including the fetal alcohol syndrome.**
  Author(s): Maykut MO.
  Source: Prog Neuropsychopharmacol. 1979; 3(5-6): 465-81. Review.
  http://www.ncbi.nlm.nih.gov:80/entrez/query.fcgi?cmd=Retrieve&db=PubMed&list_uids=401350&dopt=Abstract

- **Contingent negative variation in the fetal alcohol syndrome: a preliminary report.**
  Author(s): Buffington V, Martin DC, Streissguth AP, Smith DW.
  Source: Neurobehav Toxicol Teratol. 1981 Summer; 3(2): 183-5.
  http://www.ncbi.nlm.nih.gov:80/entrez/query.fcgi?cmd=Retrieve&db=PubMed&list_uids=7195995&dopt=Abstract

- **Contribution of fetal alcohol syndrome to mental retardation.**
  Author(s): Livingston J, Lyall H.
  Source: Lancet. 1986 December 6; 2(8519): 1337-8.
  http://www.ncbi.nlm.nih.gov:80/entrez/query.fcgi?cmd=Retrieve&db=PubMed&list_uids=2878206&dopt=Abstract

- **Contribution to first-pass metabolism of ethanol and inhibition by ethanol for retinol oxidation in human alcohol dehydrogenase family--implications for etiology of fetal alcohol syndrome and alcohol-related diseases.**
  Author(s): Han CL, Liao CS, Wu CW, Hwong CL, Lee AR, Yin SJ.
  Source: European Journal of Biochemistry / Febs. 1998 May 15; 254(1): 25-31.
  http://www.ncbi.nlm.nih.gov:80/entrez/query.fcgi?cmd=Retrieve&db=PubMed&list_uids=9652389&dopt=Abstract

- **Contribution to the etiopathogenesis of the fetal alcohol syndrome.**
  Author(s): Ticha R, Santavy J, Matlocha Z.
  Source: Acta Univ Palacki Olomuc Fac Med. 1984; 106: 133-8. No Abstract Available.
  http://www.ncbi.nlm.nih.gov:80/entrez/query.fcgi?cmd=Retrieve&db=PubMed&list_uids=6085906&dopt=Abstract

- **Corneal curvature in the fetal alcohol syndrome: preliminary report.**
  Author(s): Garber JM.
  Source: J Am Optom Assoc. 1982 August; 53(8): 641-4.
  http://www.ncbi.nlm.nih.gov:80/entrez/query.fcgi?cmd=Retrieve&db=PubMed&list_uids=7130605&dopt=Abstract

- **Corneal endothelial anomalies in the fetal alcohol syndrome.**
  Author(s): Carones F, Brancato R, Venturi E, Bianchi S, Magni R.
  Source: Archives of Ophthalmology. 1992 August; 110(8): 1128-31.
  http://www.ncbi.nlm.nih.gov:80/entrez/query.fcgi?cmd=Retrieve&db=PubMed&list_uids=1497528&dopt=Abstract

- **Correlates of psychopathology and intelligence in children with fetal alcohol syndrome.**
  Author(s): Steinhausen HC, Willms J, Spohr HL.
  Source: Journal of Child Psychology and Psychiatry, and Allied Disciplines. 1994 February; 35(2): 323-31.
  http://www.ncbi.nlm.nih.gov:80/entrez/query.fcgi?cmd=Retrieve&db=PubMed&list_uids=8188802&dopt=Abstract

- **Craniofacial and oral manifestations of fetal alcohol syndrome.**
  Author(s): Jackson IT, Hussain K.
  Source: Plastic and Reconstructive Surgery. 1990 April; 85(4): 505-12.
  http://www.ncbi.nlm.nih.gov:80/entrez/query.fcgi?cmd=Retrieve&db=PubMed&list_uids=2315390&dopt=Abstract

- **Dendritic spine anomalies in fetal alcohol syndrome.**
  Author(s): Ferrer I, Galofre E.
  Source: Neuropediatrics. 1987 August; 18(3): 161-3.
  http://www.ncbi.nlm.nih.gov:80/entrez/query.fcgi?cmd=Retrieve&db=PubMed&list_uids=3683757&dopt=Abstract

- **Derangement of pyruvate dehydrogenase activity in circulating lymphocytes of a newborn with fetal alcohol syndrome.**
  Author(s): Ferraris S, Mostert M, Rabbone I, Cerutti F, Borgione S, Curto M, Mioletti S, Ponzone A, Silvestro L, Rinaudo MT.
  Source: Acta Paediatrica (Oslo, Norway : 1992). 1996 May; 85(5): 640.
  http://www.ncbi.nlm.nih.gov:80/entrez/query.fcgi?cmd=Retrieve&db=PubMed&list_uids=8827118&dopt=Abstract

- **Dermatoglyphic abnormalities in the fetal alcohol syndrome.**
  Author(s): Qazi QH, Masakawa A, McGann B, Woods J.
  Source: Teratology. 1980 April; 21(2): 157-60.
  http://www.ncbi.nlm.nih.gov:80/entrez/query.fcgi?cmd=Retrieve&db=PubMed&list_uids=7394718&dopt=Abstract

- **Dermatoglyphic asymmetry in fetal alcohol syndrome.**
  Author(s): Wilber E, Newell-Morris L, Streissguth AP.
  Source: Biology of the Neonate. 1993; 64(1): 1-6.
  http://www.ncbi.nlm.nih.gov:80/entrez/query.fcgi?cmd=Retrieve&db=PubMed&list_uids=8399794&dopt=Abstract

- **Development and psychopathology of children with the fetal alcohol syndrome.**
  Author(s): Steinhausen HC, Nestler V, Spohr HL.
  Source: Journal of Developmental and Behavioral Pediatrics : Jdbp. 1982 June; 3(2): 49-54.
  http://www.ncbi.nlm.nih.gov:80/entrez/query.fcgi?cmd=Retrieve&db=PubMed&list_uids=7202020&dopt=Abstract

- **Development of psychopathology of children with the fetal alcohol syndrome.**
  Author(s): Steinhausen HC, Nestler V, Spohr HL.
  Source: Journal of Developmental and Behavioral Pediatrics : Jdbp. 1982 June; 3(2): 49-54.
  http://www.ncbi.nlm.nih.gov:80/entrez/query.fcgi?cmd=Retrieve&db=PubMed&list_uids=6179968&dopt=Abstract

- **Developmental neurotoxicity: do similar phenotypes indicate a common mode of action? A comparison of fetal alcohol syndrome, toluene embryopathy and maternal phenylketonuria.**
  Author(s): Costa LG, Guizzetti M, Burry M, Oberdoerster J.
  Source: Toxicology Letters. 2002 February 28; 127(1-3): 197-205.
  http://www.ncbi.nlm.nih.gov:80/entrez/query.fcgi?cmd=Retrieve&db=PubMed&list_uids=12052659&dopt=Abstract

- **Diagnosing moral disorder: the discovery and evolution of fetal alcohol syndrome.**
  Author(s): Armstrong EM.
  Source: Social Science & Medicine (1982). 1998 December; 47(12): 2025-42.
  http://www.ncbi.nlm.nih.gov:80/entrez/query.fcgi?cmd=Retrieve&db=PubMed&list_uids=10075244&dopt=Abstract

- **Differential expression of c-fos in a mouse model of fetal alcohol syndrome.**
  Author(s): Poggi SH, Goodwin KM, Hill JM, Brenneman DE, Tendi E, Schninelli S, Spong CY.
  Source: American Journal of Obstetrics and Gynecology. 2003 September; 189(3): 786-9.
  http://www.ncbi.nlm.nih.gov:80/entrez/query.fcgi?cmd=Retrieve&db=PubMed&list_uids=14526314&dopt=Abstract

- **Diffuse corneal clouding in siblings with fetal alcohol syndrome.**
  Author(s): Edward DP, Li J, Sawaguchi S, Sugar J, Yue BY, Tso MO.
  Source: American Journal of Ophthalmology. 1993 April 15; 115(4): 484-93.
  http://www.ncbi.nlm.nih.gov:80/entrez/query.fcgi?cmd=Retrieve&db=PubMed&list_uids=8470721&dopt=Abstract

- **DiGeorge's syndrome and fetal alcohol syndrome.**
  Author(s): Cavdar AO.
  Source: Am J Dis Child. 1983 August; 137(8): 806-7. No Abstract Available.
  http://www.ncbi.nlm.nih.gov:80/entrez/query.fcgi?cmd=Retrieve&db=PubMed&list_uids=6683466&dopt=Abstract

- **Down's syndrome, fetal alcohol syndrome, and upper airway obstruction.**
  Author(s): Levine OR.
  Source: Am J Dis Child. 1987 May; 141(5): 478. No Abstract Available.
  http://www.ncbi.nlm.nih.gov:80/entrez/query.fcgi?cmd=Retrieve&db=PubMed&list_uids=2953233&dopt=Abstract

- **Drinking and pregnancy; preventing fetal alcohol syndrome.**
  Author(s): Blume SB.
  Source: N Y State J Med. 1981 January; 81(1): 95-8. No Abstract Available.
  http://www.ncbi.nlm.nih.gov:80/entrez/query.fcgi?cmd=Retrieve&db=PubMed&list_uids=6936627&dopt=Abstract

- **Duane's retraction syndrome in the fetal alcohol syndrome.**
  Author(s): Holzman AE, Chrousos GA, Kozma C, Traboulsi EI.
  Source: American Journal of Ophthalmology. 1990 November 15; 110(5): 565-6.
  http://www.ncbi.nlm.nih.gov:80/entrez/query.fcgi?cmd=Retrieve&db=PubMed&list_uids=2240143&dopt=Abstract

- **E.E.G. component of fetal alcohol syndrome.**
  Author(s): Havlicek V, Childaeva R.
  Source: Lancet. 1976 August 21; 1(7982): 477.
  http://www.ncbi.nlm.nih.gov:80/entrez/query.fcgi?cmd=Retrieve&db=PubMed&list_uids=73786&dopt=Abstract

- **EEG findings in fetal alcohol syndrome and Down syndrome children.**
  Author(s): Kaneko WM, Phillips EL, Riley EP, Ehlers CL.
  Source: Electroencephalography and Clinical Neurophysiology. 1996 January; 98(1): 20-8.
  http://www.ncbi.nlm.nih.gov:80/entrez/query.fcgi?cmd=Retrieve&db=PubMed&list_uids=8689990&dopt=Abstract

- **Effectiveness of methylphenidate in Native American children with fetal alcohol syndrome and attention deficit/hyperactivity disorder: a controlled pilot study.**
  Author(s): Oesterheld JR, Kofoed L, Tervo R, Fogas B, Wilson A, Fiechtner H.
  Source: Journal of Child and Adolescent Psychopharmacology. 1998; 8(1): 39-48.
  http://www.ncbi.nlm.nih.gov:80/entrez/query.fcgi?cmd=Retrieve&db=PubMed&list_uids=9639078&dopt=Abstract

- **Endocrine balance as a factor in the etiology of the fetal alcohol syndrome.**
  Author(s): Anderson RA Jr.
  Source: Neurobehav Toxicol Teratol. 1981 Summer; 3(2): 89-104.
  http://www.ncbi.nlm.nih.gov:80/entrez/query.fcgi?cmd=Retrieve&db=PubMed&list_uids=7019743&dopt=Abstract

- **Epidemiological appraisal of the literature on the fetal alcohol syndrome in humans.**
  Author(s): Neugut RH.
  Source: Early Human Development. 1981 September; 5(4): 411-29. Review.
  http://www.ncbi.nlm.nih.gov:80/entrez/query.fcgi?cmd=Retrieve&db=PubMed&list_uids=7026219&dopt=Abstract

- **Epidemiology of fetal alcohol syndrome among American Indians of the Southwest.**
  Author(s): May PA, Hymbaugh KJ, Aase JM, Samet JM.
  Source: Soc Biol. 1983 Winter; 30(4): 374-87. No Abstract Available.
  http://www.ncbi.nlm.nih.gov:80/entrez/query.fcgi?cmd=Retrieve&db=PubMed&list_uids=6336013&dopt=Abstract

- **Epidemiology of fetal alcohol syndrome in a South African community in the Western Cape Province.**
  Author(s): May PA, Brooke L, Gossage JP, Croxford J, Adnams C, Jones KL, Robinson L, Viljoen D.
  Source: American Journal of Public Health. 2000 December; 90(12): 1905-12.
  http://www.ncbi.nlm.nih.gov:80/entrez/query.fcgi?cmd=Retrieve&db=PubMed&list_uids=11111264&dopt=Abstract

- **Epidemiology of fetal alcohol syndrome in American Indians, Alaskan Natives, and Canadian Aboriginal peoples: a review of the literature.**
  Author(s): Burd L, Moffatt ME.
  Source: Public Health Reports (Washington, D.C. : 1974). 1994 September-October; 109(5): 688-93. Review.
  http://www.ncbi.nlm.nih.gov:80/entrez/query.fcgi?cmd=Retrieve&db=PubMed&list_uids=7938391&dopt=Abstract

- **Erroneous diagnosis of fetal alcohol syndrome in a patient with ring chromosome 6.**
  Author(s): Romke C, Heyne K, Stewens J, Schwinger E.
  Source: European Journal of Pediatrics. 1987 July; 146(4): 443.
  http://www.ncbi.nlm.nih.gov:80/entrez/query.fcgi?cmd=Retrieve&db=PubMed&list_uids=3653144&dopt=Abstract

- **Estimating the prevalence of fetal alcohol syndrome. A summary.**
  Author(s): May PA, Gossage JP.
  Source: Alcohol Research & Health : the Journal of the National Institute on Alcohol Abuse and Alcoholism. 2001; 25(3): 159-67. Review.
  http://www.ncbi.nlm.nih.gov:80/entrez/query.fcgi?cmd=Retrieve&db=PubMed&list_uids=11810953&dopt=Abstract

- **Ethanol inhibits C6 cell growth: fetal alcohol syndrome model.**
  Author(s): Isenberg K, Zhou X, Moore BW.
  Source: Alcoholism, Clinical and Experimental Research. 1992 August; 16(4): 695-9.
  http://www.ncbi.nlm.nih.gov:80/entrez/query.fcgi?cmd=Retrieve&db=PubMed&list_uids=1530131&dopt=Abstract

- **Ethanol-associated selective fetal malnutrition: a contributing factor in the fetal alcohol syndrome.**
  Author(s): Fisher SE, Atkinson M, Burnap JK, Jacobson S, Sehgal PK, Scott W, Van Thiel DH.
  Source: Alcoholism, Clinical and Experimental Research. 1982 Spring; 6(2): 197-201. Review.
  http://www.ncbi.nlm.nih.gov:80/entrez/query.fcgi?cmd=Retrieve&db=PubMed&list_uids=7048972&dopt=Abstract

- **Ethanol-induced apoptotic neurodegeneration and fetal alcohol syndrome.**
  Author(s): Ikonomidou C, Bittigau P, Ishimaru MJ, Wozniak DF, Koch C, Genz K, Price MT, Stefovska V, Horster F, Tenkova T, Dikranian K, Olney JW.
  Source: Science. 2000 February 11; 287(5455): 1056-60.
  http://www.ncbi.nlm.nih.gov:80/entrez/query.fcgi?cmd=Retrieve&db=PubMed&list_uids=10669420&dopt=Abstract

- **Expression of CYP2E1 during embryogenesis and fetogenesis in human cephalic tissues: implications for the fetal alcohol syndrome.**
  Author(s): Boutelet-Bochan H, Huang Y, Juchau MR.
  Source: Biochemical and Biophysical Research Communications. 1997 September 18; 238(2): 443-7.
  http://www.ncbi.nlm.nih.gov:80/entrez/query.fcgi?cmd=Retrieve&db=PubMed&list_uids=9299528&dopt=Abstract

- **Extrahepatic biliary atresia and renal anomalies in fetal alcohol syndrome.**
  Author(s): Dunigan TH, Werlin SL.
  Source: Am J Dis Child. 1981 November; 135(11): 1067-8. No Abstract Available.
  http://www.ncbi.nlm.nih.gov:80/entrez/query.fcgi?cmd=Retrieve&db=PubMed&list_uids=7294014&dopt=Abstract

- **Eye feature extraction for diagnosing the facial phenotype associated with fetal alcohol syndrome.**
  Author(s): Douglas TS, Martinez F, Meintjes EM, Vaughan CL, Viljoen DL.
  Source: Medical & Biological Engineering & Computing. 2003 January; 41(1): 101-6.
  http://www.ncbi.nlm.nih.gov:80/entrez/query.fcgi?cmd=Retrieve&db=PubMed&list_uids=12572754&dopt=Abstract

- **Eye size in healthy Swedish children and in children with fetal alcohol syndrome.**
  Author(s): Hellstrom A, Svensson E, Stromland K.
  Source: Acta Ophthalmologica Scandinavica. 1997 August; 75(4): 423-8. Review.
  http://www.ncbi.nlm.nih.gov:80/entrez/query.fcgi?cmd=Retrieve&db=PubMed&list_
  uids=9374253&dopt=Abstract

- **Eyeground malformations in the fetal alcohol syndrome.**
  Author(s): Stromland K.
  Source: Neuropediatrics. 1981 February; 12(1): 97-8.
  http://www.ncbi.nlm.nih.gov:80/entrez/query.fcgi?cmd=Retrieve&db=PubMed&list_
  uids=6789226&dopt=Abstract

- **Eyeground malformations in the fetal alcohol syndrome.**
  Author(s): Stromland K.
  Source: Birth Defects Orig Artic Ser. 1982; 18(6): 651-5.
  http://www.ncbi.nlm.nih.gov:80/entrez/query.fcgi?cmd=Retrieve&db=PubMed&list_
  uids=6890860&dopt=Abstract

- **Factors predisposing, enabling and reinforcing routine screening of patients for preventing fetal alcohol syndrome: a survey of New Jersey physicians.**
  Author(s): Donovan CL.
  Source: Journal of Drug Education. 1991; 21(1): 35-42.
  http://www.ncbi.nlm.nih.gov:80/entrez/query.fcgi?cmd=Retrieve&db=PubMed&list_
  uids=2016663&dopt=Abstract

- **Fetal alcohol syndrome and bilateral tibial exostoses. A case report.**
  Author(s): Azouz EM, Kavianian G, Der Kaloustian VM.
  Source: Pediatric Radiology. 1993; 23(8): 615-6.
  http://www.ncbi.nlm.nih.gov:80/entrez/query.fcgi?cmd=Retrieve&db=PubMed&list_
  uids=8152879&dopt=Abstract

- **Fetal alcohol syndrome and fatty acid ethyl esters.**
  Author(s): Bearer CF, Gould S, Emerson R, Kinnunen P, Cook CS.
  Source: Pediatric Research. 1992 May; 31(5): 492-5.
  http://www.ncbi.nlm.nih.gov:80/entrez/query.fcgi?cmd=Retrieve&db=PubMed&list_
  uids=1603626&dopt=Abstract

- **Fetal alcohol syndrome and fetal alcohol effects. The University of Minnesota experience.**
  Author(s): Caruso K, ten Bensel R.
  Source: Minn Med. 1993 April; 76(4): 25-9.
  http://www.ncbi.nlm.nih.gov:80/entrez/query.fcgi?cmd=Retrieve&db=PubMed&list_
  uids=8515733&dopt=Abstract

- **Fetal alcohol syndrome and insulin-like growth factors.**
  Author(s): Krishna A, Phillips LS.
  Source: The Journal of Laboratory and Clinical Medicine. 1994 August; 124(2): 149-51.
  http://www.ncbi.nlm.nih.gov:80/entrez/query.fcgi?cmd=Retrieve&db=PubMed&list_
  uids=8051475&dopt=Abstract

- **Fetal alcohol syndrome and its implications for the day care provider.**
  Author(s): Henke C.
  Source: Prairie Rose. 1992 June-August; 61(2): 16-7. No Abstract Available.
  http://www.ncbi.nlm.nih.gov:80/entrez/query.fcgi?cmd=Retrieve&db=PubMed&list_uids=1635902&dopt=Abstract

- **Fetal alcohol syndrome and malignant disease: a case report.**
  Author(s): Battisti L, Degani D, Rugolotto S, Borgna-Pignatti C.
  Source: Am J Pediatr Hematol Oncol. 1993 February; 15(1): 136-7. No Abstract Available.
  http://www.ncbi.nlm.nih.gov:80/entrez/query.fcgi?cmd=Retrieve&db=PubMed&list_uids=8447557&dopt=Abstract

- **Fetal alcohol syndrome at the turn of the 20th century. An unexpected explanation of the Kallikak family.**
  Author(s): Karp RJ, Qazi QH, Moller KA, Angelo WA, Davis JM.
  Source: Archives of Pediatrics & Adolescent Medicine. 1995 January; 149(1): 45-8.
  http://www.ncbi.nlm.nih.gov:80/entrez/query.fcgi?cmd=Retrieve&db=PubMed&list_uids=7827659&dopt=Abstract

- **Fetal alcohol syndrome in adolescents and adults.**
  Author(s): Streissguth AP, Aase JM, Clarren SK, Randels SP, LaDue RA, Smith DF.
  Source: Jama : the Journal of the American Medical Association. 1991 April 17; 265(15): 1961-7.
  http://www.ncbi.nlm.nih.gov:80/entrez/query.fcgi?cmd=Retrieve&db=PubMed&list_uids=2008025&dopt=Abstract

- **Fetal alcohol syndrome in developmental age. Neuropsychiatric aspects.**
  Author(s): Roccella M, Testa D.
  Source: Minerva Pediatr. 2003 February; 55(1): 63-9, 69-74. English, Italian.
  http://www.ncbi.nlm.nih.gov:80/entrez/query.fcgi?cmd=Retrieve&db=PubMed&list_uids=12660628&dopt=Abstract

- **Fetal alcohol syndrome in older patients.**
  Author(s): Streissguth AP.
  Source: Alcohol Alcohol Suppl. 1993; 2: 209-12. Review.
  http://www.ncbi.nlm.nih.gov:80/entrez/query.fcgi?cmd=Retrieve&db=PubMed&list_uids=7748302&dopt=Abstract

- **Fetal alcohol syndrome in twins of alcoholic mothers: concordance of diagnosis and IQ.**
  Author(s): Streissguth AP, Dehaene P.
  Source: American Journal of Medical Genetics. 1993 November 1; 47(6): 857-61.
  http://www.ncbi.nlm.nih.gov:80/entrez/query.fcgi?cmd=Retrieve&db=PubMed&list_uids=8279483&dopt=Abstract

- **Fetal alcohol syndrome prevention research.**
  Author(s): Hankin JR.
  Source: Alcohol Research & Health : the Journal of the National Institute on Alcohol Abuse and Alcoholism. 2002; 26(1): 58-65. Review.
  http://www.ncbi.nlm.nih.gov:80/entrez/query.fcgi?cmd=Retrieve&db=PubMed&list_uids=12154653&dopt=Abstract

- **Fetal alcohol syndrome.**
  Author(s): Atkinson L.
  Source: Journal of the American Academy of Child and Adolescent Psychiatry. 1992 May; 31(3): 563-4.
  http://www.ncbi.nlm.nih.gov:80/entrez/query.fcgi?cmd=Retrieve&db=PubMed&list_uids=1510772&dopt=Abstract

- **Fetal alcohol syndrome.**
  Author(s): Ward KA, Caselli MA.
  Source: Journal of the American Podiatric Medical Association. 1991 August; 81(8): 454.
  http://www.ncbi.nlm.nih.gov:80/entrez/query.fcgi?cmd=Retrieve&db=PubMed&list_uids=1920109&dopt=Abstract

- **Fetal alcohol syndrome.**
  Author(s): Lewis DD, Woods SE.
  Source: American Family Physician. 1994 October; 50(5): 1025-32, 1035-6. Review.
  http://www.ncbi.nlm.nih.gov:80/entrez/query.fcgi?cmd=Retrieve&db=PubMed&list_uids=7942401&dopt=Abstract

- **Fetal alcohol syndrome.**
  Author(s): Jones MW, Bass WT.
  Source: Neonatal Netw. 2003 May-June; 22(3): 63-70. Review. No Abstract Available.
  http://www.ncbi.nlm.nih.gov:80/entrez/query.fcgi?cmd=Retrieve&db=PubMed&list_uids=12795509&dopt=Abstract

- **Fetal alcohol syndrome: a case report of neuropsychological, MRI and EEG assessment of two children.**
  Author(s): Mattson SN, Riley EP, Jernigan TL, Ehlers CL, Delis DC, Jones KL, Stern C, Johnson KA, Hesselink JR, Bellugi U.
  Source: Alcoholism, Clinical and Experimental Research. 1992 October; 16(5): 1001-3.
  http://www.ncbi.nlm.nih.gov:80/entrez/query.fcgi?cmd=Retrieve&db=PubMed&list_uids=1443415&dopt=Abstract

- **Fetal alcohol syndrome: a growing concern for health care professionals.**
  Author(s): Eustace LW, Kang DH, Coombs D.
  Source: Journal of Obstetric, Gynecologic, and Neonatal Nursing : Jognn / Naacog. 2003 March-April; 32(2): 215-21. Review.
  http://www.ncbi.nlm.nih.gov:80/entrez/query.fcgi?cmd=Retrieve&db=PubMed&list_uids=12685673&dopt=Abstract

- **Fetal alcohol syndrome: a nursing concern.**
  Author(s): Tanner M.
  Source: Mna Accent. 1992 June; 64(5): 7-8. No Abstract Available.
  http://www.ncbi.nlm.nih.gov:80/entrez/query.fcgi?cmd=Retrieve&db=PubMed&list_uids=1525500&dopt=Abstract

- **Fetal alcohol syndrome: an international perspective.**
  Author(s): Warren KR, Calhoun FJ, May PA, Viljoen DL, Li TK, Tanaka H, Marinicheva GS, Robinson LK, Mundle G.
  Source: Alcoholism, Clinical and Experimental Research. 2001 May; 25(5 Suppl Isbra): 202S-206S. Review.
  http://www.ncbi.nlm.nih.gov:80/entrez/query.fcgi?cmd=Retrieve&db=PubMed&list_uids=11391072&dopt=Abstract

- **Fetal alcohol syndrome: early and long-term consequences.**
  Author(s): Streissguth AP.
  Source: Nida Res Monogr. 1992; 119: 126-30. Review. No Abstract Available.
  http://www.ncbi.nlm.nih.gov:80/entrez/query.fcgi?cmd=Retrieve&db=PubMed&list_uids=1435967&dopt=Abstract

- **Fetal alcohol syndrome: misplaced emphasis.**
  Author(s): Hess KW.
  Source: Am J Dis Child. 1991 July; 145(7): 721. No Abstract Available.
  http://www.ncbi.nlm.nih.gov:80/entrez/query.fcgi?cmd=Retrieve&db=PubMed&list_uids=2058598&dopt=Abstract

- **Fetal alcohol syndrome: report of a case.**
  Author(s): Lin YS, Chang FM, Liu CH.
  Source: J Formos Med Assoc. 1991 April; 90(4): 411-4.
  http://www.ncbi.nlm.nih.gov:80/entrez/query.fcgi?cmd=Retrieve&db=PubMed&list_uids=1680974&dopt=Abstract

- **Fetal alcohol syndrome: report of three siblings.**
  Author(s): Haddad J, Messer J.
  Source: Neuropediatrics. 1994 April; 25(2): 109-11.
  http://www.ncbi.nlm.nih.gov:80/entrez/query.fcgi?cmd=Retrieve&db=PubMed&list_uids=8072675&dopt=Abstract

- **Fetal alcohol syndrome: review of the literature and case report.**
  Author(s): Nelson JA, Miller DJ, Cardo VA Jr, Zambito RF.
  Source: The New York State Dental Journal. 1990 December; 56(10): 24-7. Review.
  http://www.ncbi.nlm.nih.gov:80/entrez/query.fcgi?cmd=Retrieve&db=PubMed&list_uids=2150432&dopt=Abstract

- **Fetal alcohol syndrome: review of the literature with implications for physical therapists.**
  Author(s): Osborn JA, Harris SR, Weinberg J.
  Source: Physical Therapy. 1993 September; 73(9): 599-607. Review.
  http://www.ncbi.nlm.nih.gov:80/entrez/query.fcgi?cmd=Retrieve&db=PubMed&list_uids=7689232&dopt=Abstract

- **Fetal alcohol syndrome: the vulnerability of the developing brain and possible mechanisms of damage.**
  Author(s): West JR, Chen WJ, Pantazis NJ.
  Source: Metabolic Brain Disease. 1994 December; 9(4): 291-322. Review.
  http://www.ncbi.nlm.nih.gov:80/entrez/query.fcgi?cmd=Retrieve&db=PubMed&list_uids=7898398&dopt=Abstract

- **Fetal alcohol syndrome—South Africa, 2001.**
  Author(s): Centers for Disease Control and Prevention (CDC).
  Source: Mmwr. Morbidity and Mortality Weekly Report. 2003 July 18; 52(28): 660-2.
  http://www.ncbi.nlm.nih.gov:80/entrez/query.fcgi?cmd=Retrieve&db=PubMed&list_uids=12869904&dopt=Abstract

- **From recognition to responsibility: Josef Warkany, David Smith, and the fetal alcohol syndrome in the 21st century.**
  Author(s): Jones KL.
  Source: Birth Defects Research. Part A, Clinical and Molecular Teratology. 2003 January; 67(1): 13-20.
  http://www.ncbi.nlm.nih.gov:80/entrez/query.fcgi?cmd=Retrieve&db=PubMed&list_uids=12749380&dopt=Abstract

- **Gilles de la Tourette's syndrome in a girl with fetal alcohol syndrome.**
  Author(s): von Gontard A, Deget F.
  Source: J Stud Alcohol. 1996 March; 57(2): 219-20. No Abstract Available.
  http://www.ncbi.nlm.nih.gov:80/entrez/query.fcgi?cmd=Retrieve&db=PubMed&list_uids=8683972&dopt=Abstract

- **Gin Lane: did Hogarth know about fetal alcohol syndrome?**
  Author(s): Abel EL.
  Source: Alcohol and Alcoholism (Oxford, Oxfordshire). 2001 March-April; 36(2): 131-4.
  http://www.ncbi.nlm.nih.gov:80/entrez/query.fcgi?cmd=Retrieve&db=PubMed&list_uids=11259209&dopt=Abstract

- **Glia and fetal alcohol syndrome.**
  Author(s): Guerri C, Pascual M, Renau-Piqueras J.
  Source: Neurotoxicology. 2001 October; 22(5): 593-9. Review.
  http://www.ncbi.nlm.nih.gov:80/entrez/query.fcgi?cmd=Retrieve&db=PubMed&list_uids=11770880&dopt=Abstract

- **Glutamate signaling and the fetal alcohol syndrome.**
  Author(s): Olney JW, Wozniak DF, Jevtovic-Todorovic V, Ikonomidou C.
  Source: Mental Retardation and Developmental Disabilities Research Reviews. 2001; 7(4): 267-75. Review.
  http://www.ncbi.nlm.nih.gov:80/entrez/query.fcgi?cmd=Retrieve&db=PubMed&list_uids=11754521&dopt=Abstract

- **Growing up with fetal alcohol syndrome.**
  Author(s): Russell M.
  Source: Nida Res Monogr. 1988; 81: 368-78. Review. No Abstract Available.
  http://www.ncbi.nlm.nih.gov:80/entrez/query.fcgi?cmd=Retrieve&db=PubMed&list_uids=3136373&dopt=Abstract

- **Growth hormone response in fetal alcohol syndrome.**
  Author(s): Tze WJ, Friesen HG, MacLeod PM.
  Source: Archives of Disease in Childhood. 1976 September; 51(9): 703-6.
  http://www.ncbi.nlm.nih.gov:80/entrez/query.fcgi?cmd=Retrieve&db=PubMed&list_uids=999327&dopt=Abstract

- **Growth hormone status in six children with fetal alcohol syndrome.**
  Author(s): Hellstrom A, Jansson C, Boguszewski M, Olegard R, Laegreid L, Albertsson-Wikland K.
  Source: Acta Paediatrica (Oslo, Norway : 1992). 1996 December; 85(12): 1456-62.
  http://www.ncbi.nlm.nih.gov:80/entrez/query.fcgi?cmd=Retrieve&db=PubMed&list_uids=9001658&dopt=Abstract

- **Growth retardation in fetal alcohol syndrome. Unresponsiveness to growth-promoting hormones.**
  Author(s): Castells S, Mark E, Abaci F, Schwartz E.
  Source: Dev Pharmacol Ther. 1981; 3(4): 232-41.
  http://www.ncbi.nlm.nih.gov:80/entrez/query.fcgi?cmd=Retrieve&db=PubMed&list_uids=7201377&dopt=Abstract

- **Hearing disorders in children with fetal alcohol syndrome: findings from case reports.**
  Author(s): Church MW, Gerkin KP.
  Source: Pediatrics. 1988 August; 82(2): 147-54.
  http://www.ncbi.nlm.nih.gov:80/entrez/query.fcgi?cmd=Retrieve&db=PubMed&list_uids=3399287&dopt=Abstract

- **Hearing, language, speech, vestibular, and dentofacial disorders in fetal alcohol syndrome.**
  Author(s): Church MW, Eldis F, Blakley BW, Bawle EV.
  Source: Alcoholism, Clinical and Experimental Research. 1997 April; 21(2): 227-37.
  http://www.ncbi.nlm.nih.gov:80/entrez/query.fcgi?cmd=Retrieve&db=PubMed&list_uids=9113257&dopt=Abstract

- **Hearing, speech, language, and vestibular disorders in the fetal alcohol syndrome: a literature review.**
  Author(s): Church MW, Kaltenbach JA.
  Source: Alcoholism, Clinical and Experimental Research. 1997 May; 21(3): 495-512. Review.
  http://www.ncbi.nlm.nih.gov:80/entrez/query.fcgi?cmd=Retrieve&db=PubMed&list_uids=9161611&dopt=Abstract

- **Heavy prenatal alcohol exposure with or without physical features of fetal alcohol syndrome leads to IQ deficits.**
  Author(s): Mattson SN, Riley EP, Gramling L, Delis DC, Jones KL.
  Source: The Journal of Pediatrics. 1997 November; 131(5): 718-21.
  http://www.ncbi.nlm.nih.gov:80/entrez/query.fcgi?cmd=Retrieve&db=PubMed&list_uids=9403652&dopt=Abstract

- **Hepatic dysfunction in patient with fetal alcohol syndrome.**
  Author(s): Mooller J, Brandt NJ, Tygstrup I.
  Source: Lancet. 1979 March 17; 1(8116): 605-6.
  http://www.ncbi.nlm.nih.gov:80/entrez/query.fcgi?cmd=Retrieve&db=PubMed&list_uids=85183&dopt=Abstract

- **Hepatic fibrosis in fetal alcohol syndrome. Pathologic similarities to adult alcoholic liver disease.**
  Author(s): Lefkowitch JH, Rushton AR, Feng-Chen KC.
  Source: Gastroenterology. 1983 October; 85(4): 951-7.
  http://www.ncbi.nlm.nih.gov:80/entrez/query.fcgi?cmd=Retrieve&db=PubMed&list_uids=6684069&dopt=Abstract

- **Hepatoblastoma in child with fetal alcohol syndrome.**
  Author(s): Khan A, Bader JL, Hoy GR, Sinks LF.
  Source: Lancet. 1979 June 30; 1(8131): 1403-4.
  http://www.ncbi.nlm.nih.gov:80/entrez/query.fcgi?cmd=Retrieve&db=PubMed&list_uids=87858&dopt=Abstract

- **Hospital utilization of Saskatchewan people with fetal alcohol syndrome.**
  Author(s): Loney EA, Habbick BF, Nanson JL.
  Source: Canadian Journal of Public Health. Revue Canadienne De Sante Publique. 1998 September-October; 89(5): 333-6.
  http://www.ncbi.nlm.nih.gov:80/entrez/query.fcgi?cmd=Retrieve&db=PubMed&list_uids=9813924&dopt=Abstract

- **Hypothalamic-pituitary function in the fetal alcohol syndrome.**
  Author(s): Root AW, Reiter EO, Andriola M, Duckett G.
  Source: The Journal of Pediatrics. 1975 October; 87(4): 585-8.
  http://www.ncbi.nlm.nih.gov:80/entrez/query.fcgi?cmd=Retrieve&db=PubMed&list_uids=1159590&dopt=Abstract

- **Identifying fetal alcohol syndrome among youth in the criminal justice system.**
  Author(s): Fast DK, Conry J, Loock CA.
  Source: Journal of Developmental and Behavioral Pediatrics : Jdbp. 1999 October; 20(5): 370-2.
  http://www.ncbi.nlm.nih.gov:80/entrez/query.fcgi?cmd=Retrieve&db=PubMed&list_uids=10533996&dopt=Abstract

- **Immune deficiency in fetal alcohol syndrome.**
  Author(s): Johnson S, Knight R, Marmer DJ, Steele RW.
  Source: Pediatric Research. 1981 June; 15(6): 908-11.
  http://www.ncbi.nlm.nih.gov:80/entrez/query.fcgi?cmd=Retrieve&db=PubMed&list_uids=7195540&dopt=Abstract

- **Impaired renal acidification in infants with fetal alcohol syndrome.**
  Author(s): Assadi FK, Ziai M.
  Source: Pediatric Research. 1985 August; 19(8): 850-3.
  http://www.ncbi.nlm.nih.gov:80/entrez/query.fcgi?cmd=Retrieve&db=PubMed&list_uids=4041029&dopt=Abstract

- **Incidence of fetal alcohol syndrome and economic impact of FAS-related anomalies.**
  Author(s): Abel EL, Sokol RJ.
  Source: Drug and Alcohol Dependence. 1987 January; 19(1): 51-70. Review.
  http://www.ncbi.nlm.nih.gov:80/entrez/query.fcgi?cmd=Retrieve&db=PubMed&list_uids=3545731&dopt=Abstract

- **Incidence of fetal alcohol syndrome and prevalence of alcohol-related neurodevelopmental disorder.**
  Author(s): Sampson PD, Streissguth AP, Bookstein FL, Little RE, Clarren SK, Dehaene P, Hanson JW, Graham JM Jr.
  Source: Teratology. 1997 November; 56(5): 317-26. Review.
  http://www.ncbi.nlm.nih.gov:80/entrez/query.fcgi?cmd=Retrieve&db=PubMed&list_uids=9451756&dopt=Abstract

- **Incidence of fetal alcohol syndrome in northeastern Manitoba.**
  Author(s): Williams RJ, Odaibo FS, McGee JM.
  Source: Canadian Journal of Public Health. Revue Canadienne De Sante Publique. 1999 May-June; 90(3): 192-4.
  http://www.ncbi.nlm.nih.gov:80/entrez/query.fcgi?cmd=Retrieve&db=PubMed&list_uids=10401171&dopt=Abstract

- **Incidence of fetal alcohol syndrome on the southern part of Reunion Island (France)**
  Author(s): Maillard T, Lamblin D, Lesure JF, Fourmaintraux A.
  Source: Teratology. 1999 August; 60(2): 51-2.
  http://www.ncbi.nlm.nih.gov:80/entrez/query.fcgi?cmd=Retrieve&db=PubMed&list_uids=10440770&dopt=Abstract

- **Information service on fetal alcohol syndrome launched.**
  Author(s): Julien C.
  Source: Cmaj : Canadian Medical Association Journal = Journal De L'association Medicale Canadienne. 1995 February 15; 152(4): 470-1.
  http://www.ncbi.nlm.nih.gov:80/entrez/query.fcgi?cmd=Retrieve&db=PubMed&list_uids=7859194&dopt=Abstract

- **Inhibition of muscarinic receptor-induced proliferation of astroglial cells by ethanol: mechanisms and implications for the fetal alcohol syndrome.**
  Author(s): Costa LG, Guizzetti M.
  Source: Neurotoxicology. 2002 December; 23(6): 685-91. Review.
  http://www.ncbi.nlm.nih.gov:80/entrez/query.fcgi?cmd=Retrieve&db=PubMed&list_uids=12520758&dopt=Abstract

- **Inhibition of retinoic acid synthesis and its implications in fetal alcohol syndrome (FAS)**
  Author(s): Zachman RD, Grummer MA.
  Source: Alcoholism, Clinical and Experimental Research. 1992 February; 16(1): 141.
  http://www.ncbi.nlm.nih.gov:80/entrez/query.fcgi?cmd=Retrieve&db=PubMed&list_uids=1558296&dopt=Abstract

- **Inhibition of retinoic acid synthesis and its implications in fetal alcohol syndrome.**
  Author(s): Keir WJ.
  Source: Alcoholism, Clinical and Experimental Research. 1991 June; 15(3): 560-4. Review.
  http://www.ncbi.nlm.nih.gov:80/entrez/query.fcgi?cmd=Retrieve&db=PubMed&list_uids=1877744&dopt=Abstract

- **Intelligence, behavior, and dysmorphogenesis in the fetal alcohol syndrome: a report on 20 patients.**
  Author(s): Streissguth AP, Herman CS, Smith DW.
  Source: The Journal of Pediatrics. 1978 March; 92(3): 363-7.
  http://www.ncbi.nlm.nih.gov:80/entrez/query.fcgi?cmd=Retrieve&db=PubMed&list_uids=632974&dopt=Abstract

- **Intrinsic defects in the fetal alcohol syndrome: studies on 76 cases from British Columbia and the Yukon Territory.**
  Author(s): Smith DF, Sandor GG, MacLeod PM, Tredwell S, Wood B, Newman DE.
  Source: Neurobehav Toxicol Teratol. 1981 Summer; 3(2): 145-52.
  http://www.ncbi.nlm.nih.gov:80/entrez/query.fcgi?cmd=Retrieve&db=PubMed&list_uids=7195990&dopt=Abstract

- **Introduction to fetal alcohol syndrome.**
  Author(s): Randall CL.
  Source: Curr Alcohol. 1979; 5: 119-21. No Abstract Available.
  http://www.ncbi.nlm.nih.gov:80/entrez/query.fcgi?cmd=Retrieve&db=PubMed&list_uids=755616&dopt=Abstract

- **Introduction: a teratologist's view of the fetal alcohol syndrome.**
  Author(s): Chernoff GF.
  Source: Curr Alcohol. 1979; 7: 7-13. No Abstract Available.
  http://www.ncbi.nlm.nih.gov:80/entrez/query.fcgi?cmd=Retrieve&db=PubMed&list_uids=552350&dopt=Abstract

- **Involvement of free radical mechanism in the toxic effects of alcohol: implications for fetal alcohol syndrome.**
  Author(s): Guerri C, Montoliu C, Renau-Piqueras J.
  Source: Advances in Experimental Medicine and Biology. 1994; 366: 291-305. Review.
  http://www.ncbi.nlm.nih.gov:80/entrez/query.fcgi?cmd=Retrieve&db=PubMed&list_uids=7771260&dopt=Abstract

- **Is fetal alcohol syndrome completely irreversible?**
  Author(s): Barbour BG.
  Source: Mcn. the American Journal of Maternal Child Nursing. 1989 January-February; 14(1): 44-6.
  http://www.ncbi.nlm.nih.gov:80/entrez/query.fcgi?cmd=Retrieve&db=PubMed&list_uids=2494409&dopt=Abstract

- **Is genotype important in predicting the fetal alcohol syndrome?**
  Author(s): Chambers CD, Jones KL.
  Source: The Journal of Pediatrics. 2002 December; 141(6): 751-2.
  http://www.ncbi.nlm.nih.gov:80/entrez/query.fcgi?cmd=Retrieve&db=PubMed&list_uids=12461486&dopt=Abstract

- **Is 'herbal health tonic' safe in pregnancy; fetal alcohol syndrome revisited.**
  Author(s): Pradeepkumar VK, Tan KW, Ivy NG.
  Source: The Australian & New Zealand Journal of Obstetrics & Gynaecology. 1996 November; 36(4): 420-3.
  http://www.ncbi.nlm.nih.gov:80/entrez/query.fcgi?cmd=Retrieve&db=PubMed&list_uids=9006825&dopt=Abstract

- **Is moderate alcohol intake in pregnancy associated with the craniofacial features related to the fetal alcohol syndrome?**
  Author(s): Olsen J, Tuntiseranee P.
  Source: Scand J Soc Med. 1995 September; 23(3): 156-61.
  http://www.ncbi.nlm.nih.gov:80/entrez/query.fcgi?cmd=Retrieve&db=PubMed&list_uids=8602484&dopt=Abstract

- **Is there evidence to show that fetal alcohol syndrome can be prevented?**
  Author(s): Murphy-Brennan MG, Oei TP.
  Source: Journal of Drug Education. 1999; 29(1): 5-24. Review.
  http://www.ncbi.nlm.nih.gov:80/entrez/query.fcgi?cmd=Retrieve&db=PubMed&list_uids=10349824&dopt=Abstract

- **Isospora belli infection and chronic electrolyte disturbance in a child with fetal alcohol syndrome.**
  Author(s): Bucens IK, King RO.
  Source: The Medical Journal of Australia. 2000 September; 173(5): 252-5.
  http://www.ncbi.nlm.nih.gov:80/entrez/query.fcgi?cmd=Retrieve&db=PubMed&list_uids=11130350&dopt=Abstract

- **Klippel-Feil anomaly combined with fetal alcohol syndrome.**
  Author(s): Schilgen M, Loeser H.
  Source: European Spine Journal : Official Publication of the European Spine Society, the European Spinal Deformity Society, and the European Section of the Cervical Spine Research Society. 1994; 3(5): 289-90.
  http://www.ncbi.nlm.nih.gov:80/entrez/query.fcgi?cmd=Retrieve&db=PubMed&list_uids=7866854&dopt=Abstract

- **Klippel-Feil malformation complex in fetal alcohol syndrome.**
  Author(s): Neidengard L, Carter TE, Smith DW.
  Source: Am J Dis Child. 1978 September; 132(9): 929-30. No Abstract Available.
  http://www.ncbi.nlm.nih.gov:80/entrez/query.fcgi?cmd=Retrieve&db=PubMed&list_uids=685915&dopt=Abstract

- **Knowledge of fetal alcohol syndrome (FAS) among natives in Northern Manitoba.**
  Author(s): Williams RJ, Gloster SP.
  Source: J Stud Alcohol. 1999 November; 60(6): 833-6.
  http://www.ncbi.nlm.nih.gov:80/entrez/query.fcgi?cmd=Retrieve&db=PubMed&list_uids=10606496&dopt=Abstract

- **Knowledge of fetal alcohol syndrome among Native Indians.**
  Author(s): Robinson GC, Armstrong RW, Moczuk IB, Loock CA.
  Source: Canadian Journal of Public Health. Revue Canadienne De Sante Publique. 1992 September-October; 83(5): 337-8.
  http://www.ncbi.nlm.nih.gov:80/entrez/query.fcgi?cmd=Retrieve&db=PubMed&list_uids=1473057&dopt=Abstract

- **Letter: Fetal alcohol syndrome.**
  Author(s): Ferrier PE, Nicod I, Ferrier S.
  Source: Lancet. 1973 December 29; 2(7844): 1496.
  http://www.ncbi.nlm.nih.gov:80/entrez/query.fcgi?cmd=Retrieve&db=PubMed&list_uids=4129335&dopt=Abstract

- **Letter: Noonan syndrome and fetal alcohol syndrome.**
  Author(s): Bianchine JW, Taylor BD.
  Source: Lancet. 1974 May 11; 1(7863): 933.
  http://www.ncbi.nlm.nih.gov:80/entrez/query.fcgi?cmd=Retrieve&db=PubMed&list_uids=4133456&dopt=Abstract

- **Letter: The fetal alcohol syndrome.**
  Author(s): Mankad VN, Choksi RM.
  Source: Jama : the Journal of the American Medical Association. 1976 September 6; 236(10): 1114.
  http://www.ncbi.nlm.nih.gov:80/entrez/query.fcgi?cmd=Retrieve&db=PubMed&list_uids=988860&dopt=Abstract

- **Liver abnormalities in three patients with fetal alcohol syndrome.**
  Author(s): Habbick BF, Zaleski WA, Casey R, Murphy F.
  Source: Lancet. 1979 March 17; 1(8116): 580-1.
  http://www.ncbi.nlm.nih.gov:80/entrez/query.fcgi?cmd=Retrieve&db=PubMed&list_uids=85166&dopt=Abstract

- **Living with a child with fetal alcohol syndrome.**
  Author(s): Gardner J.
  Source: Mcn. the American Journal of Maternal Child Nursing. 2000 September-October; 25(5): 252-7.
  http://www.ncbi.nlm.nih.gov:80/entrez/query.fcgi?cmd=Retrieve&db=PubMed&list_uids=10992738&dopt=Abstract

- **Long-term follow-up of three siblings with fetal alcohol syndrome.**
  Author(s): Iosub S, Fuchs M, Bingol N, Stone RK, Gromisch DS.
  Source: Alcoholism, Clinical and Experimental Research. 1981 Fall; 5(4): 523-7.
  http://www.ncbi.nlm.nih.gov:80/entrez/query.fcgi?cmd=Retrieve&db=PubMed&list_uids=7030107&dopt=Abstract

- **Long-term outcome of children with fetal alcohol syndrome: psychopathology, behavior, and intelligence.**
  Author(s): Steinhausen HC, Spohr HL.
  Source: Alcoholism, Clinical and Experimental Research. 1998 April; 22(2): 334-8.
  http://www.ncbi.nlm.nih.gov:80/entrez/query.fcgi?cmd=Retrieve&db=PubMed&list_uids=9581637&dopt=Abstract

- **Long-term psychopathological and cognitive outcome of children with fetal alcohol syndrome.**
  Author(s): Steinhausen HC, Willms J, Spohr HL.
  Source: Journal of the American Academy of Child and Adolescent Psychiatry. 1993 September; 32(5): 990-4.
  http://www.ncbi.nlm.nih.gov:80/entrez/query.fcgi?cmd=Retrieve&db=PubMed&list_uids=8407775&dopt=Abstract

- **Magnetic resonance imaging of brain anomalies in fetal alcohol syndrome.**
  Author(s): Swayze VW 2nd, Johnson VP, Hanson JW, Piven J, Sato Y, Giedd JN, Mosnik D, Andreasen NC.
  Source: Pediatrics. 1997 February; 99(2): 232-40.
  http://www.ncbi.nlm.nih.gov:80/entrez/query.fcgi?cmd=Retrieve&db=PubMed&list_uids=9024452&dopt=Abstract

- **Major skeletal defects in the fetal alcohol syndrome. A case report.**
  Author(s): van Rensburg LJ.
  Source: South African Medical Journal. Suid-Afrikaanse Tydskrif Vir Geneeskunde. 1981 May 2; 59(19): 687-8.
  http://www.ncbi.nlm.nih.gov:80/entrez/query.fcgi?cmd=Retrieve&db=PubMed&list_uids=7194516&dopt=Abstract

- **Management of severe feeding dysfunction in children with fetal alcohol syndrome.**
  Author(s): Van Dyke DC, Mackay L, Ziaylek EN.
  Source: Clinical Pediatrics. 1982 June; 21(6): 336-9.
  http://www.ncbi.nlm.nih.gov:80/entrez/query.fcgi?cmd=Retrieve&db=PubMed&list_
  uids=6804149&dopt=Abstract

- **Maternal alcoholism and fetal alcohol syndrome.**
  Author(s): Luke B.
  Source: The American Journal of Nursing. 1977 December; 77(12): 1924-6.
  http://www.ncbi.nlm.nih.gov:80/entrez/query.fcgi?cmd=Retrieve&db=PubMed&list_
  uids=244255&dopt=Abstract

- **Maternal ethanol ingestion effects on fetal rat brain vitamin A as a model for fetal alcohol syndrome.**
  Author(s): Grummer MA, Langhough RE, Zachman RD.
  Source: Alcoholism, Clinical and Experimental Research. 1993 June; 17(3): 592-7.
  http://www.ncbi.nlm.nih.gov:80/entrez/query.fcgi?cmd=Retrieve&db=PubMed&list_
  uids=8333589&dopt=Abstract

- **Maternal risk factors in fetal alcohol syndrome: provocative and permissive influences.**
  Author(s): Abel EL, Hannigan JH.
  Source: Neurotoxicology and Teratology. 1995 July-August; 17(4): 445-62. Review.
  Erratum In: Neurotoxicol Teratol 1995 November-December; 17(6): 689.
  http://www.ncbi.nlm.nih.gov:80/entrez/query.fcgi?cmd=Retrieve&db=PubMed&list_
  uids=7565491&dopt=Abstract

- **Mental illness in adults with fetal alcohol syndrome or fetal alcohol effects.**
  Author(s): Famy C, Streissguth AP, Unis AS.
  Source: The American Journal of Psychiatry. 1998 April; 155(4): 552-4.
  http://www.ncbi.nlm.nih.gov:80/entrez/query.fcgi?cmd=Retrieve&db=PubMed&list_
  uids=9546004&dopt=Abstract

- **Metabolic and mitotic changes associated with the fetal alcohol syndrome.**
  Author(s): Shibley IA Jr, Pennington SN.
  Source: Alcohol and Alcoholism (Oxford, Oxfordshire). 1997 July-August; 32(4): 423-34. Review.
  http://www.ncbi.nlm.nih.gov:80/entrez/query.fcgi?cmd=Retrieve&db=PubMed&list_
  uids=9269850&dopt=Abstract

- **Metronidazole and the fetal alcohol syndrome.**
  Author(s): Dunn PM, Stewart-Brown S, Peel R.
  Source: Lancet. 1979 July 21; 2(8134): 144.
  http://www.ncbi.nlm.nih.gov:80/entrez/query.fcgi?cmd=Retrieve&db=PubMed&list_
  uids=88568&dopt=Abstract

- **Microcephaly and fetal alcohol syndrome.**
  Author(s): Hanley WB.
  Source: The Journal of Pediatrics. 2002 September; 141(3): 449; Author Reply 449.
  http://www.ncbi.nlm.nih.gov:80/entrez/query.fcgi?cmd=Retrieve&db=PubMed&list_uids=12219073&dopt=Abstract

- **Midaortic syndrome associated with fetal alcohol syndrome.**
  Author(s): Cura MA, Bugnone A, Becker GJ.
  Source: Journal of Vascular and Interventional Radiology : Jvir. 2002 November; 13(11): 1167-70.
  http://www.ncbi.nlm.nih.gov:80/entrez/query.fcgi?cmd=Retrieve&db=PubMed&list_uids=12427818&dopt=Abstract

- **Minnesota responds to fetal alcohol syndrome.**
  Author(s): Lussky R.
  Source: Minn Med. 1998 August; 81(8): 35-8. No Abstract Available.
  http://www.ncbi.nlm.nih.gov:80/entrez/query.fcgi?cmd=Retrieve&db=PubMed&list_uids=9715628&dopt=Abstract

- **Morphometry of the neonatal fetal alcohol syndrome face from 'snapshots'.**
  Author(s): Sokol RJ, Chik L, Martier SS, Salari V.
  Source: Alcohol Alcohol Suppl. 1991; 1: 531-4.
  http://www.ncbi.nlm.nih.gov:80/entrez/query.fcgi?cmd=Retrieve&db=PubMed&list_uids=1845594&dopt=Abstract

- **Multilevel intervention for prevention of fetal alcohol syndrome and effects of prenatal alcohol exposure.**
  Author(s): Smith IE, Coles CD.
  Source: Recent Dev Alcohol. 1991; 9: 165-80. Review.
  http://www.ncbi.nlm.nih.gov:80/entrez/query.fcgi?cmd=Retrieve&db=PubMed&list_uids=1758982&dopt=Abstract

- **Nail dysplasia and fetal alcohol syndrome. Case report of a heteropaternal sibship.**
  Author(s): Crain LS, Fitzmaurice NE, Mondry C.
  Source: Am J Dis Child. 1983 November; 137(11): 1069-72.
  http://www.ncbi.nlm.nih.gov:80/entrez/query.fcgi?cmd=Retrieve&db=PubMed&list_uids=6685432&dopt=Abstract

- **National Task Force on Fetal Alcohol Syndrome and Fetal Alcohol Effect: defining the national agenda for fetal alcohol syndrome and other prenatal alcohol-related effects.**
  Author(s): Weber MK, Floyd RL, Riley EP, Snider DE Jr; National Task Force on Fetal Alcohol Syndrome and Fetal Alcohol Effect.
  Source: Mmwr. Recommendations and Reports : Morbidity and Mortality Weekly Report. Recommendations and Reports / Centers for Disease Control. 2002 September 20; 51(Rr-14): 9-12.
  http://www.ncbi.nlm.nih.gov:80/entrez/query.fcgi?cmd=Retrieve&db=PubMed&list_uids=12572781&dopt=Abstract

- **Native American adolescents' views of fetal alcohol syndrome prevention in schools.**
  Author(s): Ma GX, Toubbeh J, Cline J, Chisholm A.
  Source: The Journal of School Health. 1998 April; 68(4): 131-6.
  http://www.ncbi.nlm.nih.gov:80/entrez/query.fcgi?cmd=Retrieve&db=PubMed&list_uids=9644604&dopt=Abstract

- **Natural history of the fetal alcohol syndrome: a 10-year follow-up of eleven patients.**
  Author(s): Streissguth AP, Clarren SK, Jones KL.
  Source: Lancet. 1985 July 13; 2(8446): 85-91.
  http://www.ncbi.nlm.nih.gov:80/entrez/query.fcgi?cmd=Retrieve&db=PubMed&list_uids=2861535&dopt=Abstract

- **Neonatal and maternal hair zinc levels in a nonhuman primate model of the fetal alcohol syndrome.**
  Author(s): Fisher SE, Alcock NW, Amirian J, Altshuler HL.
  Source: Alcoholism, Clinical and Experimental Research. 1988 June; 12(3): 417-21.
  http://www.ncbi.nlm.nih.gov:80/entrez/query.fcgi?cmd=Retrieve&db=PubMed&list_uids=3044173&dopt=Abstract

- **Neonatal diagnosis of fetal alcohol syndrome: not necessarily a hopeless prognosis.**
  Author(s): Ernhart CB, Greene T, Sokol RJ, Martier S, Boyd TA, Ager J.
  Source: Alcoholism, Clinical and Experimental Research. 1995 December; 19(6): 1550-7.
  http://www.ncbi.nlm.nih.gov:80/entrez/query.fcgi?cmd=Retrieve&db=PubMed&list_uids=8749826&dopt=Abstract

- **Neural tube defect and renal anomalies in a child with fetal alcohol syndrome.**
  Author(s): Goldstein G, Arulanantham K.
  Source: The Journal of Pediatrics. 1978 October; 93(4): 636-7.
  http://www.ncbi.nlm.nih.gov:80/entrez/query.fcgi?cmd=Retrieve&db=PubMed&list_uids=568174&dopt=Abstract

- **Neuroblastoma in a child with the hydantoin and fetal alcohol syndrome. The radiographic features.**
  Author(s): Ramilo J, Harris VJ.
  Source: The British Journal of Radiology. 1979 December; 52(624): 993-5.
  http://www.ncbi.nlm.nih.gov:80/entrez/query.fcgi?cmd=Retrieve&db=PubMed&list_uids=526805&dopt=Abstract

- **Neurological findings in the fetal alcohol syndrome.**
  Author(s): Marcus JC.
  Source: Neuropediatrics. 1987 August; 18(3): 158-60.
  http://www.ncbi.nlm.nih.gov:80/entrez/query.fcgi?cmd=Retrieve&db=PubMed&list_uids=3683756&dopt=Abstract

- **Neuropsychological comparison of alcohol-exposed children with or without physical features of fetal alcohol syndrome.**
  Author(s): Mattson SN, Riley EP, Gramling L, Delis DC, Jones KL.
  Source: Neuropsychology. 1998 January; 12(1): 146-53.
  http://www.ncbi.nlm.nih.gov:80/entrez/query.fcgi?cmd=Retrieve&db=PubMed&list_uids=9460742&dopt=Abstract

- **Neuropsychological deficits in adolescents with fetal alcohol syndrome: clinical findings.**
  Author(s): Olson HC, Feldman JJ, Streissguth AP, Sampson PD, Bookstein FL.
  Source: Alcoholism, Clinical and Experimental Research. 1998 December; 22(9): 1998-2012.
  http://www.ncbi.nlm.nih.gov:80/entrez/query.fcgi?cmd=Retrieve&db=PubMed&list_uids=9884144&dopt=Abstract

- **Neuropsychological deficits in fetal alcohol syndrome and fetal alcohol effects.**
  Author(s): Conry J.
  Source: Alcoholism, Clinical and Experimental Research. 1990 October; 14(5): 650-5.
  http://www.ncbi.nlm.nih.gov:80/entrez/query.fcgi?cmd=Retrieve&db=PubMed&list_uids=2264592&dopt=Abstract

- **Neuropsychological evaluation of preschoolers with fetal alcohol syndrome.**
  Author(s): Janzen LA, Nanson JL, Block GW.
  Source: Neurotoxicology and Teratology. 1995 May-June; 17(3): 273-9.
  http://www.ncbi.nlm.nih.gov:80/entrez/query.fcgi?cmd=Retrieve&db=PubMed&list_uids=7623737&dopt=Abstract

- **New directions in fetal alcohol syndrome research.**
  Author(s): Weinberg J.
  Source: Alcoholism, Clinical and Experimental Research. 1996 November; 20(8 Suppl): 72A-77A.
  http://www.ncbi.nlm.nih.gov:80/entrez/query.fcgi?cmd=Retrieve&db=PubMed&list_uids=8947239&dopt=Abstract

- **New ophthalmic findings in fetal alcohol syndrome.**
  Author(s): Gonzalez ER.
  Source: Jama : the Journal of the American Medical Association. 1981 January 9; 245(2): 108.
  http://www.ncbi.nlm.nih.gov:80/entrez/query.fcgi?cmd=Retrieve&db=PubMed&list_uids=7452823&dopt=Abstract

- **New perspectives on the face in fetal alcohol syndrome: what anthropometry tells us.**
  Author(s): Moore ES, Ward RE, Jamison PL, Morris CA, Bader PI, Hall BD.
  Source: American Journal of Medical Genetics. 2002 May 15; 109(4): 249-60.
  http://www.ncbi.nlm.nih.gov:80/entrez/query.fcgi?cmd=Retrieve&db=PubMed&list_uids=11992478&dopt=Abstract

- **Nursing Mirror midwifery forum. 9. Fetal alcohol syndrome.**
  Author(s): Saul P.
  Source: Nurs Mirror. 1983 October 5; 157(14): Iv-Vi. No Abstract Available.
  http://www.ncbi.nlm.nih.gov:80/entrez/query.fcgi?cmd=Retrieve&db=PubMed&list_uids=6556598&dopt=Abstract

- **Nutritional factors underlying the expression of the fetal alcohol syndrome.**
  Author(s): Dreosti IE.
  Source: Annals of the New York Academy of Sciences. 1993 March 15; 678: 193-204. Review.
  http://www.ncbi.nlm.nih.gov:80/entrez/query.fcgi?cmd=Retrieve&db=PubMed&list_uids=8494262&dopt=Abstract

- **Ocular abnormalities in the fetal alcohol syndrome.**
  Author(s): Stromland K.
  Source: Acta Ophthalmol Suppl. 1985; 171: 1-50.
  http://www.ncbi.nlm.nih.gov:80/entrez/query.fcgi?cmd=Retrieve&db=PubMed&list_uids=2988263&dopt=Abstract

- **Ocular involvement in the fetal alcohol syndrome.**
  Author(s): Stromland K.
  Source: Survey of Ophthalmology. 1987 January-February; 31(4): 277-84. Review.
  http://www.ncbi.nlm.nih.gov:80/entrez/query.fcgi?cmd=Retrieve&db=PubMed&list_uids=3107154&dopt=Abstract

- **Ocular manifestations in fetal alcohol syndrome.**
  Author(s): Chan T, Bowell R, O'Keefe M, Lanigan B.
  Source: The British Journal of Ophthalmology. 1991 September; 75(9): 524-6.
  http://www.ncbi.nlm.nih.gov:80/entrez/query.fcgi?cmd=Retrieve&db=PubMed&list_uids=1911652&dopt=Abstract

- **Of mice and women, and alcohol: a fractal history of fetal alcohol syndrome research.**
  Author(s): Hannigan JH.
  Source: Developmental Psychobiology. 1996 July; 29(5): 398-400.
  http://www.ncbi.nlm.nih.gov:80/entrez/query.fcgi?cmd=Retrieve&db=PubMed&list_uids=8809490&dopt=Abstract

- **Ophthalmic involvement in the fetal alcohol syndrome: clinical and animal model studies.**
  Author(s): Stromland K, Pinazo-Duran MD.
  Source: Alcohol and Alcoholism (Oxford, Oxfordshire). 2002 January-February; 37(1): 2-8. Review.
  http://www.ncbi.nlm.nih.gov:80/entrez/query.fcgi?cmd=Retrieve&db=PubMed&list_uids=11825849&dopt=Abstract

- **Optic nerve hypoplasia in fetal alcohol syndrome: an update.**
  Author(s): Pinazo-Duran MD, Renau-Piqueras J, Guerri C, Stromland K.
  Source: Eur J Ophthalmol. 1997 July-September; 7(3): 262-70.
  http://www.ncbi.nlm.nih.gov:80/entrez/query.fcgi?cmd=Retrieve&db=PubMed&list_uids=9352281&dopt=Abstract

- **Oral findings of fetal alcohol syndrome patients.**
  Author(s): Riekman GA.
  Source: Journal (Canadian Dental Association). 1984 November; 50(11): 841-2.
  http://www.ncbi.nlm.nih.gov:80/entrez/query.fcgi?cmd=Retrieve&db=PubMed&list_uids=6391625&dopt=Abstract

- **Organization battles fetal alcohol syndrome.**
  Author(s): Helmlinger CS.
  Source: Naacog Newsl. 1992 October; 19(10): 1, 4-5. No Abstract Available.
  http://www.ncbi.nlm.nih.gov:80/entrez/query.fcgi?cmd=Retrieve&db=PubMed&list_uids=1435845&dopt=Abstract

- **Patterns of cognitive-motor development in children with fetal alcohol syndrome from a community in South Africa.**
  Author(s): Adnams CM, Kodituwakku PW, Hay A, Molteno CD, Viljoen D, May PA.
  Source: Alcoholism, Clinical and Experimental Research. 2001 April; 25(4): 557-62. Erratum In: Alcohol Clin Exp Res 2001 August; 25(8): 1187.
  http://www.ncbi.nlm.nih.gov:80/entrez/query.fcgi?cmd=Retrieve&db=PubMed&list_uids=11329496&dopt=Abstract

- **Pediatricians' perspectives on fetal alcohol syndrome.**
  Author(s): Morse BA, Idelson RK, Sachs WH, Weiner L, Kaplan LC.
  Source: Journal of Substance Abuse. 1992; 4(2): 187-95.
  http://www.ncbi.nlm.nih.gov:80/entrez/query.fcgi?cmd=Retrieve&db=PubMed&list_uids=1504642&dopt=Abstract

- **Performance of American Indian children with fetal alcohol syndrome on the test of language development.**
  Author(s): Carney LJ, Chermak GD.
  Source: Journal of Communication Disorders. 1991 April; 24(2): 123-34.
  http://www.ncbi.nlm.nih.gov:80/entrez/query.fcgi?cmd=Retrieve&db=PubMed&list_uids=2066470&dopt=Abstract

- **Perspectives on the cause and frequency of the fetal alcohol syndrome.**
  Author(s): Smith DW, Jones KL, Hanson JW.
  Source: Annals of the New York Academy of Sciences. 1976; 273: 138-9.
  http://www.ncbi.nlm.nih.gov:80/entrez/query.fcgi?cmd=Retrieve&db=PubMed&list_uids=1072342&dopt=Abstract

- **Perspectives on the pathophysiology of fetal alcohol syndrome.**
  Author(s): Randall CL, Ekblad U, Anton RF.
  Source: Alcoholism, Clinical and Experimental Research. 1990 December; 14(6): 807-12. Review.
  http://www.ncbi.nlm.nih.gov:80/entrez/query.fcgi?cmd=Retrieve&db=PubMed&list_uids=2088115&dopt=Abstract

- **Physician awareness and screening for fetal alcohol syndrome.**
  Author(s): Conrad C.
  Source: Journal of Health and Human Services Administration. 2000 Winter; 22(3): 257-76.
  http://www.ncbi.nlm.nih.gov:80/entrez/query.fcgi?cmd=Retrieve&db=PubMed&list_uids=11010122&dopt=Abstract

- **Physician awareness of fetal alcohol syndrome: a survey of pediatricians and general practitioners.**
  Author(s): Nanson JL, Bolaria R, Snyder RE, Morse BA, Weiner L.
  Source: Cmaj : Canadian Medical Association Journal = Journal De L'association Medicale Canadienne. 1995 April 1; 152(7): 1071-6.
  http://www.ncbi.nlm.nih.gov:80/entrez/query.fcgi?cmd=Retrieve&db=PubMed&list_uids=7712419&dopt=Abstract

- **Polythelia: a marker of fetal alcohol syndrome and a clue for familial ethilism.**
  Author(s): Urbani CE, Betti R.
  Source: Pediatric Dermatology. 1995 June; 12(2): 197.
  http://www.ncbi.nlm.nih.gov:80/entrez/query.fcgi?cmd=Retrieve&db=PubMed&list_uids=7659654&dopt=Abstract

- **Possible maternal auto-immune component in the etiology of the fetal alcohol syndrome.**
  Author(s): Foster JW.
  Source: Developmental Medicine and Child Neurology. 1986 October; 28(5): 654-6.
  http://www.ncbi.nlm.nih.gov:80/entrez/query.fcgi?cmd=Retrieve&db=PubMed&list_uids=3781107&dopt=Abstract

- **Prediction of fetal alcohol syndrome by maternal alpha fetoprotein, human placental lactogen and pregnancy specific beta 1-glycoprotein.**
  Author(s): Halmesmaki E, Autti I, Granstrom ML, Heikinheimo M, Raivio KO, Ylikorkala O.
  Source: Alcohol and Alcoholism (Oxford, Oxfordshire). 1987; Suppl 1: 473-6.
  http://www.ncbi.nlm.nih.gov:80/entrez/query.fcgi?cmd=Retrieve&db=PubMed&list_uids=2447904&dopt=Abstract

- **Prenatal factors including fetal alcohol syndrome.**
  Author(s): Olegard R, Laegreid L, Wahlstrom J, Conradi N.
  Source: Ups J Med Sci Suppl. 1987; 44: 169-72. Review.
  http://www.ncbi.nlm.nih.gov:80/entrez/query.fcgi?cmd=Retrieve&db=PubMed&list_uids=2895525&dopt=Abstract

- **Present state of the fetal alcohol syndrome.**
  Author(s): Stromland K.
  Source: Acta Ophthalmologica Scandinavica. Supplement. 1996; (219): 10-2. Review.
  http://www.ncbi.nlm.nih.gov:80/entrez/query.fcgi?cmd=Retrieve&db=PubMed&list_uids=8741106&dopt=Abstract

- **Prevalence of fetal alcohol syndrome largely unknown.**
  Author(s): Wallace P.
  Source: Iowa Med. 1991 September; 81(9): 381. No Abstract Available.
  http://www.ncbi.nlm.nih.gov:80/entrez/query.fcgi?cmd=Retrieve&db=PubMed&list_uids=1743929&dopt=Abstract

- **Preventing fetal alcohol syndrome.**
  Author(s): Mitchell KT, Donaldson T.
  Source: Journal of Pediatric Health Care : Official Publication of National Association of Pediatric Nurse Associates & Practitioners. 1999 March-April; 13(2): 87-9.
  http://www.ncbi.nlm.nih.gov:80/entrez/query.fcgi?cmd=Retrieve&db=PubMed&list_uids=10382471&dopt=Abstract

- **Preventing fetal alcohol syndrome: where are we now?**
  Author(s): Blume SB.
  Source: Addiction (Abingdon, England). 1996 April; 91(4): 473-5.
  http://www.ncbi.nlm.nih.gov:80/entrez/query.fcgi?cmd=Retrieve&db=PubMed&list_uids=8857368&dopt=Abstract

- **Prevention of fetal alcohol syndrome.**
  Author(s): Colmorgen GH.
  Source: Del Med J. 1986 August; 58(8): 544-5. No Abstract Available.
  http://www.ncbi.nlm.nih.gov:80/entrez/query.fcgi?cmd=Retrieve&db=PubMed&list_uids=3758435&dopt=Abstract

- **Prevention of fetal alcohol syndrome.**
  Author(s): Alpert JJ, Zuckerman BS.
  Source: Pediatrics. 1993 November; 92(5): 739; Author Reply 739-40.
  http://www.ncbi.nlm.nih.gov:80/entrez/query.fcgi?cmd=Retrieve&db=PubMed&list_uids=8414873&dopt=Abstract

- **Prevention of fetal alcohol syndrome.**
  Author(s): Shoemaker FW.
  Source: Pediatrics. 1993 November; 92(5): 738-9; Author Reply 739-40.
  http://www.ncbi.nlm.nih.gov:80/entrez/query.fcgi?cmd=Retrieve&db=PubMed&list_uids=8414872&dopt=Abstract

- **Prevention of Fetal Alcohol Syndrome: a model program.**
  Author(s): Little RE, Streissguth AP, Guzinski GM.
  Source: Alcoholism, Clinical and Experimental Research. 1980 April; 4(2): 185-9.
  http://www.ncbi.nlm.nih.gov:80/entrez/query.fcgi?cmd=Retrieve&db=PubMed&list_uids=6990821&dopt=Abstract

- **Psychologic handicaps in children with the fetal alcohol syndrome.**
  Author(s): Streissguth AP.
  Source: Annals of the New York Academy of Sciences. 1976; 273: 140-5.
  http://www.ncbi.nlm.nih.gov:80/entrez/query.fcgi?cmd=Retrieve&db=PubMed&list_uids=1072343&dopt=Abstract

- **Psychostimulant clinical response in fetal alcohol syndrome.**
  Author(s): O'Malley KD, Koplin B, Dohner VA.
  Source: Canadian Journal of Psychiatry. Revue Canadienne De Psychiatrie. 2000 February; 45(1): 90-1.
  http://www.ncbi.nlm.nih.gov:80/entrez/query.fcgi?cmd=Retrieve&db=PubMed&list_uids=10696504&dopt=Abstract

- **Public attitudes to and awareness of fetal alcohol syndrome in young adults.**
  Author(s): Oei TP, Anderson L, Wilks J.
  Source: Journal of Drug Education. 1986; 16(2): 135-47.
  http://www.ncbi.nlm.nih.gov:80/entrez/query.fcgi?cmd=Retrieve&db=PubMed&list_uids=3735023&dopt=Abstract

- **Radiological aspects of the fetal alcohol syndrome.**
  Author(s): Cremin BJ, Jaffer Z.
  Source: Pediatric Radiology. 1981; 11(3): 151-3.
  http://www.ncbi.nlm.nih.gov:80/entrez/query.fcgi?cmd=Retrieve&db=PubMed&list_uids=7198770&dopt=Abstract

- **Ratings of fetal alcohol syndrome facial features by medical providers and biomedical scientists.**
  Author(s): Abel EL, Martier S, Kruger M, Ager J, Sokol RJ.
  Source: Alcoholism, Clinical and Experimental Research. 1993 June; 17(3): 717-21.
  http://www.ncbi.nlm.nih.gov:80/entrez/query.fcgi?cmd=Retrieve&db=PubMed&list_uids=8333606&dopt=Abstract

- **Reassessment of patients with the diagnosis of fetal alcohol syndrome.**
  Author(s): Stoler JM.
  Source: Pediatrics. 1999 June; 103(6 Pt 1): 1313-5.
  http://www.ncbi.nlm.nih.gov:80/entrez/query.fcgi?cmd=Retrieve&db=PubMed&list_uids=10400526&dopt=Abstract

- **Recognition and prevention of fetal alcohol syndrome.**
  Author(s): Hogan M.
  Source: Aarn News Lett. 1992 May; 48(5): 14-6. No Abstract Available.
  http://www.ncbi.nlm.nih.gov:80/entrez/query.fcgi?cmd=Retrieve&db=PubMed&list_uids=1609558&dopt=Abstract

- **Recognition of fetal alcohol syndrome.**
  Author(s): Clarren SK.
  Source: Jama : the Journal of the American Medical Association. 1981 June 19; 245(23): 2436-9.
  http://www.ncbi.nlm.nih.gov:80/entrez/query.fcgi?cmd=Retrieve&db=PubMed&list_uids=7230482&dopt=Abstract

- **Recognition of the fetal alcohol syndrome in early infancy.**
  Author(s): Jones KL, Smith DW.
  Source: Lancet. 1973 November 3; 2(7836): 999-1001.
  http://www.ncbi.nlm.nih.gov:80/entrez/query.fcgi?cmd=Retrieve&db=PubMed&list_uids=4127281&dopt=Abstract

- **Recognizing fetal alcohol syndrome in the nursery.**
  Author(s): Bartlett D, Davis A.
  Source: Jogn Nurs. 1980 July-August; 9(4): 223-5. No Abstract Available.
  http://www.ncbi.nlm.nih.gov:80/entrez/query.fcgi?cmd=Retrieve&db=PubMed&list_uids=6903634&dopt=Abstract

- **Renal anomalies in fetal alcohol syndrome.**
  Author(s): Qazi Q, Masakawa A, Milman D, McGann B, Chua A, Haller J.
  Source: Pediatrics. 1979 June; 63(6): 886-9.
  http://www.ncbi.nlm.nih.gov:80/entrez/query.fcgi?cmd=Retrieve&db=PubMed&list_uids=450525&dopt=Abstract

- **Renal anomalies in the fetal alcohol syndrome.**
  Author(s): DeBeukelaer MM, Randall CL, Stroud DR.
  Source: The Journal of Pediatrics. 1977 November; 91(5): 759-60.
  http://www.ncbi.nlm.nih.gov:80/entrez/query.fcgi?cmd=Retrieve&db=PubMed&list_uids=909015&dopt=Abstract

- **Renal tubular dysfunction in fetal alcohol syndrome.**
  Author(s): Assadi FK.
  Source: Pediatric Nephrology (Berlin, Germany). 1990 January; 4(1): 48-51.
  http://www.ncbi.nlm.nih.gov:80/entrez/query.fcgi?cmd=Retrieve&db=PubMed&list_uids=2206881&dopt=Abstract

- **Screening for fetal alcohol syndrome in primary schools: a feasibility study.**
  Author(s): Clarren SK, Randels SP, Sanderson M, Fineman RM.
  Source: Teratology. 2001 January; 63(1): 3-10.
  http://www.ncbi.nlm.nih.gov:80/entrez/query.fcgi?cmd=Retrieve&db=PubMed&list_uids=11169548&dopt=Abstract

- **Selective fetal malnutrition: the fetal alcohol syndrome.**
  Author(s): Fisher SE.
  Source: Journal of the American College of Nutrition. 1988 April; 7(2): 101-6. Review.
  http://www.ncbi.nlm.nih.gov:80/entrez/query.fcgi?cmd=Retrieve&db=PubMed&list_uids=3283194&dopt=Abstract

- **Sex ratio in fetal alcohol syndrome.**
  Author(s): Abel EL.
  Source: Lancet. 1979 July 14; 2(8133): 105.
  http://www.ncbi.nlm.nih.gov:80/entrez/query.fcgi?cmd=Retrieve&db=PubMed&list_uids=87958&dopt=Abstract

- **She can't help it. Fetal alcohol syndrome haunts those who watch but can't change things.**
  Author(s): Justin RG.
  Source: Postgraduate Medicine. 1998 March; 103(3): 27-8.
  http://www.ncbi.nlm.nih.gov:80/entrez/query.fcgi?cmd=Retrieve&db=PubMed&list_uids=9547175&dopt=Abstract

- **Simultaneous occurrence of extrahepatic biliary atresia and fetal alcohol syndrome.**
  Author(s): Newman SL, Flannery DB, Caplan DB.
  Source: Am J Dis Child. 1979 January; 133(1): 101. No Abstract Available.
  http://www.ncbi.nlm.nih.gov:80/entrez/query.fcgi?cmd=Retrieve&db=PubMed&list_uids=760506&dopt=Abstract

- **Skeletal defects and fetal alcohol syndrome.**
  Author(s): Gonzalez ER.
  Source: Archives of Internal Medicine. 1979 September; 139(9): 959.
  http://www.ncbi.nlm.nih.gov:80/entrez/query.fcgi?cmd=Retrieve&db=PubMed&list_
  uids=475531&dopt=Abstract

- **Spatial but not object memory impairments in children with fetal alcohol syndrome.**
  Author(s): Uecker A, Nadel L.
  Source: Am J Ment Retard. 1998 July; 103(1): 12-8.
  http://www.ncbi.nlm.nih.gov:80/entrez/query.fcgi?cmd=Retrieve&db=PubMed&list_
  uids=9678226&dopt=Abstract

- **Spatial locations gone awry: object and spatial memory deficits in children with fetal alcohol syndrome.**
  Author(s): Uecker A, Nadel L.
  Source: Neuropsychologia. 1996 March; 34(3): 209-23.
  http://www.ncbi.nlm.nih.gov:80/entrez/query.fcgi?cmd=Retrieve&db=PubMed&list_
  uids=8868278&dopt=Abstract

- **Speech & language in fetal alcohol syndrome.**
  Author(s): Sparks SN.
  Source: Asha. 1984 February; 26(2): 27-31. Review.
  http://www.ncbi.nlm.nih.gov:80/entrez/query.fcgi?cmd=Retrieve&db=PubMed&list_
  uids=6367760&dopt=Abstract

- **Stability of intelligence in the fetal alcohol syndrome: a preliminary report.**
  Author(s): Streissguth AP, Herman CS, Smith DW.
  Source: Alcoholism, Clinical and Experimental Research. 1978 April; 2(2): 165-70.
  http://www.ncbi.nlm.nih.gov:80/entrez/query.fcgi?cmd=Retrieve&db=PubMed&list_
  uids=350080&dopt=Abstract

- **Statement of the Public Affairs Committee of the Teratology Society on the fetal alcohol syndrome.**
  Author(s): Adams J, Bittner P, Buttar HS, Chambers CD, Collins TF, Daston GP, Filkins K, Flynn TJ, Graham JM Jr, Lyons Jones K, Kimmel C, Lammer E, Librizzi R, Mitala J, Polifka JE.
  Source: Teratology. 2002 December; 66(6): 344-7.
  http://www.ncbi.nlm.nih.gov:80/entrez/query.fcgi?cmd=Retrieve&db=PubMed&list_
  uids=12486768&dopt=Abstract

- **Steep corneal curvature: a fetal alcohol syndrome landmark.**
  Author(s): Garber JM.
  Source: J Am Optom Assoc. 1984 August; 55(8): 595-8.
  http://www.ncbi.nlm.nih.gov:80/entrez/query.fcgi?cmd=Retrieve&db=PubMed&list_
  uids=6541235&dopt=Abstract

- **Stippled epiphyses in fetal alcohol syndrome.**
  Author(s): Leicher-Duber A, Schumacher R, Spranger J.
  Source: Pediatric Radiology. 1990; 20(5): 369-70. Review.
  http://www.ncbi.nlm.nih.gov:80/entrez/query.fcgi?cmd=Retrieve&db=PubMed&list_uids=2190164&dopt=Abstract

- **Structural and functional brain integrity of fetal alcohol syndrome in nonretarded cases.**
  Author(s): Clark CM, Li D, Conry J, Conry R, Loock C.
  Source: Pediatrics. 2000 May; 105(5): 1096-9.
  http://www.ncbi.nlm.nih.gov:80/entrez/query.fcgi?cmd=Retrieve&db=PubMed&list_uids=10790468&dopt=Abstract

- **Studying alcohol teratogenesis from the perspective of the fetal alcohol syndrome: methodological and statistical issues.**
  Author(s): Streissguth AP, Sampson PD, Barr HM, Clarren SK, Martin DC.
  Source: Annals of the New York Academy of Sciences. 1986; 477: 63-86.
  http://www.ncbi.nlm.nih.gov:80/entrez/query.fcgi?cmd=Retrieve&db=PubMed&list_uids=3468839&dopt=Abstract

- **Suicide prevention training for Aboriginal young adults with learning disabilities from Fetal Alcohol Syndrome/Fetal Alcohol Effects (FAS/FAE).**
  Author(s): Devlin RE.
  Source: Int J Circumpolar Health. 2001 November; 60(4): 564-79. Review. No Abstract Available.
  http://www.ncbi.nlm.nih.gov:80/entrez/query.fcgi?cmd=Retrieve&db=PubMed&list_uids=11768436&dopt=Abstract

- **Surveillance for fetal alcohol syndrome in Colorado.**
  Author(s): Miller LA, Shaikh T, Stanton C, Montgomery A, Rickard R, Keefer S, Hoffman R.
  Source: Public Health Reports (Washington, D.C. : 1974). 1995 November-December; 110(6): 690-7.
  http://www.ncbi.nlm.nih.gov:80/entrez/query.fcgi?cmd=Retrieve&db=PubMed&list_uids=8570819&dopt=Abstract

- **Teratologists, the fetal alcohol syndrome, and alcohol addiction: are we doing enough?**
  Author(s): Brent RL.
  Source: Teratology. 1990 April; 41(4): 491-3.
  http://www.ncbi.nlm.nih.gov:80/entrez/query.fcgi?cmd=Retrieve&db=PubMed&list_uids=2339327&dopt=Abstract

- **The Alcoholic Beverages Labeling Act of 1988. A preemptive shield against fetal alcohol syndrome claims?**
  Author(s): Wagner EN.
  Source: The Journal of Legal Medicine. 1991 June; 12(2): 167-200.
  http://www.ncbi.nlm.nih.gov:80/entrez/query.fcgi?cmd=Retrieve&db=PubMed&list_uids=1885938&dopt=Abstract

- **The fetal alcohol syndrome and fetal alcohol effects on immune competence.**
  Author(s): Chiappelli F, Taylor AN.
  Source: Alcohol and Alcoholism (Oxford, Oxfordshire). 1995 March; 30(2): 259-62.
  http://www.ncbi.nlm.nih.gov:80/entrez/query.fcgi?cmd=Retrieve&db=PubMed&list_uids=7662046&dopt=Abstract

- **The fetal alcohol syndrome in adolescence.**
  Author(s): Spohr HL, Willms J, Steinhausen HC.
  Source: Acta Paediatrica (Oslo, Norway : 1992). Supplement. 1994 November; 404: 19-26.
  http://www.ncbi.nlm.nih.gov:80/entrez/query.fcgi?cmd=Retrieve&db=PubMed&list_uids=7531038&dopt=Abstract

- **The fetal alcohol syndrome in Australia.**
  Author(s): Lipson T.
  Source: The Medical Journal of Australia. 1994 October 17; 161(8): 461-2.
  http://www.ncbi.nlm.nih.gov:80/entrez/query.fcgi?cmd=Retrieve&db=PubMed&list_uids=7935115&dopt=Abstract

- **The fetal alcohol syndrome.**
  Author(s): Galea P, Goel K.
  Source: Scott Med J. 1989 August; 34(4): 505. No Abstract Available.
  http://www.ncbi.nlm.nih.gov:80/entrez/query.fcgi?cmd=Retrieve&db=PubMed&list_uids=2799376&dopt=Abstract

- **The fetal alcohol syndrome.**
  Author(s): Van Demark RE.
  Source: S D J Med. 1988 April; 41(4): 19. No Abstract Available.
  http://www.ncbi.nlm.nih.gov:80/entrez/query.fcgi?cmd=Retrieve&db=PubMed&list_uids=3375803&dopt=Abstract

- **The fetal alcohol syndrome.**
  Author(s): Cooper S.
  Source: Journal of Child Psychology and Psychiatry, and Allied Disciplines. 1987 March; 28(2): 223-7.
  http://www.ncbi.nlm.nih.gov:80/entrez/query.fcgi?cmd=Retrieve&db=PubMed&list_uids=3584293&dopt=Abstract

- **The fetal alcohol syndrome.**
  Author(s): Ouellette EM.
  Source: Bol Asoc Med P R. 1984 November; 76(11): 492-4. No Abstract Available.
  http://www.ncbi.nlm.nih.gov:80/entrez/query.fcgi?cmd=Retrieve&db=PubMed&list_uids=6596112&dopt=Abstract

- **The fetal alcohol syndrome: a multihandicapped child.**
  Author(s): Hill RM, Hegemier S, Tennyson LM.
  Source: Neurotoxicology. 1989 Fall; 10(3): 585-95. Review.
  http://www.ncbi.nlm.nih.gov:80/entrez/query.fcgi?cmd=Retrieve&db=PubMed&list_uids=2696901&dopt=Abstract

- **The incidence of fetal alcohol syndrome in New Zealand.**
  Author(s): Glasgow G.
  Source: N Z Med J. 1996 January 26; 109(1014): 18. No Abstract Available.
  http://www.ncbi.nlm.nih.gov:80/entrez/query.fcgi?cmd=Retrieve&db=PubMed&list_uids=8628531&dopt=Abstract

- **The influence of socioeconomic factors on the occurrence of fetal alcohol syndrome.**
  Author(s): Bingol N, Schuster C, Fuchs M, Iosub S, Turner G, Stone RK, Gromisch DS.
  Source: Adv Alcohol Subst Abuse. 1987 Summer; 6(4): 105-18.
  http://www.ncbi.nlm.nih.gov:80/entrez/query.fcgi?cmd=Retrieve&db=PubMed&list_uids=3425475&dopt=Abstract

- **The interaction of ethanol and vitamin A as a potential mechanism for the pathogenesis of Fetal Alcohol syndrome.**
  Author(s): Zachman RD, Grummer MA.
  Source: Alcoholism, Clinical and Experimental Research. 1998 October; 22(7): 1544-56. Review.
  http://www.ncbi.nlm.nih.gov:80/entrez/query.fcgi?cmd=Retrieve&db=PubMed&list_uids=9802541&dopt=Abstract

- **The lasting impact of fetal alcohol syndrome and fetal alcohol effect on children and adolescents.**
  Author(s): Smitherman CH.
  Source: Journal of Pediatric Health Care : Official Publication of National Association of Pediatric Nurse Associates & Practitioners. 1994 May-June; 8(3): 121-6.
  http://www.ncbi.nlm.nih.gov:80/entrez/query.fcgi?cmd=Retrieve&db=PubMed&list_uids=7799176&dopt=Abstract

- **The metabolic basis of the fetal alcohol syndrome.**
  Author(s): Luke B.
  Source: Int J Fertil. 1990 November-December; 35(6): 333-7. Review. No Abstract Available.
  http://www.ncbi.nlm.nih.gov:80/entrez/query.fcgi?cmd=Retrieve&db=PubMed&list_uids=1981207&dopt=Abstract

- **The prevalence of fetal alcohol syndrome in New Zealand.**
  Author(s): Leversha AM, Marks RE.
  Source: N Z Med J. 1995 December 8; 108(1013): 502-5.
  http://www.ncbi.nlm.nih.gov:80/entrez/query.fcgi?cmd=Retrieve&db=PubMed&list_uids=8532234&dopt=Abstract

- **The role of alcohol dehydrogenase in retinoic acid homeostasis and fetal alcohol syndrome.**
  Author(s): Shean ML, Duester G.
  Source: Alcohol Alcohol Suppl. 1993; 2: 51-6.
  http://www.ncbi.nlm.nih.gov:80/entrez/query.fcgi?cmd=Retrieve&db=PubMed&list_uids=7748347&dopt=Abstract

- **The role of docosahexaenoic acid in brain development and fetal alcohol syndrome.**
  Author(s): Burdge GC.
  Source: Biochemical Society Transactions. 1998 May; 26(2): 246-52. Review.
  http://www.ncbi.nlm.nih.gov:80/entrez/query.fcgi?cmd=Retrieve&db=PubMed&list_
  uids=9649756&dopt=Abstract

- **The role of the genetic counselor in fetal alcohol syndrome prevention.**
  Author(s): Belsky R.
  Source: Birth Defects Orig Artic Ser. 1987; 23(6): 111-4. No Abstract Available.
  http://www.ncbi.nlm.nih.gov:80/entrez/query.fcgi?cmd=Retrieve&db=PubMed&list_
  uids=3435750&dopt=Abstract

- **Toluene embryopathy: delineation of the phenotype and comparison with fetal alcohol syndrome.**
  Author(s): Pearson MA, Hoyme HE, Seaver LH, Rimsza ME.
  Source: Pediatrics. 1994 February; 93(2): 211-5. Review.
  http://www.ncbi.nlm.nih.gov:80/entrez/query.fcgi?cmd=Retrieve&db=PubMed&list_
  uids=7510061&dopt=Abstract

- **Tuning our 'clinical antenna' to fetal alcohol syndrome.**
  Author(s): Marino RV.
  Source: J Am Osteopath Assoc. 1996 April; 96(4): 221-2. No Abstract Available.
  http://www.ncbi.nlm.nih.gov:80/entrez/query.fcgi?cmd=Retrieve&db=PubMed&list_
  uids=8935426&dopt=Abstract

- **Two-dimensional protein electrophoresis and multiple hypothesis testing to detect potential serum protein biomarkers in children with fetal alcohol syndrome.**
  Author(s): Robinson MK, Myrick JE, Henderson LO, Coles CD, Powell MK, Orr GA, Lemkin PF.
  Source: Electrophoresis. 1995 July; 16(7): 1176-83.
  http://www.ncbi.nlm.nih.gov:80/entrez/query.fcgi?cmd=Retrieve&db=PubMed&list_
  uids=7498162&dopt=Abstract

- **Unilateral retinoschisis in fetal alcohol syndrome.**
  Author(s): Desai UR, Raman VR, Dennehy P.
  Source: Retina (Philadelphia, Pa.). 2000; 20(6): 676-8.
  http://www.ncbi.nlm.nih.gov:80/entrez/query.fcgi?cmd=Retrieve&db=PubMed&list_
  uids=11131427&dopt=Abstract

- **Upper airway obstruction in infants with fetal alcohol syndrome.**
  Author(s): Usowicz AG, Golabi M, Curry C.
  Source: Am J Dis Child. 1986 October; 140(10): 1039-41.
  http://www.ncbi.nlm.nih.gov:80/entrez/query.fcgi?cmd=Retrieve&db=PubMed&list_
  uids=3752013&dopt=Abstract

- **Use of capture-recapture analyses in fetal alcohol syndrome surveillance in Alaska.**
  Author(s): Egeland GM, Perham-Hester KA, Hook EB.
  Source: American Journal of Epidemiology. 1995 February 15; 141(4): 335-41.
  http://www.ncbi.nlm.nih.gov:80/entrez/query.fcgi?cmd=Retrieve&db=PubMed&list_
  uids=7840111&dopt=Abstract

- **Vanished twin and fetal alcohol syndrome in the surviving twin. A case report.**
  Author(s): Mathelier AC, Karachorlu K.
  Source: J Reprod Med. 1999 April; 44(4): 394-8.
  http://www.ncbi.nlm.nih.gov:80/entrez/query.fcgi?cmd=Retrieve&db=PubMed&list_uids=10319316&dopt=Abstract

- **Variation in induction of human placental CYP2E1: possible role in susceptibility to fetal alcohol syndrome?**
  Author(s): Rasheed A, Hines RN, McCarver-May DG.
  Source: Toxicology and Applied Pharmacology. 1997 June; 144(2): 396-400.
  http://www.ncbi.nlm.nih.gov:80/entrez/query.fcgi?cmd=Retrieve&db=PubMed&list_uids=9194424&dopt=Abstract

- **Verbal learning and memory in children with fetal alcohol syndrome.**
  Author(s): Mattson SN, Riley EP, Delis DC, Stern C, Jones KL.
  Source: Alcoholism, Clinical and Experimental Research. 1996 August; 20(5): 810-6.
  http://www.ncbi.nlm.nih.gov:80/entrez/query.fcgi?cmd=Retrieve&db=PubMed&list_uids=8865953&dopt=Abstract

- **Was the fetal alcohol syndrome recognized by the Greeks and Romans?**
  Author(s): Abel EL.
  Source: Alcohol and Alcoholism (Oxford, Oxfordshire). 1999 November-December; 34(6): 868-72.
  http://www.ncbi.nlm.nih.gov:80/entrez/query.fcgi?cmd=Retrieve&db=PubMed&list_uids=10659722&dopt=Abstract

- **Was the fetal alcohol syndrome recognized in the ancient Near East?**
  Author(s): Abel EL.
  Source: Alcohol and Alcoholism (Oxford, Oxfordshire). 1997 January-February; 32(1): 3-7.
  http://www.ncbi.nlm.nih.gov:80/entrez/query.fcgi?cmd=Retrieve&db=PubMed&list_uids=9131889&dopt=Abstract

- **What do physicians know and say about fetal alcohol syndrome: a survey of obstetricians, pediatricians, and family medicine physicians.**
  Author(s): Abel EL, Kruger M.
  Source: Alcoholism, Clinical and Experimental Research. 1998 December; 22(9): 1951-4.
  http://www.ncbi.nlm.nih.gov:80/entrez/query.fcgi?cmd=Retrieve&db=PubMed&list_uids=9884137&dopt=Abstract

- **What syndrome is this? Fetal alcohol syndrome.**
  Author(s): Bertucci V, Krafchik BR.
  Source: Pediatric Dermatology. 1994 June; 11(2): 178-80.
  http://www.ncbi.nlm.nih.gov:80/entrez/query.fcgi?cmd=Retrieve&db=PubMed&list_uids=8041663&dopt=Abstract

- **Withdrawal symptoms in infants with the fetal alcohol syndrome.**
  Author(s): Pierog S, Chandavasu O, Wexler I.
  Source: The Journal of Pediatrics. 1977 April; 90(4): 630-3.
  http://www.ncbi.nlm.nih.gov:80/entrez/query.fcgi?cmd=Retrieve&db=PubMed&list_uids=839382&dopt=Abstract

- **Zinc deficiency and the fetal alcohol syndrome.**
  Author(s): Dreosti IE.
  Source: The Medical Journal of Australia. 1981 July 11; 2(1): 3-4.
  http://www.ncbi.nlm.nih.gov:80/entrez/query.fcgi?cmd=Retrieve&db=PubMed&list_uids=7278770&dopt=Abstract

Chapter 2. Nutrition and Fetal Alcohol Syndrome

Overview

In this chapter, we will show you how to find studies dedicated specifically to nutrition and fetal alcohol syndrome.

Finding Nutrition Studies on Fetal Alcohol Syndrome

The National Institutes of Health's Office of Dietary Supplements (ODS) offers a searchable bibliographic database called the IBIDS (International Bibliographic Information on Dietary Supplements; National Institutes of Health, Building 31, Room 1B29, 31 Center Drive, MSC 2086, Bethesda, Maryland 20892-2086, Tel: 301-435-2920, Fax: 301-480-1845, E-mail: ods@nih.gov). The IBIDS contains over 460,000 scientific citations and summaries about dietary supplements and nutrition as well as references to published international, scientific literature on dietary supplements such as vitamins, minerals, and botanicals.[4] The IBIDS includes references and citations to both human and animal research studies.

As a service of the ODS, access to the IBIDS database is available free of charge at the following Web address: **http://ods.od.nih.gov/databases/ibids.html**. After entering the search area, you have three choices: (1) IBIDS Consumer Database, (2) Full IBIDS Database, or (3) Peer Reviewed Citations Only.

Now that you have selected a database, click on the "Advanced" tab. An advanced search allows you to retrieve up to 100 fully explained references in a comprehensive format. Type "fetal alcohol syndrome" (or synonyms) into the search box, and click "Go." To narrow the search, you can also select the "Title" field.

---

[4] Adapted from **http://ods.od.nih.gov**. IBIDS is produced by the Office of Dietary Supplements (ODS) at the National Institutes of Health to assist the public, healthcare providers, educators, and researchers in locating credible, scientific information on dietary supplements. IBIDS was developed and will be maintained through an interagency partnership with the Food and Nutrition Information Center of the National Agricultural Library, U.S. Department of Agriculture.

The following information is typical of that found when using the "Full IBIDS Database" to search for "fetal alcohol syndrome" (or a synonym):

- **Altered mineral metabolism as a mechanism underlying the expression of fetal alcohol syndrome in rats.**
  Source: Zidenberg Cherr, S. Rosenbaum, J. Keen, C.L. Trace elements in man and animals 6 / edited by Lucille S. Hurley,. [et al.]. New York : Plenum Press, c1988. page 613-614. ISBN: 0306430045

- **Blackcurrant seed oil, zinc, and fetal alcohol syndrome.**
  Author(s): Institute of Nutrition, University of L'Aquila.
  Source: Seri, S D'Alessandro, A Boll-Soc-Ital-Biol-Sper. 1997 Jan-February; 73(1-2): 15-21 0037-8771

- **Contribution to first-pass metabolism of ethanol and inhibition by ethanol for retinol oxidation in human alcohol dehydrogenase family–implications for etiology of fetal alcohol syndrome and alcohol-related diseases.**
  Author(s): Graduate Institute of Life Sciences, National Defense Medical Center, Taipei, Taiwan, Republic of China.
  Source: Han, C L Liao, C S Wu, C W Hwong, C L Lee, A R Yin, S J Eur-J-Biochem. 1998 May 15; 254(1): 25-31 0014-2956

- **Developmental neurotoxicity: do similar phenotypes indicate a common mode of action? A comparison of fetal alcohol syndrome, toluene embryopathy and maternal phenylketonuria.**
  Author(s): Toxicology Program, University of Washington, 4225 Roosevelt Way NE, #100, Seattle 98105-6099, USA. lgosta@u.washington.edu
  Source: Costa, L G Guizzetti, M Burry, M Oberdoerster, J Toxicol-Lett. 2002 February 28; 127(1-3): 197-205 0378-4274

- **Fetal alcohol syndrome: a role for zinc? Implications for intervention.**
  Source: Ouellette, M D J-Pediatr-Perinat-Nutr. 1987 Spring-Summer; 1(1): 1-12 8756-6206

- **Flow cytometric and histological analysis of mouse thymus in fetal alcohol syndrome.**
  Author(s): Department of Microbiology, Montana State University, Bozeman 59717.
  Source: Ewald, S J Walden, S M J-Leukoc-Biol. 1988 November; 44(5): 434-40 0741-5400

- **In utero ethanol suppresses cerebellar activator protein-1 and nuclear factor-kappa B transcriptional activation in a rat fetal alcohol syndrome model.**
  Author(s): Division of Pharmacology and Toxicology, College of Pharmacy, and the Waggoner Center for Alcohol and Addiction Research, The University of Texas at Austin, Austin, Texas, USA. George.Acquaah-Mensah@uchsc.edu
  Source: Acquaah Mensah, George K Kehrer, James P Leslie, Steven W J-Pharmacol-Exp-Ther. 2002 April; 301(1): 277-83 0022-3565

- **Liver development in a rat model of fetal alcohol syndrome.**
  Author(s): Department of Medicine & Pharmacology, University of Manitoba, Winnipeg, Canada.
  Source: Meyers, A F A Gong, Y Zhang, M Casiro, O G Battistuzzi, S Pettigrew, N Minuk, G Y Dig-Dis-Sci. 2002 April; 47(4): 767-72 0163-2116

- **Optic nerve hypoplasia in fetal alcohol syndrome: an update.**
  Author(s): Institute of Cytological Research and Investigation Center, University Hospital La Fe, Valencia, Spain.
  Source: Pinazo Duran, M D Renau Piqueras, J Guerri, C Stromland, K Eur-J-Ophthalmol. 1997 Jul-September; 7(3): 262-70 1120-6721

- **The Alcoholic Beverages Labeling Act of 1988. A preemptive shield against fetal alcohol syndrome claims?**
  Source: Wagner, E N J-Leg-Med. 1991 June; 12(2): 167-200 0194-7648

- **The interaction of ethanol and vitamin A as a potential mechanism for the pathogenesis of Fetal Alcohol syndrome.**
  Author(s): Department of Pediatrics and Nutritional Science, University of Wisconsin, Madison 53715, USA.
  Source: Zachman, R D Grummer, M A Alcohol-Clin-Exp-Res. 1998 October; 22(7): 1544-56 0145-6008

- **The role of alcohol dehydrogenase in retinoic acid homeostasis and fetal alcohol syndrome.**
  Author(s): Department of Biochemistry, Colorado State University, Fort Collins 80523, USA.
  Source: Shean, M L Duester, G Alcohol-Alcohol-Suppl. 1993; 251-6 1358-6173

- **The role of docosahexaenoic acid in brain development and fetal alcohol syndrome.**
  Author(s): University of Southampton, Southampton General Hospital, U.K.
  Source: Burdge, G C Biochem-Soc-Trans. 1998 May; 26(2): 246-52 0300-5127

- **Vitamin E and beta-carotene protect against ethanol combined with ischemia in an embryonic rat hippocampal culture model of fetal alcohol syndrome.**
  Author(s): University of Florida Brain Institute, Center for Alcohol Research, Department of Neuroscience, University of Florida College of Medicine, Gainesville 32610-0244, USA. mitchell@ufbi.ufl.edu
  Source: Mitchell, J J Paiva, M Heaton, M B Neurosci-Lett. 1999 March 26; 263(2-3): 189-92 0304-3940

- **Zinc and fetal alcohol syndrome: another dimension.**
  Source: Beaton, G.H. Nutr-Rev. Washington, D.C. : Nutrition Foundation. November 1986. volume 44 (11) page 359-360. 0029-6643

- **Zinc nutrition in fetal alcohol syndrome.**
  Author(s): Department of Pediatrics, University of Arkansas for Medical Sciences, Little Rock 72205.
  Source: Keppen, L D Moore, D J Cannon, D J Neurotoxicology. 1990 Summer; 11(2): 375-80 0161-813X

Federal Resources on Nutrition

In addition to the IBIDS, the United States Department of Health and Human Services (HHS) and the United States Department of Agriculture (USDA) provide many sources of information on general nutrition and health. Recommended resources include:

- healthfinder®, HHS's gateway to health information, including diet and nutrition: **http://www.healthfinder.gov/scripts/SearchContext.asp?topic=238&page=0**

- The United States Department of Agriculture's Web site dedicated to nutrition information: **www.nutrition.gov**

- The Food and Drug Administration's Web site for federal food safety information: **www.foodsafety.gov**

- The National Action Plan on Overweight and Obesity sponsored by the United States Surgeon General: **http://www.surgeongeneral.gov/topics/obesity/**

- The Center for Food Safety and Applied Nutrition has an Internet site sponsored by the Food and Drug Administration and the Department of Health and Human Services: **http://vm.cfsan.fda.gov/**

- Center for Nutrition Policy and Promotion sponsored by the United States Department of Agriculture: **http://www.usda.gov/cnpp/**

- Food and Nutrition Information Center, National Agricultural Library sponsored by the United States Department of Agriculture: **http://www.nal.usda.gov/fnic/**

- Food and Nutrition Service sponsored by the United States Department of Agriculture: **http://www.fns.usda.gov/fns/**

Additional Web Resources

A number of additional Web sites offer encyclopedic information covering food and nutrition. The following is a representative sample:

- AOL: **http://search.aol.com/cat.adp?id=174&layer=&from=subcats**

- Family Village: **http://www.familyvillage.wisc.edu/med_nutrition.html**

- Google: **http://directory.google.com/Top/Health/Nutrition/**

- Healthnotes: **http://www.healthnotes.com/**

- Open Directory Project: **http://dmoz.org/Health/Nutrition/**

- Yahoo.com: **http://dir.yahoo.com/Health/Nutrition/**

- WebMD®Health: **http://my.webmd.com/nutrition**

- WholeHealthMD.com: **http://www.wholehealthmd.com/reflib/0,1529,00.html**

CHAPTER 3. ALTERNATIVE MEDICINE AND FETAL ALCOHOL SYNDROME

Overview

In this chapter, we will begin by introducing you to official information sources on complementary and alternative medicine (CAM) relating to fetal alcohol syndrome. At the conclusion of this chapter, we will provide additional sources.

National Center for Complementary and Alternative Medicine

The National Center for Complementary and Alternative Medicine (NCCAM) of the National Institutes of Health (**http://nccam.nih.gov/**) has created a link to the National Library of Medicine's databases to facilitate research for articles that specifically relate to fetal alcohol syndrome and complementary medicine. To search the database, go to the following Web site: **http://www.nlm.nih.gov/nccam/camonpubmed.html**. Select "CAM on PubMed." Enter "fetal alcohol syndrome" (or synonyms) into the search box. Click "Go." The following references provide information on particular aspects of complementary and alternative medicine that are related to fetal alcohol syndrome:

- **Alcohol, deafness, epilepsy, and autism.**
  Author(s): Gordon AG.
  Source: Alcoholism, Clinical and Experimental Research. 1993 August; 17(4): 926-8.
  http://www.ncbi.nlm.nih.gov:80/entrez/query.fcgi?cmd=Retrieve&db=PubMed&list_uids=8214437&dopt=Abstract

- **Auditory and visual sustained attention in adolescents prenatally exposed to alcohol.**
  Author(s): Coles CD, Platzman KA, Lynch ME, Freides D.
  Source: Alcoholism, Clinical and Experimental Research. 2002 February; 26(2): 263-71.
  http://www.ncbi.nlm.nih.gov:80/entrez/query.fcgi?cmd=Retrieve&db=PubMed&list_uids=11964567&dopt=Abstract

- **Development of glial cells cultured from prenatally alcohol treated rat brain: effect of supplementation of the maternal alcohol diet with a grape extract.**
  Author(s): Ledig M, Holownia A, Copin JC, Tholey G, Anokhina I.

Source: Neurochemical Research. 1996 March; 21(3): 313-7.
http://www.ncbi.nlm.nih.gov:80/entrez/query.fcgi?cmd=Retrieve&db=PubMed&list_uids=9139236&dopt=Abstract

- **Dietary fatty acids and alcohol: effects on cellular membranes.**
  Author(s): Wainwright PE.
  Source: Alcohol and Alcoholism (Oxford, Oxfordshire). 1993 September; 28(5): 607-8.
  http://www.ncbi.nlm.nih.gov:80/entrez/query.fcgi?cmd=Retrieve&db=PubMed&list_uids=8274186&dopt=Abstract

- **Effect of maternal ethanol consumption during pregnancy on the phospholipid molecular species composition of fetal guinea-pig brain, liver and plasma.**
  Author(s): Burdge GC, Postle AD.
  Source: Biochimica Et Biophysica Acta. 1995 June 6; 1256(3): 346-52. Erratum In: Biochim Biophys Acta 1995 November 16; 1259(2): 197.
  http://www.ncbi.nlm.nih.gov:80/entrez/query.fcgi?cmd=Retrieve&db=PubMed&list_uids=7786898&dopt=Abstract

- **Effects of an oil enriched in gamma linolenic acid on locomotor activity and behaviour in the Morris Maze, following in utero ethanol exposure in rats.**
  Author(s): Duffy O, Menez JF, Leonard BE.
  Source: Drug and Alcohol Dependence. 1992 April; 30(1): 65-70.
  http://www.ncbi.nlm.nih.gov:80/entrez/query.fcgi?cmd=Retrieve&db=PubMed&list_uids=1317288&dopt=Abstract

- **Effects of prenatal ethanol and long-chain n-3 fatty acid supplementation on development in mice. 1. Body and brain growth, sensorimotor development, and water T-maze reversal learning.**
  Author(s): Wainwright PE, Ward GR, Winfield D, Huang YS, Mills DE, Ward RP, McCutcheon D.
  Source: Alcoholism, Clinical and Experimental Research. 1990 June; 14(3): 405-12.
  http://www.ncbi.nlm.nih.gov:80/entrez/query.fcgi?cmd=Retrieve&db=PubMed&list_uids=2378425&dopt=Abstract

- **Effects of prenatal ethanol and long-chain n-3 fatty acid supplementation on development in mice. 2. Fatty acid composition of brain membrane phospholipids.**
  Author(s): Wainwright PE, Huang YS, Simmons V, Mills DE, Ward RP, Ward GR, Winfield D, McCutcheon D.
  Source: Alcoholism, Clinical and Experimental Research. 1990 June; 14(3): 413-20.
  http://www.ncbi.nlm.nih.gov:80/entrez/query.fcgi?cmd=Retrieve&db=PubMed&list_uids=2143055&dopt=Abstract

- **Effects of prenatal stress and ethanol on cerebellar fiber tract maturation in B6D2F2 mice: an image analysis study.**
  Author(s): Ward GR, Wainwright PE.
  Source: Neurotoxicology. 1991 Winter; 12(4): 665-76.
  http://www.ncbi.nlm.nih.gov:80/entrez/query.fcgi?cmd=Retrieve&db=PubMed&list_uids=1795894&dopt=Abstract

- **Ethanol inhibits astroglial cell proliferation by disruption of phospholipase D-mediated signaling.**
  Author(s): Kotter K, Klein J.
  Source: Journal of Neurochemistry. 1999 December; 73(6): 2517-23.
  http://www.ncbi.nlm.nih.gov:80/entrez/query.fcgi?cmd=Retrieve&db=PubMed&list_uids=10582613&dopt=Abstract

- **Families caring for children with fetal alcohol syndrome: the nurse's role in early identification and intervention.**
  Author(s): Hess DJ, Kenner C.
  Source: Holistic Nursing Practice. 1998 April; 12(3): 47-54. Review.
  http://www.ncbi.nlm.nih.gov:80/entrez/query.fcgi?cmd=Retrieve&db=PubMed&list_uids=9624957&dopt=Abstract

- **Fear conditioning-induced alterations of phospholipase C-beta1a protein level and enzyme activity in rat hippocampal formation and medial frontal cortex.**
  Author(s): Weeber EJ, Savage DD, Sutherland RJ, Caldwell KK.
  Source: Neurobiology of Learning and Memory. 2001 September; 76(2): 151-82.
  http://www.ncbi.nlm.nih.gov:80/entrez/query.fcgi?cmd=Retrieve&db=PubMed&list_uids=11502147&dopt=Abstract

- **Fetal alcohol syndrome: failure of zinc supplementation to reverse the effect of ethanol on placental transport of zinc.**
  Author(s): Ghishan FK, Greene HL.
  Source: Pediatric Research. 1983 July; 17(7): 529-31.
  http://www.ncbi.nlm.nih.gov:80/entrez/query.fcgi?cmd=Retrieve&db=PubMed&list_uids=6622095&dopt=Abstract

- **Fetoprotectivity of the flavanolignan compound siliphos against ethanol-induced toxicity.**
  Author(s): Edwards J, Grange LL, Wang M, Reyes E.
  Source: Phytotherapy Research : Ptr. 2000 November; 14(7): 517-21.
  http://www.ncbi.nlm.nih.gov:80/entrez/query.fcgi?cmd=Retrieve&db=PubMed&list_uids=11054841&dopt=Abstract

- **Health benefits of docosahexaenoic acid (DHA)**
  Author(s): Horrocks LA, Yeo YK.
  Source: Pharmacological Research : the Official Journal of the Italian Pharmacological Society. 1999 September; 40(3): 211-25. Review.
  http://www.ncbi.nlm.nih.gov:80/entrez/query.fcgi?cmd=Retrieve&db=PubMed&list_uids=10479465&dopt=Abstract

- **Hearing, speech, language, and vestibular disorders in the fetal alcohol syndrome: a literature review.**
  Author(s): Church MW, Kaltenbach JA.
  Source: Alcoholism, Clinical and Experimental Research. 1997 May; 21(3): 495-512. Review.
  http://www.ncbi.nlm.nih.gov:80/entrez/query.fcgi?cmd=Retrieve&db=PubMed&list_uids=9161611&dopt=Abstract

- **In utero alcohol heightens juvenile reactivity.**
  Author(s): Anandam N, Felegi W, Stern JM.
  Source: Pharmacology, Biochemistry, and Behavior. 1980 October; 13(4): 531-5.
  http://www.ncbi.nlm.nih.gov:80/entrez/query.fcgi?cmd=Retrieve&db=PubMed&list_uids=7433484&dopt=Abstract

- **Independent dysmorphology evaluations at birth and 4 years of age for children exposed to varying amounts of alcohol in utero.**
  Author(s): Graham JM Jr, Hanson JW, Darby BL, Barr HM, Streissguth AP.
  Source: Pediatrics. 1988 June; 81(6): 772-8.
  http://www.ncbi.nlm.nih.gov:80/entrez/query.fcgi?cmd=Retrieve&db=PubMed&list_uids=3368276&dopt=Abstract

- **Is 'herbal health tonic' safe in pregnancy; fetal alcohol syndrome revisited.**
  Author(s): Pradeepkumar VK, Tan KW, Ivy NG.
  Source: The Australian & New Zealand Journal of Obstetrics & Gynaecology. 1996 November; 36(4): 420-3.
  http://www.ncbi.nlm.nih.gov:80/entrez/query.fcgi?cmd=Retrieve&db=PubMed&list_uids=9006825&dopt=Abstract

- **Long-term effects of developmental exposure to alcohol.**
  Author(s): West JR.
  Source: Neurotoxicology. 1986 Summer; 7(2): 245-56.
  http://www.ncbi.nlm.nih.gov:80/entrez/query.fcgi?cmd=Retrieve&db=PubMed&list_uids=3785751&dopt=Abstract

- **Multidisciplinary approaches in behavioral technology.**
  Author(s): Riley EP.
  Source: Developmental Psychobiology. 1996 July; 29(5): 400-1.
  http://www.ncbi.nlm.nih.gov:80/entrez/query.fcgi?cmd=Retrieve&db=PubMed&list_uids=8809491&dopt=Abstract

- **Mutual support groups to reduce alcohol consumption by pregnant women: marketing implications.**
  Author(s): Coleman MA, Coleman NC, Murray JP.
  Source: Health Marketing Quarterly. 1990; 7(3-4): 47-63.
  http://www.ncbi.nlm.nih.gov:80/entrez/query.fcgi?cmd=Retrieve&db=PubMed&list_uids=10105907&dopt=Abstract

- **Neuropsychiatric implications and long-term consequences of fetal alcohol spectrum disorders.**
  Author(s): Streissguth AP, O'Malley K.
  Source: Semin Clin Neuropsychiatry. 2000 July; 5(3): 177-90. Review.
  http://www.ncbi.nlm.nih.gov:80/entrez/query.fcgi?cmd=Retrieve&db=PubMed&list_uids=11291013&dopt=Abstract

- **Of mice and women, and alcohol: a fractal history of fetal alcohol syndrome research.**
  Author(s): Hannigan JH.

Source: Developmental Psychobiology. 1996 July; 29(5): 398-400.
http://www.ncbi.nlm.nih.gov:80/entrez/query.fcgi?cmd=Retrieve&db=PubMed&list_
uids=8809490&dopt=Abstract

- **Prenatal ethanol exposure alters ventricular myocyte contractile function in the offspring of rats: influence of maternal Mg2+ supplementation.**
  Author(s): Wold LE, Norby FL, Hintz KK, Colligan PB, Epstein PN, Ren J.
  Source: Cardiovascular Toxicology. 2001; 1(3): 215-24.
  http://www.ncbi.nlm.nih.gov:80/entrez/query.fcgi?cmd=Retrieve&db=PubMed&list_
  uids=12213974&dopt=Abstract

- **Prevention by a silymarin/phospholipid compound of ethanol-induced social learning deficits in rats.**
  Author(s): Reid C, Edwards J, Wang M, Manybeads Y, Mike L, Martinez N, La Grange L, Reyes E.
  Source: Planta Medica. 1999 June; 65(5): 421-4.
  http://www.ncbi.nlm.nih.gov:80/entrez/query.fcgi?cmd=Retrieve&db=PubMed&list_
  uids=10418328&dopt=Abstract

- **Protective effect of Liv.52 on alcohol-induced fetotoxicity.**
  Author(s): Gopumadhavan S, Jagadeesh S, Chauhan BL, Kulkarni RD.
  Source: Alcoholism, Clinical and Experimental Research. 1993 October; 17(5): 1089-92.
  http://www.ncbi.nlm.nih.gov:80/entrez/query.fcgi?cmd=Retrieve&db=PubMed&list_
  uids=8279671&dopt=Abstract

- **Protective effects of the flavonoid mixture, silymarin, on fetal rat brain and liver.**
  Author(s): La Grange L, Wang M, Watkins R, Ortiz D, Sanchez ME, Konst J, Lee C, Reyes E.
  Source: Journal of Ethnopharmacology. 1999 April; 65(1): 53-61.
  http://www.ncbi.nlm.nih.gov:80/entrez/query.fcgi?cmd=Retrieve&db=PubMed&list_
  uids=10350368&dopt=Abstract

- **Substance abuse: infant and childhood outcomes.**
  Author(s): D'Apolito K.
  Source: Journal of Pediatric Nursing. 1998 October; 13(5): 307-16. Review.
  http://www.ncbi.nlm.nih.gov:80/entrez/query.fcgi?cmd=Retrieve&db=PubMed&list_
  uids=9798367&dopt=Abstract

- **The fetus and alcohol.**
  Author(s): Davis VE.
  Source: The Medical Journal of Australia. 1980 May 31; 1(11): 558.
  http://www.ncbi.nlm.nih.gov:80/entrez/query.fcgi?cmd=Retrieve&db=PubMed&list_
  uids=7393048&dopt=Abstract

- **The incidence of renal anomalies at full term in fetal rats is synergistically increased by estradiol (but not testosterone) supplementation on day 18 of alcoholic gestation.**
  Author(s): Calvano CJ, LeFevre R, Mankes RF, Reddy PP, Moran ME, Hoar RM, Mandell J.

Source: Journal of Pediatric Surgery. 1997 September; 32(9): 1302-6.
http://www.ncbi.nlm.nih.gov:80/entrez/query.fcgi?cmd=Retrieve&db=PubMed&list_uids=9314248&dopt=Abstract

- **The role of docosahexaenoic acid in brain development and fetal alcohol syndrome.**
  Author(s): Burdge GC.
  Source: Biochemical Society Transactions. 1998 May; 26(2): 246-52. Review.
  http://www.ncbi.nlm.nih.gov:80/entrez/query.fcgi?cmd=Retrieve&db=PubMed&list_uids=9649756&dopt=Abstract

- **The role of the expanded function nurse in fertility preservation.**
  Author(s): Keating CE.
  Source: Naacogs Clin Issu Perinat Womens Health Nurs. 1992; 3(2): 293-300.
  http://www.ncbi.nlm.nih.gov:80/entrez/query.fcgi?cmd=Retrieve&db=PubMed&list_uids=1596437&dopt=Abstract

- **Three-year outcome of children exposed prenatally to drugs.**
  Author(s): Griffith DR, Azuma SD, Chasnoff IJ.
  Source: Journal of the American Academy of Child and Adolescent Psychiatry. 1994 January; 33(1): 20-7.
  http://www.ncbi.nlm.nih.gov:80/entrez/query.fcgi?cmd=Retrieve&db=PubMed&list_uids=7511139&dopt=Abstract

- **Was the fetal alcohol syndrome recognized in the ancient Near East?**
  Author(s): Abel EL.
  Source: Alcohol and Alcoholism (Oxford, Oxfordshire). 1997 January-February; 32(1): 3-7.
  http://www.ncbi.nlm.nih.gov:80/entrez/query.fcgi?cmd=Retrieve&db=PubMed&list_uids=9131889&dopt=Abstract

- **Zinc supplementation does not attenuate alcohol-induced cerebellar Purkinje cell loss during the brain growth spurt period.**
  Author(s): Chen WJ, Berryhill EC, West JR.
  Source: Alcoholism, Clinical and Experimental Research. 2001 April; 25(4): 600-5.
  http://www.ncbi.nlm.nih.gov:80/entrez/query.fcgi?cmd=Retrieve&db=PubMed&list_uids=11329502&dopt=Abstract

- **Zinc supplementation in ethanol-treated pregnant rats increases the metabolic activity in the fetal hippocampus.**
  Author(s): Tanaka H, Inomata K, Arima M.
  Source: Brain & Development. 1983; 5(6): 549-54.
  http://www.ncbi.nlm.nih.gov:80/entrez/query.fcgi?cmd=Retrieve&db=PubMed&list_uids=6199999&dopt=Abstract

Additional Web Resources

A number of additional Web sites offer encyclopedic information covering CAM and related topics. The following is a representative sample:

- Alternative Medicine Foundation, Inc.: **http://www.herbmed.org/**

- AOL: **http://search.aol.com/cat.adp?id=169&layer=&from=subcats**

- Chinese Medicine: **http://www.newcenturynutrition.com/**

- drkoop.com®: **http://www.drkoop.com/InteractiveMedicine/IndexC.html**

- Family Village: **http://www.familyvillage.wisc.edu/med_altn.htm**

- Google: **http://directory.google.com/Top/Health/Alternative/**

- Healthnotes: **http://www.healthnotes.com/**

- MedWebPlus:
  http://medwebplus.com/subject/Alternative_and_Complementary_Medicine

- Open Directory Project: **http://dmoz.org/Health/Alternative/**

- HealthGate: **http://www.tnp.com/**

- WebMD®Health: **http://my.webmd.com/drugs_and_herbs**

- WholeHealthMD.com: **http://www.wholehealthmd.com/reflib/0,1529,00.html**

- Yahoo.com: **http://dir.yahoo.com/Health/Alternative_Medicine/**

The following is a specific Web list relating to fetal alcohol syndrome; please note that any particular subject below may indicate either a therapeutic use, or a contraindication (potential danger), and does not reflect an official recommendation:

- **General Overview**

  Birth Defects Prevention
  Source: Healthnotes, Inc.; www.healthnotes.com

General References

A good place to find general background information on CAM is the National Library of Medicine. It has prepared within the MEDLINEplus system an information topic page dedicated to complementary and alternative medicine. To access this page, go to the MEDLINEplus site at **http://www.nlm.nih.gov/medlineplus/alternativemedicine.html** This Web site provides a general overview of various topics and can lead to a number of general sources.

CHAPTER 4. DISSERTATIONS ON FETAL ALCOHOL SYNDROME

Overview

In this chapter, we will give you a bibliography on recent dissertations relating to fetal alcohol syndrome. We will also provide you with information on how to use the Internet to stay current on dissertations. **IMPORTANT NOTE:** When following the search strategy described below, you may discover <u>non-medical dissertations</u> that use the generic term "fetal alcohol syndrome" (or a synonym) in their titles. To accurately reflect the results that you might find while conducting research on fetal alcohol syndrome, <u>we have not necessarily excluded non-medical dissertations</u> in this bibliography.

Dissertations on Fetal Alcohol Syndrome

ProQuest Digital Dissertations, the largest archive of academic dissertations available, is located at the following Web address: **http://wwwlib.umi.com/dissertations**. From this archive, we have compiled the following list covering dissertations devoted to fetal alcohol syndrome. You will see that the information provided includes the dissertation's title, its author, and the institution with which the author is associated. The following covers recent dissertations found when using this search procedure:

- **A Comparative Analysis of Language Competency in Native American Children with Fetal Alcohol Syndrome and Their Culturally Matched Peers** by Engelhart, Ellen Mardel Janis, EDD from University of South Dakota, 1992, 133 pages
  http://wwwlib.umi.com/dissertations/fullcit/9238483

- **Alcohol-related Birth Defects (ARBD): Perspectives of Early-childhood Educators in South Dakota (Fetal Alcohol Syndrome)** by Boettcher, Lynn Marie, EDD from University of South Dakota, 1995, 156 pages
  http://wwwlib.umi.com/dissertations/fullcit/9542564

- **Fetal Alcohol Syndrome and Fetal Alcohol Effects: Implications for Educators** by Herbst, Karen Croffoot, EDD from University of La Verne, 1995, 242 pages
  http://wwwlib.umi.com/dissertations/fullcit/9606386

- **Fetal Alcohol Syndrome/fetal Alcohol Effects: a Survey of Alaskan Educators** by Binns, Wayne R.; PhD from The University of Utah, 2000, 217 pages
  http://wwwlib.umi.com/dissertations/fullcit/9977467

- **Fetal Alcohol Syndrome: Designing and Implementing a Training Program for Teaching Nursing Students and Other Healthcare Professionals to Understand the Impact of Alcohol Use during Pregnancy on Fetal Development** by Davis, Melvin, PhD from The Union Institute, 1993, 80 pages
  http://wwwlib.umi.com/dissertations/fullcit/9410244

- **Fetal Alcohol Syndrome: How Diagnosis Affects Families and Services** by Hess, Deborah Jean, PhD from University of Cincinnati, 1996, 192 pages
  http://wwwlib.umi.com/dissertations/fullcit/9713451

- **Issues of Communication and Miscommunication among Parents, Physicians, and Teachers about Fetal Alcohol Syndrome/fetal Alcohol Effects** by Kapp, Frances M. E.; PhD from Gonzaga University, 2000, 272 pages
  http://wwwlib.umi.com/dissertations/fullcit/9978100

- **Linguistic Abilities of Children with Fetal Alcohol Syndrome** by Hamilton, Marilyn Ann, PhD from University of Washington, 1981, 83 pages
  http://wwwlib.umi.com/dissertations/fullcit/8212547

- **Navajo Children and Families Living with Fetal Alcohol Syndrome/Fetal Alcohol Effects** by Beckett, Cynthia Diane; PhD from The University of Arizona, 2002, 289 pages
  http://wwwlib.umi.com/dissertations/fullcit/3073191

- **Postnatal Development of the Rat Cerebellar Cortex in Fetal Alcohol Syndrome a Light, Electron Microscopic and Morphometric Study** by Mohamed, Sana A; PhD from The University of Manitoba (canada), 1986
  http://wwwlib.umi.com/dissertations/fullcit/NL33842

- **Raising a Child with Fetal Alcohol Syndrome: Effects on Family Functioning** by Wilton, Georgiana; PhD from The University of Wisconsin - Madison, 2002, 124 pages
  http://wwwlib.umi.com/dissertations/fullcit/3072762

- **Reading and Fetal Alcohol Syndrome in a Male Child: A Case Study** by Porter-Larsen, Jodi Elnora; Edd from University of South Dakota, 2000, 123 pages
  http://wwwlib.umi.com/dissertations/fullcit/9991660

- **Revolving Door: Young Offender Activity and Adolescents with Fetal Alcohol Syndrome/Fetal Alcohol Effect** by Tanchak, Sherri Lynn; MSW from University of Calgary (Canada), 2002, 216 pages
  http://wwwlib.umi.com/dissertations/fullcit/MQ76300

- **The Educational Status of Fetal Alcohol Syndrome** by Wentz, Thomas Lee, PhD from The University of North Dakota, 1995, 138 pages
  http://wwwlib.umi.com/dissertations/fullcit/9605484

- **The Effect of Information and Influence on Health Beliefs Regarding the Fetal Alcohol Syndrome of Pregnant Women Receiving Prenatal Care in a Medical Care Center** by Vaughn, Janice Singleton, PhD from University of Pittsburgh, 1979, 207 pages
  http://wwwlib.umi.com/dissertations/fullcit/8004841

- **The Face and Form in Fetal Alcohol Syndrome: Use of Anthropometry to Assess Growth and Objectify the Diagnosis** by McGhehey Moore, Elizabeth Sue, PhD from Indiana University, 1998, 231 pages
  http://wwwlib.umi.com/dissertations/fullcit/9919475

- **The Fetal Alcohol Syndrome in Mice: an Animal Model** by Chernoff, Gerald F; PhD from The University of British Columbia (Canada), 1978
  http://wwwlib.umi.com/dissertations/fullcit/NK37587

Keeping Current

Ask the medical librarian at your library if it has full and unlimited access to the *ProQuest Digital Dissertations* database. From the library, you should be able to do more complete searches via **http://wwwlib.umi.com/dissertations**.

CHAPTER 5. PATENTS ON FETAL ALCOHOL SYNDROME

Overview

Patents can be physical innovations (e.g. chemicals, pharmaceuticals, medical equipment) or processes (e.g. treatments or diagnostic procedures). The United States Patent and Trademark Office defines a patent as a grant of a property right to the inventor, issued by the Patent and Trademark Office.[5] Patents, therefore, are intellectual property. For the United States, the term of a new patent is 20 years from the date when the patent application was filed. If the inventor wishes to receive economic benefits, it is likely that the invention will become commercially available within 20 years of the initial filing. It is important to understand, therefore, that an inventor's patent does not indicate that a product or service is or will be commercially available. The patent implies only that the inventor has "the right to exclude others from making, using, offering for sale, or selling" the invention in the United States. While this relates to U.S. patents, similar rules govern foreign patents.

In this chapter, we show you how to locate information on patents and their inventors. If you find a patent that is particularly interesting to you, contact the inventor or the assignee for further information. **IMPORTANT NOTE:** When following the search strategy described below, you may discover <u>non-medical patents</u> that use the generic term "fetal alcohol syndrome" (or a synonym) in their titles. To accurately reflect the results that you might find while conducting research on fetal alcohol syndrome, <u>we have not necessarily excluded non-medical patents</u> in this bibliography.

Patent Applications on Fetal Alcohol Syndrome

As of December 2000, U.S. patent applications are open to public viewing.[6] Applications are patent requests which have yet to be granted. (The process to achieve a patent can take several years.) The following patent applications have been filed since December 2000 relating to fetal alcohol syndrome:

---

[5] Adapted from the United States Patent and Trademark Office:
http://www.uspto.gov/web/offices/pac/doc/general/whatis.htm.

[6] This has been a common practice outside the United States prior to December 2000.

- **PREVENTION OF FETAL ALCOHOL SYNDROME AND NEURONAL CELL DEATH WITH ADNF POLYPEPTIDES**

Inventor(s): BASSAN, MERAV; (RAMAT HASHARON, IL), BRENNEMAN, DOUGLAS E.; (DAMASCUS, MD), GOZES, ILLANA; (RAMAT HASHARON, IL), SPONG, CATHERINE Y.; (ARLINGTON, VA), ZAMOSTIANO, RACHEL; (HOD HASHARON, IL)

Correspondence: Townsend And Townsend And Crew, Llp; Two Embarcadero Center; Eighth Floor; San Francisco; CA; 94111-3834; US

Patent Application Number: 20020111301

Date filed: March 12, 1999

Abstract: This invention relates to a method for reducing a condition associated with **fetal alcohol syndrome** in a subject who is exposed to alcohol in utero with an ADNF polypeptide. In particular, the present invention relates to a method of reducing a condition associated with **fetal alcohol syndrome** in a subject who is exposed to alcohol in utero with a combination of ADNF I and ADNF III polypeptides. The present invention further relates to a method for reducing neuronal cell death by contacting neuronal cells with a combination of ADNF I and ADNF III polypeptides. Still further, the present invention relates to a pharmaceutical composition comprising a combination of ADNF I and ADNF III polypeptides.

Excerpt(s): This application is related to U.S. Ser. No. 07/871,973 filed Apr. 22, 1992, now U.S. Pat. No. 5,767,240, issued Jun. 16, 1998; U.S. Ser. No. 08/342, 297, filed Oct. 17, 1994 (published as WO96/11948); U.S. Ser. No. 60/037,404, filed Feb. 27, 1997 (published as WO98/35042); and U.S. Ser. No. 09/187,330, filed Nov. 11, 1998. All of these applications are incorporated herein by reference. Not applicable. This invention relates to a method for reducing a condition associated with **fetal alcohol syndrome** in a subject who is exposed to alcohol in utero with an ADNF polypeptide. In particular, the present invention relates to a method for reducing a condition associated with **fetal alcohol syndrome** in a subject who is exposed to alcohol in utero with a combination of ADNF I and ADNF III polypeptides. The present invention further relates to a method for reducing neuronal cell death by contacting neuronal cells with a combination of ADNF I and ADNF III polypeptides. Still further, the present invention relates to a pharmaceutical composition comprising a combination of ADNF I and ADNF III polypeptides.

Web site: http://appft1.uspto.gov/netahtml/PTO/search-bool.html

Keeping Current

In order to stay informed about patents and patent applications dealing with fetal alcohol syndrome, you can access the U.S. Patent Office archive via the Internet at the following Web address: **http://www.uspto.gov/patft/index.html**. You will see two broad options: (1) Issued Patent, and (2) Published Applications. To see a list of issued patents, perform the following steps: Under "Issued Patents," click "Quick Search." Then, type "fetal alcohol syndrome" (or synonyms) into the "Term 1" box. After clicking on the search button, scroll down to see the various patents which have been granted to date on fetal alcohol syndrome.

You can also use this procedure to view pending patent applications concerning fetal alcohol syndrome. Simply go back to **http://www.uspto.gov/patft/index.html** Select "Quick Search" under "Published Applications." Then proceed with the steps listed above.

Chapter 6. Books on Fetal Alcohol Syndrome

Overview

This chapter provides bibliographic book references relating to fetal alcohol syndrome. In addition to online booksellers such as **www.amazon.com** and **www.bn.com**, excellent sources for book titles on fetal alcohol syndrome include the Combined Health Information Database and the National Library of Medicine. Your local medical library also may have these titles available for loan.

Book Summaries: Federal Agencies

The Combined Health Information Database collects various book abstracts from a variety of healthcare institutions and federal agencies. To access these summaries, go directly to the following hyperlink: **http://chid.nih.gov/detail/detail.html**. You will need to use the "Detailed Search" option. To find book summaries, use the drop boxes at the bottom of the search page where "You may refine your search by." Select the dates and language you prefer. For the format option, select "Monograph/Book." Now type "fetal alcohol syndrome" (or synonyms) into the "For these words:" box. You should check back periodically with this database which is updated every three months. The following is a typical result when searching for books on fetal alcohol syndrome:

- **Fetal alcohol syndrome: Diagnosis, epidemiology, prevention, and treatment**

    Source: Washington, DC: National Academy Press. 1996. 213 pp., summ. (57 pp.).

    Contact: Available from National Academy Press, 2101 Constitution Avenue, N.W., Lockbox 285, Washington, DC 20002 / Web site: http://www.nap.edu. $39.95, full report, plus $4.00 shipping and handling; prepayment required by check, money order, or credit card; purchase orders accepted; discounts available for bulk orders. A limited supply of the summary is available from the Division of Biobehavioral Sciences and Mental Disorders, Institute of Medicine, 2101 Constitution Avenue, N.W., Washington, D.C., 20418. Telephone: (202) 334-3935; fax (202) 334- 2939.

    Summary: This book considers the impact of fetal alcohol syndrome (FAS) from a family perspective; it focuses on the implications for the mother, her child, and her whole family. It provides a context for the federal involvement with FAS, reviews topics affecting research in fetal alcohol effects, and presents a number personal vignettes. It devotes individual chapters to these topics: diagnosis and clinical evaluation, epidemiology and surveillance, the epidemiology of women's drinking, prevention of FAS, and intervention and treatment of the affected individual. A concluding chapter considers strategies for integrating and coordinating future activities related to fetal alcohol syndrome. The summary of the report is available on the Internet at http://www.nap/nap/online.

- **Recognizing and managing children with fetal alcohol syndrome/ fetal alcohol effects: A guide**

  Source: Washington,DC: Child Welfare League of America. 1997. 153 pp.

  Contact: Available from CWLA c/o PMDS, Child Welfare League of America, P.O. Box 2019, Annapolis Junction, MD 20701-2019. Telephone: (800) 407-6273 or (301) 617-7825 / e-mail: cwla@pmds.com. $16.95 includes shipping and handling; prepayment required.

  Summary: This book describes the incidence and symptoms of fetal alcohol syndrome, and how to work with affected children from infancy through late adolescence. It is aimed at parents and teachers, and includes case histories, and a resource list.

- **Modern concepts in fetal alcohol syndrome and fetal alcohol effects**

  Source: Laramie, WY: Creative Consultants. 1994. 204 pp.

  Contact: Available from Cheryl A. Schroeder, President, Creative Consultants, P.O. Box 6023, Laramie, WY 82070. Telephone: (307) 745- 3435 / fax: (307) 745-3435. $20.00 plus $3.50 shipping and handling.

  Summary: This book focuses on the prevention of and education about fetal alcohol syndrome (FAS) and fetal alcohol effects (FAE). Some of the areas covered in this book include: 1) the history of FAS, 2) the effects of teratogens in general and alcohol specifically, 3) the need for preconceptual health care, 4) the physical, behavioral, and social characteristics of FAS/FAE, 5) education characteristics, issues, and strategies, 6) psychosocial issues, 7) working with community and state agencies, and 8) networking and coalition building. A listing of resources available regarding FAS/FAE is provided at the end of the book.

- **Maternal risk assessment for fetal alcohol syndrome and alcohol related birth defects and neurodevelopmental disorders**

  Source: Grand Forks, ND: North Dakota Fetal Alcohol Syndrome Center. (between 1997 and 2002?). 29 pp.

  Contact: Available from North Dakota Fetal Alcohol Syndrome Center, 501 North Columbia Road, Grand Forks, ND 58203. Telephone: (701) 777-3683 / Web site: http://www.online-clinic.com. Contact for cost information.

  Summary: This report describes a method for assessing pregnant women at increased risk of having a baby with fetal alcohol syndrome (FAS). Topics include risk and exposure assessments; risk stratification; clinical implications and services; and prevention strategies. The report also contains score sheets and questionnaires for the clinician to use in assessing risk before and during pregnancy. Charts and graphs illustrate the model and other statistical data relating to FAS. Also provided are pocket guides to aid in screening for alcohol abuse and potential fetal exposure.

Book Summaries: Online Booksellers

Commercial Internet-based booksellers, such as Amazon.com and Barnes&Noble.com, offer summaries which have been supplied by each title's publisher. Some summaries also include customer reviews. Your local bookseller may have access to in-house and commercial databases that index all published books (e.g. Books in Print®). **IMPORTANT NOTE:** Online booksellers typically produce search results for medical and non-medical books. When searching for "fetal alcohol syndrome" at online booksellers' Web sites, you may discover <u>non-medical books</u> that use the generic term "fetal alcohol syndrome" (or a synonym) in their titles. The following is indicative of the results you might find when searching for "fetal alcohol syndrome" (sorted alphabetically by title; follow the hyperlink to view more details at Amazon.com):

- **Alcohol and Birth Defects: The Fetal Alcohol Syndrome and Related Disorders** by Peter L. Petrakis; ISBN: 9999539599;
  http://www.amazon.com/exec/obidos/ASIN/9999539599/icongroupinterna

- **Alcohol and Pregnancy: A Retrieval Index and Bibliography of the Fetal Alcohol Syndrome** by Leslie P. Gartner (1984); ISBN: 0910841039;
  http://www.amazon.com/exec/obidos/ASIN/0910841039/icongroupinterna

- **Alcohol, Pregnancy and the Developing Child : Fetal Alcohol Syndrome** by Hans-Ludwig Spohr (Editor), Hans-Christoph Steinhausen (Editor) (1996); ISBN: 0521564263;
  http://www.amazon.com/exec/obidos/ASIN/0521564263/icongroupinterna

- **Conceiving Risk, Bearing Responsibility: Fetal Alcohol Syndrome & the Diagnosis of Moral Disorder** by Elizabeth M. Armstrong (2003); ISBN: 0801873452;
  http://www.amazon.com/exec/obidos/ASIN/0801873452/icongroupinterna

- **Drinking and Pregnancy: Preventing Fetal Alcohol Syndrome** by Sheila B Blume; ISBN: 0935908161;
  http://www.amazon.com/exec/obidos/ASIN/0935908161/icongroupinterna

- **Fantastic Antone Grows Up: Adolescents and Adults With Fetal Alcohol Syndrome** by Judith Kleinfeld (Editor), et al (2000); ISBN: 1889963119;
  http://www.amazon.com/exec/obidos/ASIN/1889963119/icongroupinterna

- **Fetal Alcohol Syndrome** by Abel (1981); ISBN: 0849361923;
  http://www.amazon.com/exec/obidos/ASIN/0849361923/icongroupinterna

- **Fetal Alcohol Syndrome (Revised)(Drug Abuse Prevention)** by Amy Nevitt; ISBN: 0823928292;
  http://www.amazon.com/exec/obidos/ASIN/0823928292/icongroupinterna

- **Fetal alcohol syndrome : hearing before the Subcommittee on Social Security and Family Policy of the Committee on Finance, United States Senate, One Hundred First Congress, second session, December 10, 1990 (SuDoc Y 4.F 49:S.hrg.101-1262)**; ISBN: B000106UIA;
  http://www.amazon.com/exec/obidos/ASIN/B000106UIA/icongroupinterna

- **Fetal alcohol syndrome a training manual to aid in vocational rehabilitation and other non-medical services (SuDoc ED 1.310/2:434789)** by U.S. Dept of Education; ISBN: B000113BDQ;
  http://www.amazon.com/exec/obidos/ASIN/B000113BDQ/icongroupinterna

- **Fetal Alcohol Syndrome and Fetal Alcohol Effects** by Ernest L. Abel (1984); ISBN: 0306414279;
  http://www.amazon.com/exec/obidos/ASIN/0306414279/icongroupinterna

- **Fetal Alcohol Syndrome Information Packet: Early Childhood Research Project** by Enoch Gordis (Editor); ISBN: 0788189069;
  http://www.amazon.com/exec/obidos/ASIN/0788189069/icongroupinterna

- **Fetal Alcohol Syndrome, Fetal Alcohol Effects: Strategies for Professionals** by Diane Malbin, Hazelden Educational Materials (1996); ISBN: 0894869515;
  http://www.amazon.com/exec/obidos/ASIN/0894869515/icongroupinterna

- **Fetal Alcohol Syndrome/Effect: Developing a Community Response** by Jeanette Turpin, eds. Glend Schmidt (1999); ISBN: 1552660117;
  http://www.amazon.com/exec/obidos/ASIN/1552660117/icongroupinterna

- **Fetal Alcohol Syndrome: A Guide for Families and Communities** by Ann Pytkowicz Streissguth; ISBN: 1557662835;
  http://www.amazon.com/exec/obidos/ASIN/1557662835/icongroupinterna

- **Fetal Alcohol Syndrome: Diagnosis, Epidemiology, Prevention, and Treatment** by Kathleen Stratton (Editor), et al; ISBN: 0309052920;
  http://www.amazon.com/exec/obidos/ASIN/0309052920/icongroupinterna

- **Fetal Alcohol Syndrome: From Mechanism to Prevention** by Ernest L. Abel (Editor); ISBN: 0849376858;
  http://www.amazon.com/exec/obidos/ASIN/0849376858/icongroupinterna

- **Indian Fetal Alcohol Syndrome Prevention and Treatment Act : hearing before the Committee on Interior and Insular Affairs, House of Representatives, One Hundred Second Congress, second session, on H.R. 1322. hearingnpm held in Washington, DC, March 5, 1992 (SuDoc Y 4.IN 8/14:102-52)**; ISBN: 0160392187;
  http://www.amazon.com/exec/obidos/ASIN/0160392187/icongroupinterna

- **Prenatal Exposure to Drugs/Alcohol: Characteristics and Educational Implications of Fetal Alcohol Syndrome and Cocaine - Polydrug Effects** by Jeanette M. Soby (1996); ISBN: 0398064369;
  http://www.amazon.com/exec/obidos/ASIN/0398064369/icongroupinterna

- **Program Strategies for Preventing Fetal Alcohol Syndrome and Alcohol-Related Birth Defects**; ISBN: 0318229358;
  http://www.amazon.com/exec/obidos/ASIN/0318229358/icongroupinterna

- **Recent Developments in Alcoholism: Children of Alcoholics: Genetic Predisposition, Fetal Alcohol Syndrome, Vulnerability to Disease, Social and Env** by Marc Galanter (Editor) (1991); ISBN: 0306438402;
  http://www.amazon.com/exec/obidos/ASIN/0306438402/icongroupinterna

- **Recognizing and Managing Children With Fetal Alcohol Syndrome/Fetal Alcohol Effects: A Guidebook** by Brenda McCreight (1997); ISBN: 087868607X;
  http://www.amazon.com/exec/obidos/ASIN/087868607X/icongroupinterna

- **Tad and Me: How I Found Out About Fetal Alcohol Syndrome (Hazeldens Drug Tales)** by Betsy Houlton, Eric Hanson (Illustrator); ISBN: 0894867393;
  http://www.amazon.com/exec/obidos/ASIN/0894867393/icongroupinterna

- **The Best I Can Be: Living with Fetal Alcohol Syndrome-Effects** by Liz Kulp, Jodee Kulp (2000); ISBN: 096370723X;
  http://www.amazon.com/exec/obidos/ASIN/096370723X/icongroupinterna

- **The Broken Cord: A Family's Ongoing Struggle With Fetal Alcohol Syndrome** by Michael Dorris, Louise Erdrich (Designer); ISBN: 0060160713; http://www.amazon.com/exec/obidos/ASIN/0060160713/icongroupinterna

- **The Challenge of Fetal Alcohol Syndrome: Overcoming Secondary Disabilities** by Ann Streissguth (Editor), et al (1997); ISBN: 0295976500; http://www.amazon.com/exec/obidos/ASIN/0295976500/icongroupinterna

- **What You Can Do to Prevent Fetal Alcohol Syndrome: A Professional's Guide** by Sheila B. Blume (1992); ISBN: 1562460439; http://www.amazon.com/exec/obidos/ASIN/1562460439/icongroupinterna

The National Library of Medicine Book Index

The National Library of Medicine at the National Institutes of Health has a massive database of books published on healthcare and biomedicine. Go to the following Internet site, **http://locatorplus.gov/**, and then select "Search LOCATORplus." Once you are in the search area, simply type "fetal alcohol syndrome" (or synonyms) into the search box, and select "books only." From there, results can be sorted by publication date, author, or relevance. The following was recently catalogued by the National Library of Medicine:[7]

- **A manual on adolescents and adults with fetal alcohol syndrome with special reference to American Indians** Author: Streissguth, Ann Pytkowicz.; Year: 1991; [Rockville, Md.?]: U.S. Dept. of Health and Human Services, Public Health Service, Indian Health Service, [1988]

- **Maternal alcohol consumption and fetal and newborn effects, including the fetal alcohol syndrome (FAS): May 1978 through October 1983: 304 citations in English** Author: Kenton, Charlotte.; Year: 1983; [Bethesda, Md.]: U.S. Dept. of Health and Human Services, Public Health Service, National Institutes of Health, 1983

- **Maternal alcohol use and effects on the fetus and the neonate: including the fetal alcohol syndrome (FAS): January 1975 through April 1978: 128 citations** Author: National Library of Medicine (U.S.); Year: 1979; [Bethesda, Md.]: Dept. of Health, Education, and Welfare, Public Health Service, National Institutes of Health, [1978]

- **Ocular abnormalities in the fetal alcohol syndrome** Author: Strömland, Kerstin.; Year: 1987; Göteborg, Sweden: Scriptor, 1985; ISBN: 8787473895

- **Program strategies for preventing fetal alcohol syndrome and alcohol-related birth defects** Author: National Institute on Alcohol Abuse and Alcoholism (U.S.); Year: 1990; Rockville, Md.: U.S. Dept. of Health and Human Services, Public Health Service, Alcohol, Drug Abuse, and Mental Health Administration, National Institute on Alcohol Abuse and Alcoholism; Washington, D.C.: For sale by the Supt. of Docs.,U.S. G.P.O., [1987]

- **The Fetal alcohol syndrome - public awareness campaign, 1979: progress report concerning the advance notice of proposed rulemaking on warning labels on**

---

[7] In addition to LOCATORPlus, in collaboration with authors and publishers, the National Center for Biotechnology Information (NCBI) is currently adapting biomedical books for the Web. The books may be accessed in two ways: (1) by searching directly using any search term or phrase (in the same way as the bibliographic database PubMed), or (2) by following the links to PubMed abstracts. Each PubMed abstract has a "Books" button that displays a facsimile of the abstract in which some phrases are hypertext links. These phrases are also found in the books available at NCBI. Click on hyperlinked results in the list of books in which the phrase is found. Currently, the majority of the links are between the books and PubMed. In the future, more links will be created between the books and other types of information, such as gene and protein sequences and macromolecular structures. See http://www.ncbi.nlm.nih.gov/entrez/query.fcgi?db=Books.

containers of alcoholic beverages and addendum. Author: National Institute on Alcohol Abuse and Alcoholism (U.S.); Year: 9999; Washington: Dept. of Treasury, Bureau of Alcohol, Tobacco, and Firearms; for sale by the Supt. of Docs., U. S. Govt. Print. Off., 1979

Chapters on Fetal Alcohol Syndrome

In order to find chapters that specifically relate to fetal alcohol syndrome, an excellent source of abstracts is the Combined Health Information Database. You will need to limit your search to book chapters and fetal alcohol syndrome using the "Detailed Search" option. Go to the following hyperlink: **http://chid.nih.gov/detail/detail.html**. To find book chapters, use the drop boxes at the bottom of the search page where "You may refine your search by." Select the dates and language you prefer, and the format option "Book Chapter." Type "fetal alcohol syndrome" (or synonyms) into the "For these words:" box. The following is a typical result when searching for book chapters on fetal alcohol syndrome:

- **Alcohol: Fetal Alcohol Syndrome**

  Source: in Plumbridge, D.; et al., eds. Student with a Genetic Disorder: Educational Implications for Special Education Teachers and for Physical Therapists, Occupational Therapists, and Speech Pathologists. Springfield, IL: Charles C Thomas Publisher. 1993. p. 299-304.

  Contact: Available from Charles C Thomas Publisher. 2600 South First Street, Springfield, IL 62794-9265. (212) 789-8980; Fax (217) 789-9130. PRICE: $75.95 plus shipping and handling (cloth); $39.95 plus shipping and handling (paper). ISBN: 0398058393.

  Summary: This chapter, from a text for educators about genetic disorders, discusses fetal alcohol syndrome (FAS), caused by fetal exposure to excessive alcohol levels during pregnancy. Topics covered include characteristic features, diagnosis, and classification of type; the incidence of FAS; the cognitive profile; the behavior profile; the educational implications; physical therapy; occupational therapy; hearing and speech considerations, notably speech delays, oral motor problems, and the impact of memory problems, attention deficits, and distractibility; and psychosocial issues. 1 figure. 9 references.

Directories

In addition to the references and resources discussed earlier in this chapter, a number of directories relating to fetal alcohol syndrome have been published that consolidate information across various sources. The Combined Health Information Database lists the following, which you may wish to consult in your local medical library:[8]

---

[8] You will need to limit your search to "Directory" and "fetal alcohol syndrome" using the "Detailed Search" option. Go directly to the following hyperlink: **http://chid.nih.gov/detail/detail.html**. To find directories, use the drop boxes at the bottom of the search page where "You may refine your search by." For publication date, select "All Years." Select your preferred language and the format option "Directory." Type "fetal alcohol syndrome" (or synonyms) into the "For these words:" box. You should check back periodically with this database as it is updated every three months.

- **Charting the future: Resource directory for the diagnosis prevention and treatment of fetal alcohol syndrome**

  Source: Concord, MA: Fetal Alcohol Education Program, Boston University School of Medicine. 2000. 89 pp.

  Contact: Available from National Maternal and Child Health Clearinghouse, 2070 Chain Bridge Road, Suite 450, Vienna, VA 22182-2536. Telephone: (703) 356-1964 or (888) 434-4MCH / fax: (703) 821-2098 / e-mail: nmchc@circsol.com / Web site: http://www.nmchc.org. Available at no charge.

  Summary: This directory lists resources for the diagnosis, prevention, and treatment of fetal alcohol syndrome (FAS). It is divided into three main parts. The first section is a brief overview of fetal alcohol syndrome, including diagnosis, manifestation, treatment, and prevention. The second section lists national resources for FAS, most of which provide printed or video resources, referrals, or links to other organizations. The third and largest section is a listing for each state and trust territory of identified sources for diagnosis, support for families, treatment of FAS, community activities, and where to inquire about treatment for pregnant women with alcohol problems. [Funded by the Maternal and Child Health Bureau].

Chapter 7. Multimedia on Fetal Alcohol Syndrome

Overview

In this chapter, we show you how to keep current on multimedia sources of information on fetal alcohol syndrome. We start with sources that have been summarized by federal agencies, and then show you how to find bibliographic information catalogued by the National Library of Medicine.

Audio Recordings

The Combined Health Information Database contains abstracts on audio productions. To search CHID, go directly to the following hyperlink: **http://chid.nih.gov/detail/detail.html** To find audio productions, use the drop boxes at the bottom of the search page where "You may refine your search by." Select the dates and language you prefer, and the format option "Sound Recordings." Type "fetal alcohol syndrome" (or synonyms) into the "For these words:" box. The following is a typical result when searching for sound recordings on fetal alcohol syndrome:

- **Substance Use/Multiple Diagnosis. National Conference on Women and AIDS/HIV Infection; Washington, D.C., December 13-14, 1990**

  Contact: Triad Media Group, PO Box 778, Frederick, MD, 21701, (301) 663-1471.

  Summary: This sound recording is a presentation from the National Conference on Women and AIDS/HIV Infection held December 13-14, 1990, in Washington, D.C. It examines the relationship between substance abuse and Human immunodeficiency virus (HIV) infection. Acquired immunodeficiency syndrome (AIDS) and alcohol and drug abuse go hand-in-hand, according to the first speaker. Addiction is inherited, and the families it afflicts are dysfunctional. Women in such families need multiple, systemic, and comprehensive support services and treatment. The second speaker discusses results of antibody tests on women who came to an alcohol detoxification center. The seropositive rate was much higher than normal. Since alcohol abuse can cause liver damage, it may also prevent individuals from being treated with certain drugs which can also adversely affect liver function. Relapse after treatment for alcohol addiction and **fetal alcohol syndrome** are two other major problems. The third speaker describes HIV-brain disease, or dementia, and lists several other factors which may affect a patient's mental state. These are opportunistic infections which may affect the brain, medication side effects, and drug interactions. A good client history is useful to distinguish the cause of the problem. The fourth speaker explains the types of mental disorders common to substance abusers, the stages of addiction treatment and interventions necessary in each one, and the need for suicidal assessment and support groups.

Bibliography: Multimedia on Fetal Alcohol Syndrome

The National Library of Medicine is a rich source of information on healthcare-related multimedia productions including slides, computer software, and databases. To access the multimedia database, go to the following Web site: **http://locatorplus.gov/**. Select "Search LOCATORplus." Once in the search area, simply type in fetal alcohol syndrome (or synonyms). Then, in the option box provided below the search box, select "Audiovisuals and Computer Files." From there, you can choose to sort results by publication date, author, or relevance. The following multimedia has been indexed on fetal alcohol syndrome:

- **Alcohol and pregnancy [videorecording]: fetal alcohol syndrome and fetal alcohol effects** Source: produced by John Ralmon Productions; Year: 1992; Format: Videorecording; Chatsworth, Calif.: AIMS Media, c1992

- **Alcohol, pregnancy and the fetal alcohol syndrome [slide]** Source: [authors, Ruth E. Little, Ann Pytkowicz Streissguth]; Year: 1982; Format: Slide; Timonium, Md.: Milner-Fenwick, c1982

- **Alcohol, pregnancy, and the fetal alcohol syndrome [slide]** Source: [Ann P. Streissguth, Ruth E. Little]; Year: 1994; Format: Slide; Timonium, Md.: Milner-Fenwick, c1994

- **Fetal alcohol syndrome [electronic resource]: prevention, diagnosis, treatment: a clinical guide for obstetric and pediatric providers.** Year: 2000; Format: Electronic resource; Cambridge, MA: Vida Health Communications, [2000?]

- **Fetal alcohol syndrome [sound recording]** Source: Addiction Research Foundation; Year: 1979; Format: Sound recording; [Toronto]: The Foundation, 1979

- **Fetal alcohol syndrome [videorecording]** Source: [presented by] Films Incorporated; Year: 1975; Format: Videorecording; [New York]: National Broadcasting Company, c1975

- **Fetal alcohol syndrome [videorecording]** Source: [presented by] the Marshfield Regional Video Network, in cooperation with Marshfield Clinic & St. Joseph's Hospital; Year: 1981; Format: Videorecording; Marshfield, WI: The Network, 1981

- **Fetal alcohol syndrome [videorecording]** Source: NHV, National Health Video Inc; Year: 1998; Format: Videorecording; Los Angeles, CA: National Health Video, 1998

- **Fetal alcohol syndrome [videorecording]: life sentence** Source: a presentation of Films for the Humanities & Sciences; produced and distributed by Canadian Broadcasting Corporation; CBC News; Year: 1998; Format: Videorecording; Princeton, N.J.: Films for the Humanities & Sciences, c1998

CHAPTER 8. PERIODICALS AND NEWS ON FETAL ALCOHOL SYNDROME

Overview

In this chapter, we suggest a number of news sources and present various periodicals that cover fetal alcohol syndrome.

News Services and Press Releases

One of the simplest ways of tracking press releases on fetal alcohol syndrome is to search the news wires. In the following sample of sources, we will briefly describe how to access each service. These services only post recent news intended for public viewing.

PR Newswire

To access the PR Newswire archive, simply go to **http://www.prnewswire.com/**. Select your country. Type "fetal alcohol syndrome" (or synonyms) into the search box. You will automatically receive information on relevant news releases posted within the last 30 days. The search results are shown by order of relevance.

Reuters Health

The Reuters' Medical News and Health eLine databases can be very useful in exploring news archives relating to fetal alcohol syndrome. While some of the listed articles are free to view, others are available for purchase for a nominal fee. To access this archive, go to **http://www.reutershealth.com/en/index.html** and search by "fetal alcohol syndrome" (or synonyms). The following was recently listed in this archive for fetal alcohol syndrome:

- **Peptide's ethanol blocking effect protects against fetal alcohol syndrome**
  Source: Reuters Medical News
  Date: June 10, 2003

- **Fetal alcohol syndrome still major health concern**
  Source: Reuters Health eLine
  Date: May 23, 2002

- **Fetal alcohol syndrome continues to be a major public health concern**
  Source: Reuters Medical News
  Date: May 23, 2002

- **Long-chain alcohol blocks mechanism of fetal alcohol syndrome**
  Source: Reuters Medical News
  Date: May 21, 2001

- **Fetal alcohol syndrome damage same across cultures**
  Source: Reuters Health eLine
  Date: April 20, 2001

- **Mechanism of brain damage in fetal alcohol syndrome identified**
  Source: Reuters Medical News
  Date: February 11, 2000

- **Clinic identifies previously undiagnosed cases of fetal alcohol syndrome**
  Source: Reuters Medical News
  Date: October 16, 1998

- **Test predicts alcohol-related birth defects**
  Source: Reuters Health eLine
  Date: September 25, 1998

- **High cytokine production linked to immune dysfunction in fetal alcohol syndrome**
  Source: Reuters Medical News
  Date: September 16, 1998

- **Fetal Alcohol Syndrome Prevalence Best Determined By Multiple Surveillance**
  Source: Reuters Medical News
  Date: December 01, 1997

- **Fetal Alcohol Syndrome Leads To Lifelong Disabilities**
  Source: Reuters Medical News
  Date: September 04, 1996

- **Fetal Alcohol Syndrome Affects Adult Life**
  Source: Reuters Health eLine
  Date: September 04, 1996

- **IOM Committee Calls Fetal Alcohol Syndrome "Completely Preventable"**
  Source: Reuters Medical News
  Date: September 25, 1995

The NIH

Within MEDLINEplus, the NIH has made an agreement with the New York Times Syndicate, the AP News Service, and Reuters to deliver news that can be browsed by the public. Search news releases at **http://www.nlm.nih.gov/medlineplus/alphanews_a.html**. MEDLINEplus allows you to browse across an alphabetical index. Or you can search by date at the following Web page: **http://www.nlm.nih.gov/medlineplus/newsbydate.html**. Often, news items are indexed by MEDLINEplus within its search engine.

Business Wire

Business Wire is similar to PR Newswire. To access this archive, simply go to **http://www.businesswire.com/**. You can scan the news by industry category or company name.

Market Wire

Market Wire is more focused on technology than the other wires. To browse the latest press releases by topic, such as alternative medicine, biotechnology, fitness, healthcare, legal, nutrition, and pharmaceuticals, access Market Wire's Medical/Health channel at **http://www.marketwire.com/mw/release_index?channel=MedicalHealth**. Or simply go to Market Wire's home page at **http://www.marketwire.com/mw/home**, type "fetal alcohol syndrome" (or synonyms) into the search box, and click on "Search News." As this service is technology oriented, you may wish to use it when searching for press releases covering diagnostic procedures or tests.

Search Engines

Medical news is also available in the news sections of commercial Internet search engines. See the health news page at Yahoo (**http://dir.yahoo.com/Health/News_and_Media/**), or you can use this Web site's general news search page at **http://news.yahoo.com/**. Type in "fetal alcohol syndrome" (or synonyms). If you know the name of a company that is relevant to fetal alcohol syndrome, you can go to any stock trading Web site (such as **http://www.etrade.com/**) and search for the company name there. News items across various news sources are reported on indicated hyperlinks. Google offers a similar service at **http://news.google.com/**.

BBC

Covering news from a more European perspective, the British Broadcasting Corporation (BBC) allows the public free access to their news archive located at **http://www.bbc.co.uk/**. Search by "fetal alcohol syndrome" (or synonyms).

Academic Periodicals covering Fetal Alcohol Syndrome

Numerous periodicals are currently indexed within the National Library of Medicine's PubMed database that are known to publish articles relating to fetal alcohol syndrome. In addition to these sources, you can search for articles covering fetal alcohol syndrome that have been published by any of the periodicals listed in previous chapters. To find the latest studies published, go to **http://www.ncbi.nlm.nih.gov/pubmed**, type the name of the periodical into the search box, and click "Go."

If you want complete details about the historical contents of a journal, you can also visit the following Web site: **http://www.ncbi.nlm.nih.gov/entrez/jrbrowser.cgi**. Here, type in the name of the journal or its abbreviation, and you will receive an index of published articles. At **http://locatorplus.gov/**, you can retrieve more indexing information on medical periodicals (e.g. the name of the publisher). Select the button "Search LOCATORplus." Then type in the name of the journal and select the advanced search option "Journal Title Search."

APPENDICES

APPENDIX A. PHYSICIAN RESOURCES

Overview

In this chapter, we focus on databases and Internet-based guidelines and information resources created or written for a professional audience.

NIH Guidelines

Commonly referred to as "clinical" or "professional" guidelines, the National Institutes of Health publish physician guidelines for the most common diseases. Publications are available at the following by relevant Institute[9]:

- Office of the Director (OD); guidelines consolidated across agencies available at **http://www.nih.gov/health/consumer/conkey.htm**

- National Institute of General Medical Sciences (NIGMS); fact sheets available at **http://www.nigms.nih.gov/news/facts/**

- National Library of Medicine (NLM); extensive encyclopedia (A.D.A.M., Inc.) with guidelines: **http://www.nlm.nih.gov/medlineplus/healthtopics.html**

- National Cancer Institute (NCI); guidelines available at **http://www.cancer.gov/cancerinfo/list.aspx?viewid=5f35036e-5497-4d86-8c2c-714a9f7c8d25**

- National Eye Institute (NEI); guidelines available at **http://www.nei.nih.gov/order/index.htm**

- National Heart, Lung, and Blood Institute (NHLBI); guidelines available at **http://www.nhlbi.nih.gov/guidelines/index.htm**

- National Human Genome Research Institute (NHGRI); research available at **http://www.genome.gov/page.cfm?pageID=10000375**

- National Institute on Aging (NIA); guidelines available at **http://www.nia.nih.gov/health/**

---

[9] These publications are typically written by one or more of the various NIH Institutes.

- National Institute on Alcohol Abuse and Alcoholism (NIAAA); guidelines available at **http://www.niaaa.nih.gov/publications/publications.htm**

- National Institute of Allergy and Infectious Diseases (NIAID); guidelines available at **http://www.niaid.nih.gov/publications/**

- National Institute of Arthritis and Musculoskeletal and Skin Diseases (NIAMS); fact sheets and guidelines available at **http://www.niams.nih.gov/hi/index.htm**

- National Institute of Child Health and Human Development (NICHD); guidelines available at **http://www.nichd.nih.gov/publications/pubskey.cfm**

- National Institute on Deafness and Other Communication Disorders (NIDCD); fact sheets and guidelines at **http://www.nidcd.nih.gov/health/**

- National Institute of Dental and Craniofacial Research (NIDCR); guidelines available at **http://www.nidr.nih.gov/health/**

- National Institute of Diabetes and Digestive and Kidney Diseases (NIDDK); guidelines available at **http://www.niddk.nih.gov/health/health.htm**

- National Institute on Drug Abuse (NIDA); guidelines available at **http://www.nida.nih.gov/DrugAbuse.html**

- National Institute of Environmental Health Sciences (NIEHS); environmental health information available at **http://www.niehs.nih.gov/external/facts.htm**

- National Institute of Mental Health (NIMH); guidelines available at **http://www.nimh.nih.gov/practitioners/index.cfm**

- National Institute of Neurological Disorders and Stroke (NINDS); neurological disorder information pages available at **http://www.ninds.nih.gov/health_and_medical/disorder_index.htm**

- National Institute of Nursing Research (NINR); publications on selected illnesses at **http://www.nih.gov/ninr/news-info/publications.html**

- National Institute of Biomedical Imaging and Bioengineering; general information at **http://grants.nih.gov/grants/becon/becon_info.htm**

- Center for Information Technology (CIT); referrals to other agencies based on keyword searches available at **http://kb.nih.gov/www_query_main.asp**

- National Center for Complementary and Alternative Medicine (NCCAM); health information available at **http://nccam.nih.gov/health/**

- National Center for Research Resources (NCRR); various information directories available at **http://www.ncrr.nih.gov/publications.asp**

- Office of Rare Diseases; various fact sheets available at **http://rarediseases.info.nih.gov/html/resources/rep_pubs.html**

- Centers for Disease Control and Prevention; various fact sheets on infectious diseases available at **http://www.cdc.gov/publications.htm**

NIH Databases

In addition to the various Institutes of Health that publish professional guidelines, the NIH has designed a number of databases for professionals.[10] Physician-oriented resources provide a wide variety of information related to the biomedical and health sciences, both past and present. The format of these resources varies. Searchable databases, bibliographic citations, full-text articles (when available), archival collections, and images are all available. The following are referenced by the National Library of Medicine:[11]

- **Bioethics:** Access to published literature on the ethical, legal, and public policy issues surrounding healthcare and biomedical research. This information is provided in conjunction with the Kennedy Institute of Ethics located at Georgetown University, Washington, D.C.: **http://www.nlm.nih.gov/databases/databases_bioethics.html**

- **HIV/AIDS Resources:** Describes various links and databases dedicated to HIV/AIDS research: **http://www.nlm.nih.gov/pubs/factsheets/aidsinfs.html**

- **NLM Online Exhibitions:** Describes "Exhibitions in the History of Medicine": **http://www.nlm.nih.gov/exhibition/exhibition.html**. Additional resources for historical scholarship in medicine: **http://www.nlm.nih.gov/hmd/hmd.html**

- **Biotechnology Information:** Access to public databases. The National Center for Biotechnology Information conducts research in computational biology, develops software tools for analyzing genome data, and disseminates biomedical information for the better understanding of molecular processes affecting human health and disease: **http://www.ncbi.nlm.nih.gov/**

- **Population Information:** The National Library of Medicine provides access to worldwide coverage of population, family planning, and related health issues, including family planning technology and programs, fertility, and population law and policy: **http://www.nlm.nih.gov/databases/databases_population.html**

- **Cancer Information:** Access to cancer-oriented databases: **http://www.nlm.nih.gov/databases/databases_cancer.html**

- **Profiles in Science:** Offering the archival collections of prominent twentieth-century biomedical scientists to the public through modern digital technology: **http://www.profiles.nlm.nih.gov/**

- **Chemical Information:** Provides links to various chemical databases and references: **http://sis.nlm.nih.gov/Chem/ChemMain.html**

- **Clinical Alerts:** Reports the release of findings from the NIH-funded clinical trials where such release could significantly affect morbidity and mortality: **http://www.nlm.nih.gov/databases/alerts/clinical_alerts.html**

- **Space Life Sciences:** Provides links and information to space-based research (including NASA): **http://www.nlm.nih.gov/databases/databases_space.html**

- **MEDLINE:** Bibliographic database covering the fields of medicine, nursing, dentistry, veterinary medicine, the healthcare system, and the pre-clinical sciences: **http://www.nlm.nih.gov/databases/databases_medline.html**

---

[10] Remember, for the general public, the National Library of Medicine recommends the databases referenced in MEDLINE*plus* (**http://medlineplus.gov/** or **http://www.nlm.nih.gov/medlineplus/databases.html**).

[11] See **http://www.nlm.nih.gov/databases/databases.html**.

- **Toxicology and Environmental Health Information (TOXNET):** Databases covering toxicology and environmental health: **http://sis.nlm.nih.gov/Tox/ToxMain.html**

- **Visible Human Interface:** Anatomically detailed, three-dimensional representations of normal male and female human bodies: **http://www.nlm.nih.gov/research/visible/visible_human.html**

The Combined Health Information Database

A comprehensive source of information on clinical guidelines written for professionals is the Combined Health Information Database. You will need to limit your search to one of the following: Brochure/Pamphlet, Fact Sheet, or Information Package, and "fetal alcohol syndrome" using the "Detailed Search" option. Go directly to the following hyperlink: **http://chid.nih.gov/detail/detail.html**. To find associations, use the drop boxes at the bottom of the search page where "You may refine your search by." For the publication date, select "All Years." Select your preferred language and the format option "Fact Sheet." Type "fetal alcohol syndrome" (or synonyms) into the "For these words:" box. The following is a sample result:

- **Fetal Alcohol Syndrome, Crack and AIDS Babies - Fostering Families: A Specialized Training Program Designed for Foster Care Workers & Foster Care Parents**

   Contact: Colorado State University, Department of Social Work, Fort Collins, CO, 80523, (970) 491-6612.

   Summary: Fostering Families is a specialized foster care training program for caseworkers and foster parents. This manual examines the needs of children who have been exposed prenatally to alcohol, drugs, and/or AIDS. Specific suggestions for caseworkers and caregivers cover identifying problem areas to assist these children. Available referral services and support services are outlined. Five lecturettes present information on drug-exposed infants; fetal alcohol syndrome; cocaine and crack babies; infants with AIDS; and caring for medically fragile infants. Exercises include practice situations, which provide discussions of possible actions in real situations. This module can be used to earn partial university credit or continuing education units (CEUs).

- **Understanding the occurrence of secondary disabilities in clients with fetal alcohol syndrome and fetal alcohol effects: Final report**

   Source: Seattle, WA: Fetal Alcohol and Drug Unit, University of Washington School of Medicine. 1996. 71 pp.

   Contact: Available from University of Washington School of Medicine, Fetal Alcohol and Drug Unit, 180 Nickerson Street, Suite 309, Seattle, WA 98109. Telephone: (206) 543-7155 / fax: (206) 685-2903 / e-mail: pphipps@u.washington.edu.

   Summary: This report provides information on the types and magnitudes of secondary disabilities associated with fetal alcohol syndrome and fetal alcohol effects. It assesses the risk and protective factors that might alter the rates of occurrence of secondary disabilities. The report discusses client characteristics, primary disabilities, risk and protective factors, secondary disabilities, mental health problems, disrupted school experience, trouble with the law, confinement, inappropriate sexual behavior, alcohol and drug problems, dependent living over 21 years, problems with employment over 21 years, and problems with parenting. It ends with a list of references and a glossary.

- **Suffer the children: The preventable tragedy of fetal alcohol syndrome**

  Source: Minneapolis, MN: Minnesota Office of the Governor. 1998. 35 pp.

  Contact: Available from Minnesota Planning, 658 Cedar Street, Saint Paul, MN 55155. Telephone: (612) 296-3985 / Web site: http://www.governor.state.mn.us/new/firstlad/fas.pdf. Available from the Web site at no charge.

  Summary: This report summarizes task force findings from the public hearings of Governor Arne H. Carlson's Task Force on Fetal Alcohol Syndrome. The report looks at how fetal alcohol syndrome affects individuals, their families, and their communities, how much it costs, and what can be done to prevent it. The report recommends action steps, changes in state policy, and improved funding to prevent the harm of this condition.

The NLM Gateway[12]

The NLM (National Library of Medicine) Gateway is a Web-based system that lets users search simultaneously in multiple retrieval systems at the U.S. National Library of Medicine (NLM). It allows users of NLM services to initiate searches from one Web interface, providing one-stop searching for many of NLM's information resources or databases.[13] To use the NLM Gateway, simply go to the search site at **http://gateway.nlm.nih.gov/gw/Cmd**. Type "fetal alcohol syndrome" (or synonyms) into the search box and click "Search." The results will be presented in a tabular form, indicating the number of references in each database category.

Results Summary

Category	Items Found
Journal Articles	2531
Books / Periodicals / Audio Visual	91
Consumer Health	732
Meeting Abstracts	30
Other Collections	3
Total	3387

HSTAT[14]

HSTAT is a free, Web-based resource that provides access to full-text documents used in healthcare decision-making.[15] These documents include clinical practice guidelines, quick-reference guides for clinicians, consumer health brochures, evidence reports and technology assessments from the Agency for Healthcare Research and Quality (AHRQ), as well as AHRQ's Put Prevention Into Practice. Simply search by "fetal alcohol syndrome" (or synonyms) at the following Web site: **http://text.nlm.nih.gov**.

---

[12] Adapted from NLM: **http://gateway.nlm.nih.gov/gw/Cmd?Overview.x**.

[13] The NLM Gateway is currently being developed by the Lister Hill National Center for Biomedical Communications (LHNCBC) at the National Library of Medicine (NLM) of the National Institutes of Health (NIH).

[14] Adapted from HSTAT: **http://www.nlm.nih.gov/pubs/factsheets/hstat.html**.

[15] The HSTAT URL is **http://hstat.nlm.nih.gov/**.

Coffee Break: Tutorials for Biologists [16]

Coffee Break is a general healthcare site that takes a scientific view of the news and covers recent breakthroughs in biology that may one day assist physicians in developing treatments. Here you will find a collection of short reports on recent biological discoveries. Each report incorporates interactive tutorials that demonstrate how bioinformatics tools are used as a part of the research process. Currently, all Coffee Breaks are written by NCBI staff.[17] Each report is about 400 words and is usually based on a discovery reported in one or more articles from recently published, peer-reviewed literature.[18] This site has new articles every few weeks, so it can be considered an online magazine of sorts. It is intended for general background information. You can access the Coffee Break Web site at the following hyperlink: **http://www.ncbi.nlm.nih.gov/Coffeebreak/**.

Other Commercial Databases

In addition to resources maintained by official agencies, other databases exist that are commercial ventures addressing medical professionals. Here are some examples that may interest you:

- **CliniWeb International:** Index and table of contents to selected clinical information on the Internet; see **http://www.ohsu.edu/cliniweb/**.

- **Medical World Search:** Searches full text from thousands of selected medical sites on the Internet; see **http://www.mwsearch.com/**.

---

[16] Adapted from **http://www.ncbi.nlm.nih.gov/Coffeebreak/Archive/FAQ.html**.

[17] The figure that accompanies each article is frequently supplied by an expert external to NCBI, in which case the source of the figure is cited. The result is an interactive tutorial that tells a biological story.

[18] After a brief introduction that sets the work described into a broader context, the report focuses on how a molecular understanding can provide explanations of observed biology and lead to therapies for diseases. Each vignette is accompanied by a figure and hypertext links that lead to a series of pages that interactively show how NCBI tools and resources are used in the research process.

APPENDIX B. PATIENT RESOURCES

Overview

Official agencies, as well as federally funded institutions supported by national grants, frequently publish a variety of guidelines written with the patient in mind. These are typically called "Fact Sheets" or "Guidelines." They can take the form of a brochure, information kit, pamphlet, or flyer. Often they are only a few pages in length. Since new guidelines on fetal alcohol syndrome can appear at any moment and be published by a number of sources, the best approach to finding guidelines is to systematically scan the Internet-based services that post them.

Patient Guideline Sources

The remainder of this chapter directs you to sources which either publish or can help you find additional guidelines on topics related to fetal alcohol syndrome. Due to space limitations, these sources are listed in a concise manner. Do not hesitate to consult the following sources by either using the Internet hyperlink provided, or, in cases where the contact information is provided, contacting the publisher or author directly.

The National Institutes of Health

The NIH gateway to patients is located at **http://health.nih.gov/**. From this site, you can search across various sources and institutes, a number of which are summarized below.

Topic Pages: MEDLINEplus

The National Library of Medicine has created a vast and patient-oriented healthcare information portal called MEDLINEplus. Within this Internet-based system are "health topic pages" which list links to available materials relevant to fetal alcohol syndrome. To access this system, log on to **http://www.nlm.nih.gov/medlineplus/healthtopics.html**. From there you can either search using the alphabetical index or browse by broad topic areas. Recently, MEDLINEplus listed the following when searched for "fetal alcohol syndrome":

- Guides on fetal alcohol syndrome

    Alcohol Consumption
    http://www.nlm.nih.gov/medlineplus/alcoholconsumption.html

    Alcoholism
    http://www.nlm.nih.gov/medlineplus/alcoholism.html

- Other guides

    Birth Defects
    http://www.nlm.nih.gov/medlineplus/birthdefects.html

    Developmental Disabilities
    http://www.nlm.nih.gov/medlineplus/developmentaldisabilities.html

    Fetal Alcohol Syndrome
    http://www.nlm.nih.gov/medlineplus/fetalalcoholsyndrome.html

    Pregnancy and Substance Abuse
    http://www.nlm.nih.gov/medlineplus/pregnancyandsubstanceabuse.html

    Prenatal Care
    http://www.nlm.nih.gov/medlineplus/prenatalcare.html

Within the health topic page dedicated to fetal alcohol syndrome, the following was listed:

- General/Overviews

    Drinking Alcohol during Pregnancy
    Source: March of Dimes Birth Defects Foundation
    http://www.marchofdimes.com/professionals/681_1170.asp

    Fetal Alcohol Syndrome
    Source: Nemours Foundation
    http://kidshealth.org/parent/medical/brain/fas.html

- Specific Conditions/Aspects

    Living with Fetal Alcohol Syndrome
    http://www.cdc.gov/ncbddd/factsheets/living_fas.pdf

- From the National Institutes of Health

    Drinking and Your Pregnancy
    http://www.niaaa.nih.gov/publications/brochure.htm

- Organizations

    March of Dimes
    Source: March of Dimes Birth Defects Foundation
    http://www.marchofdimes.com/

    National Center on Birth Defects and Developmental Disabilities
    Source: Centers for Disease Control and Prevention
    http://www.cdc.gov/ncbddd/default.htm

National Clearinghouse for Alcohol and Drug Information
Source: Dept. of Health and Human Services, Substance Abuse and Mental Health
Services Administration
http://www.health.org/

National Institute on Alcohol Abuse and Alcoholism
http://www.niaaa.nih.gov/

- Pictures/Diagrams

    Areas of the Brain That Can Be Damaged in Utero by Maternal Alcohol Consumption
    Source: National Institute on Alcohol Abuse and Alcoholism
    http://www.niaaa.nih.gov/gallery/fetal/mattson.htm

    Illustration of the Craniofacial Features Associated with Fetal Alcohol Syndrome
    Source: National Institute on Alcohol Abuse and Alcoholism
    http://www.niaaa.nih.gov/gallery/fetal/faskid.htm

- Research

    Compounds Prevent Alcohol's Disruption of Important Developmental Process
    Source: National Institute on Alcohol Abuse and Alcoholism
    http://www.nih.gov/news/pr/sep2002/niaaa-18.htm

    Long-Chain Alcohol Found to Block Mechanism of Fetal Alcohol Syndrome
    Source: National Institute on Alcohol Abuse and Alcoholism
    http://www.nih.gov/news/pr/may2001/niaaa-18.htm

    Mouse Study Identifies Protective Mechanism against Alcohol-Induced Embryo Toxicity
    Source: National Institute on Alcohol Abuse and Alcoholism
    http://www.nih.gov/news/pr/jun2003/niaaa-09.htm

    Reducing the Risk of Alcohol-Exposed Pregnancies: A Study of Motivational Counseling in Community Settings
    http://www.cdc.gov/ncbddd/factsheets/pediatrics/Pediatrics_Project_CHOICES.pdf

- Statistics

    FASTATS: Pregnancy Risk Factors
    Source: National Center for Health Statistics
    http://www.cdc.gov/nchs/fastats/pregrisk.htm

    Leading Categories of Birth Defects
    Source: March of Dimes Birth Defects Foundation
    http://www.marchofdimes.com/aboutus/680_2164.asp

You may also choose to use the search utility provided by MEDLINEplus at the following Web address: **http://www.nlm.nih.gov/medlineplus/**. Simply type a keyword into the search box and click "Search." This utility is similar to the NIH search utility, with the exception that it only includes materials that are linked within the MEDLINEplus system (mostly patient-oriented information). It also has the disadvantage of generating unstructured results. We recommend, therefore, that you use this method only if you have a very targeted search.

The Combined Health Information Database (CHID)

CHID Online is a reference tool that maintains a database directory of thousands of journal articles and patient education guidelines on fetal alcohol syndrome. CHID offers summaries that describe the guidelines available, including contact information and pricing. CHID's general Web site is **http://chid.nih.gov/**. To search this database, go to **http://chid.nih.gov/detail/detail.html**. In particular, you can use the advanced search options to look up pamphlets, reports, brochures, and information kits. The following was recently posted in this archive:

- **Sacred trust: Protect your baby against fetal alcohol syndrome**

  Source: Washington, DC: Food and Consumer Service, U.S. Department of Agriculture. 1995. 12 pp.

  Contact: Available from U.S. Food and Nutrition Service, Special Supplemental Nutrition Program for Women, Infants and Children (WIC), Washington, DC 20250. Telephone: (202) 720-7327 or (202) 720-1127 TDD.

  Summary: This brochure discourages the use of alcohol during pregnancy in order to prevent fetal alcohol syndrome (FAS) in children. It goes over the symptoms of FAS and offers helpful suggestions to mothers. The pamphlet was designed for a Native American audience and contains Native American artwork.

Healthfinder™

Healthfinder™ is sponsored by the U.S. Department of Health and Human Services and offers links to hundreds of other sites that contain healthcare information. This Web site is located at **http://www.healthfinder.gov**. Again, keyword searches can be used to find guidelines. The following was recently found in this database:

- **Fetal Alcohol Syndrome Fact Sheet**

  Source: National Center on Birth Defects and Developmental Disabilities

  http://www.healthfinder.gov/scripts/recordpass.asp?RecordType=0&RecordID=5426

- **Fetal Alcohol Syndrome: Prevention Activities**

  Summary: This web page highlights CDC's partnership with state health departments and universities for the purpose of identifying FAS cases and developing prevention programs.

  Source: National Center on Birth Defects and Developmental Disabilities

  http://www.healthfinder.gov/scripts/recordpass.asp?RecordType=0&RecordID=852

- **What Is Fetal Alcohol Syndrome?**

  Summary: Describes fetal alcohol syndrome (FAS), alcohol-related neurodevelopmental disorder (ARND), and alcohol-related birth defects (ARBD).

  Source: National Organization on Fetal Alcohol Syndrome

  http://www.healthfinder.gov/scripts/recordpass.asp?RecordType=0&RecordID=6958

The NIH Search Utility

The NIH search utility allows you to search for documents on over 100 selected Web sites that comprise the NIH-WEB-SPACE. Each of these servers is "crawled" and indexed on an ongoing basis. Your search will produce a list of various documents, all of which will relate in some way to fetal alcohol syndrome. The drawbacks of this approach are that the information is not organized by theme and that the references are often a mix of information for professionals and patients. Nevertheless, a large number of the listed Web sites provide useful background information. We can only recommend this route, therefore, for relatively rare or specific disorders, or when using highly targeted searches. To use the NIH search utility, visit the following Web page: **http://search.nih.gov/index.html**

Additional Web Sources

A number of Web sites are available to the public that often link to government sites. These can also point you in the direction of essential information. The following is a representative sample:

- AOL: **http://search.aol.com/cat.adp?id=168&layer=&from=subcats**

- Family Village: **http://www.familyvillage.wisc.edu/specific.htm**

- Google: **http://directory.google.com/Top/Health/Conditions_and_Diseases/**

- Med Help International: **http://www.medhelp.org/HealthTopics/A.html**

- Open Directory Project: **http://dmoz.org/Health/Conditions_and_Diseases/**

- Yahoo.com: **http://dir.yahoo.com/Health/Diseases_and_Conditions/**

- WebMD®Health: **http://my.webmd.com/health_topics**

Associations and Fetal Alcohol Syndrome

The following is a list of associations that provide information on and resources relating to fetal alcohol syndrome:

- **National Organization on Fetal Alcohol Syndrome**

  Telephone: (202) 785-4585 Toll-free: (800) 666-6327

  Fax: (202) 466-6456

  Email: information@nofas.org

  Web Site: http://www.nofas.org

  Background: The National Organization on **Fetal Alcohol Syndrome** is a voluntary not-for-profit service agency dedicated to eliminating birth defects caused by alcohol consumption during pregnancy and improving the quality of life for all those affected by **fetal alcohol syndrome.** Established in 1990, the organization is committed to increasing public awareness of **fetal alcohol syndrome** (FAS) and fetal alcohol effects (FAE); assisting in community empowerment and the promotion of preventive education through media campaigns; and training health care professionals, educators, and community members in addressing the specialized needs of affected children. The organization is also committed to serving as a national clearinghouse for local, regional, and state **fetal alcohol syndrome** organizations to ensure the effective exchange of information and resources. In addition, it engages in patient advocacy; promotes and supports research; provides appropriate referrals; and offers educational and supportive information through its database, directory, regular newsletter, reports, and brochures.

Relevant area(s) of interest: Fetal Alcohol Syndrome

Finding Associations

There are several Internet directories that provide lists of medical associations with information on or resources relating to fetal alcohol syndrome. By consulting all of associations listed in this chapter, you will have nearly exhausted all sources for patient associations concerned with fetal alcohol syndrome.

The National Health Information Center (NHIC)

The National Health Information Center (NHIC) offers a free referral service to help people find organizations that provide information about fetal alcohol syndrome. For more information, see the NHIC's Web site at **http://www.health.gov/NHIC/** or contact an information specialist by calling 1-800-336-4797.

Directory of Health Organizations

The Directory of Health Organizations, provided by the National Library of Medicine Specialized Information Services, is a comprehensive source of information on associations. The Directory of Health Organizations database can be accessed via the Internet at **http://www.sis.nlm.nih.gov/Dir/DirMain.html**. It is composed of two parts: DIRLINE and Health Hotlines.

The DIRLINE database comprises some 10,000 records of organizations, research centers, and government institutes and associations that primarily focus on health and biomedicine. To access DIRLINE directly, go to the following Web site: **http://dirline.nlm.nih.gov/**. Simply type in "fetal alcohol syndrome" (or a synonym), and you will receive information on all relevant organizations listed in the database.

Health Hotlines directs you to toll-free numbers to over 300 organizations. You can access this database directly at **http://www.sis.nlm.nih.gov/hotlines/**. On this page, you are given the option to search by keyword or by browsing the subject list. When you have received your search results, click on the name of the organization for its description and contact information.

The Combined Health Information Database

Another comprehensive source of information on healthcare associations is the Combined Health Information Database. Using the "Detailed Search" option, you will need to limit your search to "Organizations" and "fetal alcohol syndrome". Type the following hyperlink into your Web browser: **http://chid.nih.gov/detail/detail.html**. To find associations, use the drop boxes at the bottom of the search page where "You may refine your search by." For publication date, select "All Years." Then, select your preferred language and the format option "Organization Resource Sheet." Type "fetal alcohol syndrome" (or synonyms) into the "For these words:" box. You should check back periodically with this database since it is updated every three months.

The National Organization for Rare Disorders, Inc.

The National Organization for Rare Disorders, Inc. has prepared a Web site that provides, at no charge, lists of associations organized by health topic. You can access this database at the following Web site: **http://www.rarediseases.org/search/orgsearch.html**. Type "fetal alcohol syndrome" (or a synonym) into the search box, and click "Submit Query."

APPENDIX C. FINDING MEDICAL LIBRARIES

Overview

In this Appendix, we show you how to quickly find a medical library in your area.

Preparation

Your local public library and medical libraries have interlibrary loan programs with the National Library of Medicine (NLM), one of the largest medical collections in the world. According to the NLM, most of the literature in the general and historical collections of the National Library of Medicine is available on interlibrary loan to any library. If you would like to access NLM medical literature, then visit a library in your area that can request the publications for you.[19]

Finding a Local Medical Library

The quickest method to locate medical libraries is to use the Internet-based directory published by the National Network of Libraries of Medicine (NN/LM). This network includes 4626 members and affiliates that provide many services to librarians, health professionals, and the public. To find a library in your area, simply visit **http://nnlm.gov/members/adv.html** or call 1-800-338-7657.

Medical Libraries in the U.S. and Canada

In addition to the NN/LM, the National Library of Medicine (NLM) lists a number of libraries with reference facilities that are open to the public. The following is the NLM's list and includes hyperlinks to each library's Web site. These Web pages can provide information on hours of operation and other restrictions. The list below is a small sample of

---

[19] Adapted from the NLM: **http://www.nlm.nih.gov/psd/cas/interlibrary.html**.

libraries recommended by the National Library of Medicine (sorted alphabetically by name of the U.S. state or Canadian province where the library is located)[20]:

- **Alabama:** Health InfoNet of Jefferson County (Jefferson County Library Cooperative, Lister Hill Library of the Health Sciences), **http://www.uab.edu/infonet/**

- **Alabama:** Richard M. Scrushy Library (American Sports Medicine Institute)

- **Arizona:** Samaritan Regional Medical Center: The Learning Center (Samaritan Health System, Phoenix, Arizona), **http://www.samaritan.edu/library/bannerlibs.htm**

- **California:** Kris Kelly Health Information Center (St. Joseph Health System, Humboldt), **http://www.humboldt1.com/~kkhic/index.html**

- **California:** Community Health Library of Los Gatos, **http://www.healthlib.org/orgresources.html**

- **California:** Consumer Health Program and Services (CHIPS) (County of Los Angeles Public Library, Los Angeles County Harbor-UCLA Medical Center Library) - Carson, CA, **http://www.colapublib.org/services/chips.html**

- **California:** Gateway Health Library (Sutter Gould Medical Foundation)

- **California:** Health Library (Stanford University Medical Center), **http://www-med.stanford.edu/healthlibrary/**

- **California:** Patient Education Resource Center - Health Information and Resources (University of California, San Francisco), **http://sfghdean.ucsf.edu/barnett/PERC/default.asp**

- **California:** Redwood Health Library (Petaluma Health Care District), **http://www.phcd.org/rdwdlib.html**

- **California:** Los Gatos PlaneTree Health Library, **http://planetreesanjose.org/**

- **California:** Sutter Resource Library (Sutter Hospitals Foundation, Sacramento), **http://suttermedicalcenter.org/library/**

- **California:** Health Sciences Libraries (University of California, Davis), **http://www.lib.ucdavis.edu/healthsci/**

- **California:** ValleyCare Health Library & Ryan Comer Cancer Resource Center (ValleyCare Health System, Pleasanton), **http://gaelnet.stmarys-ca.edu/other.libs/gbal/east/vchl.html**

- **California:** Washington Community Health Resource Library (Fremont), **http://www.healthlibrary.org/**

- **Colorado:** William V. Gervasini Memorial Library (Exempla Healthcare), **http://www.saintjosephdenver.org/yourhealth/libraries/**

- **Connecticut:** Hartford Hospital Health Science Libraries (Hartford Hospital), **http://www.harthosp.org/library/**

- **Connecticut:** Healthnet: Connecticut Consumer Health Information Center (University of Connecticut Health Center, Lyman Maynard Stowe Library), **http://library.uchc.edu/departm/hnet/**

---

[20] Abstracted from **http://www.nlm.nih.gov/medlineplus/libraries.html**.

- **Connecticut:** Waterbury Hospital Health Center Library (Waterbury Hospital, Waterbury), **http://www.waterburyhospital.com/library/consumer.shtml**

- **Delaware:** Consumer Health Library (Christiana Care Health System, Eugene du Pont Preventive Medicine & Rehabilitation Institute, Wilmington), **http://www.christianacare.org/health_guide/health_guide_pmri_health_info.cfm**

- **Delaware:** Lewis B. Flinn Library (Delaware Academy of Medicine, Wilmington), **http://www.delamed.org/chls.html**

- **Georgia:** Family Resource Library (Medical College of Georgia, Augusta), **http://cmc.mcg.edu/kids_families/fam_resources/fam_res_lib/frl.htm**

- **Georgia:** Health Resource Center (Medical Center of Central Georgia, Macon), **http://www.mccg.org/hrc/hrchome.asp**

- **Hawaii:** Hawaii Medical Library: Consumer Health Information Service (Hawaii Medical Library, Honolulu), **http://hml.org/CHIS/**

- **Idaho:** DeArmond Consumer Health Library (Kootenai Medical Center, Coeur d'Alene), **http://www.nicon.org/DeArmond/index.htm**

- **Illinois:** Health Learning Center of Northwestern Memorial Hospital (Chicago), **http://www.nmh.org/health_info/hlc.html**

- **Illinois:** Medical Library (OSF Saint Francis Medical Center, Peoria), **http://www.osfsaintfrancis.org/general/library/**

- **Kentucky:** Medical Library - Services for Patients, Families, Students & the Public (Central Baptist Hospital, Lexington), **http://www.centralbap.com/education/community/library.cfm**

- **Kentucky:** University of Kentucky - Health Information Library (Chandler Medical Center, Lexington), **http://www.mc.uky.edu/PatientEd/**

- **Louisiana:** Alton Ochsner Medical Foundation Library (Alton Ochsner Medical Foundation, New Orleans), **http://www.ochsner.org/library/**

- **Louisiana:** Louisiana State University Health Sciences Center Medical Library-Shreveport, **http://lib-sh.lsuhsc.edu/**

- **Maine:** Franklin Memorial Hospital Medical Library (Franklin Memorial Hospital, Farmington), **http://www.fchn.org/fmh/lib.htm**

- **Maine:** Gerrish-True Health Sciences Library (Central Maine Medical Center, Lewiston), **http://www.cmmc.org/library/library.html**

- **Maine:** Hadley Parrot Health Science Library (Eastern Maine Healthcare, Bangor), **http://www.emh.org/hll/hpl/guide.htm**

- **Maine:** Maine Medical Center Library (Maine Medical Center, Portland), **http://www.mmc.org/library/**

- **Maine:** Parkview Hospital (Brunswick), **http://www.parkviewhospital.org/**

- **Maine:** Southern Maine Medical Center Health Sciences Library (Southern Maine Medical Center, Biddeford), **http://www.smmc.org/services/service.php3?choice=10**

- **Maine:** Stephens Memorial Hospital's Health Information Library (Western Maine Health, Norway), **http://www.wmhcc.org/Library/**

- **Manitoba, Canada:** Consumer & Patient Health Information Service (University of Manitoba Libraries), **http://www.umanitoba.ca/libraries/units/health/reference/chis.html**

- **Manitoba, Canada:** J.W. Crane Memorial Library (Deer Lodge Centre, Winnipeg), **http://www.deerlodge.mb.ca/crane_library/about.asp**

- **Maryland:** Health Information Center at the Wheaton Regional Library (Montgomery County, Dept. of Public Libraries, Wheaton Regional Library), **http://www.mont.lib.md.us/healthinfo/hic.asp**

- **Massachusetts:** Baystate Medical Center Library (Baystate Health System), **http://www.baystatehealth.com/1024/**

- **Massachusetts:** Boston University Medical Center Alumni Medical Library (Boston University Medical Center), **http://med-libwww.bu.edu/library/lib.html**

- **Massachusetts:** Lowell General Hospital Health Sciences Library (Lowell General Hospital, Lowell), **http://www.lowellgeneral.org/library/HomePageLinks/WWW.htm**

- **Massachusetts:** Paul E. Woodard Health Sciences Library (New England Baptist Hospital, Boston), **http://www.nebh.org/health_lib.asp**

- **Massachusetts:** St. Luke's Hospital Health Sciences Library (St. Luke's Hospital, Southcoast Health System, New Bedford), **http://www.southcoast.org/library/**

- **Massachusetts:** Treadwell Library Consumer Health Reference Center (Massachusetts General Hospital), **http://www.mgh.harvard.edu/library/chrcindex.html**

- **Massachusetts:** UMass HealthNet (University of Massachusetts Medical School, Worchester), **http://healthnet.umassmed.edu/**

- **Michigan:** Botsford General Hospital Library - Consumer Health (Botsford General Hospital, Library & Internet Services), **http://www.botsfordlibrary.org/consumer.htm**

- **Michigan:** Helen DeRoy Medical Library (Providence Hospital and Medical Centers), **http://www.providence-hospital.org/library/**

- **Michigan:** Marquette General Hospital - Consumer Health Library (Marquette General Hospital, Health Information Center), **http://www.mgh.org/center.html**

- **Michigan:** Patient Education Resouce Center - University of Michigan Cancer Center (University of Michigan Comprehensive Cancer Center, Ann Arbor), **http://www.cancer.med.umich.edu/learn/leares.htm**

- **Michigan:** Sladen Library & Center for Health Information Resources - Consumer Health Information (Detroit), **http://www.henryford.com/body.cfm?id=39330**

- **Montana:** Center for Health Information (St. Patrick Hospital and Health Sciences Center, Missoula)

- **National:** Consumer Health Library Directory (Medical Library Association, Consumer and Patient Health Information Section), **http://caphis.mlanet.org/directory/index.html**

- **National:** National Network of Libraries of Medicine (National Library of Medicine) - provides library services for health professionals in the United States who do not have access to a medical library, **http://nnlm.gov/**

- **National:** NN/LM List of Libraries Serving the Public (National Network of Libraries of Medicine), **http://nnlm.gov/members/**

- **Nevada:** Health Science Library, West Charleston Library (Las Vegas-Clark County Library District, Las Vegas), **http://www.lvccld.org/special_collections/medical/index.htm**

- **New Hampshire:** Dartmouth Biomedical Libraries (Dartmouth College Library, Hanover), **http://www.dartmouth.edu/~biomed/resources.htmld/conshealth.htmld/**

- **New Jersey:** Consumer Health Library (Rahway Hospital, Rahway), **http://www.rahwayhospital.com/library.htm**

- **New Jersey:** Dr. Walter Phillips Health Sciences Library (Englewood Hospital and Medical Center, Englewood), **http://www.englewoodhospital.com/links/index.htm**

- **New Jersey:** Meland Foundation (Englewood Hospital and Medical Center, Englewood), **http://www.geocities.com/ResearchTriangle/9360/**

- **New York:** Choices in Health Information (New York Public Library) - NLM Consumer Pilot Project participant, **http://www.nypl.org/branch/health/links.html**

- **New York:** Health Information Center (Upstate Medical University, State University of New York, Syracuse), **http://www.upstate.edu/library/hic/**

- **New York:** Health Sciences Library (Long Island Jewish Medical Center, New Hyde Park), **http://www.lij.edu/library/library.html**

- **New York:** ViaHealth Medical Library (Rochester General Hospital), **http://www.nyam.org/library/**

- **Ohio:** Consumer Health Library (Akron General Medical Center, Medical & Consumer Health Library), **http://www.akrongeneral.org/hwlibrary.htm**

- **Oklahoma:** The Health Information Center at Saint Francis Hospital (Saint Francis Health System, Tulsa), **http://www.sfh-tulsa.com/services/healthinfo.asp**

- **Oregon:** Planetree Health Resource Center (Mid-Columbia Medical Center, The Dalles), **http://www.mcmc.net/phrc/**

- **Pennsylvania:** Community Health Information Library (Milton S. Hershey Medical Center, Hershey), **http://www.hmc.psu.edu/commhealth/**

- **Pennsylvania:** Community Health Resource Library (Geisinger Medical Center, Danville), **http://www.geisinger.edu/education/commlib.shtml**

- **Pennsylvania:** HealthInfo Library (Moses Taylor Hospital, Scranton), **http://www.mth.org/healthwellness.html**

- **Pennsylvania:** Hopwood Library (University of Pittsburgh, Health Sciences Library System, Pittsburgh), **http://www.hsls.pitt.edu/guides/chi/hopwood/index_html**

- **Pennsylvania:** Koop Community Health Information Center (College of Physicians of Philadelphia), **http://www.collphyphil.org/kooppg1.shtml**

- **Pennsylvania:** Learning Resources Center - Medical Library (Susquehanna Health System, Williamsport), **http://www.shscares.org/services/lrc/index.asp**

- **Pennsylvania:** Medical Library (UPMC Health System, Pittsburgh), **http://www.upmc.edu/passavant/library.htm**

- **Quebec, Canada:** Medical Library (Montreal General Hospital), **http://www.mghlib.mcgill.ca/**

- **South Dakota:** Rapid City Regional Hospital Medical Library (Rapid City Regional Hospital), **http://www.rcrh.org/Services/Library/Default.asp**

- **Texas:** Houston HealthWays (Houston Academy of Medicine-Texas Medical Center Library), **http://hhw.library.tmc.edu/**

- **Washington:** Community Health Library (Kittitas Valley Community Hospital), **http://www.kvch.com/**

- **Washington:** Southwest Washington Medical Center Library (Southwest Washington Medical Center, Vancouver), **http://www.swmedicalcenter.com/body.cfm?id=72**

ONLINE GLOSSARIES

The Internet provides access to a number of free-to-use medical dictionaries. The National Library of Medicine has compiled the following list of online dictionaries:

- ADAM Medical Encyclopedia (A.D.A.M., Inc.), comprehensive medical reference: **http://www.nlm.nih.gov/medlineplus/encyclopedia.html**

- MedicineNet.com Medical Dictionary (MedicineNet, Inc.): **http://www.medterms.com/Script/Main/hp.asp**

- Merriam-Webster Medical Dictionary (Inteli-Health, Inc.): **http://www.intelihealth.com/IH/**

- Multilingual Glossary of Technical and Popular Medical Terms in Eight European Languages (European Commission) - Danish, Dutch, English, French, German, Italian, Portuguese, and Spanish: **http://allserv.rug.ac.be/~rvdstich/eugloss/welcome.html**

- On-line Medical Dictionary (CancerWEB): **http://cancerweb.ncl.ac.uk/omd/**

- Rare Diseases Terms (Office of Rare Diseases): **http://ord.aspensys.com/asp/diseases/diseases.asp**

- Technology Glossary (National Library of Medicine) - Health Care Technology: **http://www.nlm.nih.gov/nichsr/ta101/ta10108.htm**

Beyond these, MEDLINEplus contains a very patient-friendly encyclopedia covering every aspect of medicine (licensed from A.D.A.M., Inc.). The ADAM Medical Encyclopedia can be accessed at **http://www.nlm.nih.gov/medlineplus/encyclopedia.html**. ADAM is also available on commercial Web sites such as drkoop.com (**http://www.drkoop.com/**) and Web MD (**http://my.webmd.com/adam/asset/adam_disease_articles/a_to_z/a**). The NIH suggests the following Web sites in the ADAM Medical Encyclopedia when searching for information on fetal alcohol syndrome:

- **Basic Guidelines for Fetal Alcohol Syndrome**

  Asd
  Web site: http://www.nlm.nih.gov/medlineplus/ency/article/000157.htm

  Fetal alcohol syndrome
  Web site: http://www.nlm.nih.gov/medlineplus/ency/article/000911.htm

  Vsd
  Web site: http://www.nlm.nih.gov/medlineplus/ency/article/001099.htm

- **Signs & Symptoms for Fetal Alcohol Syndrome**

  Agitation
  Web site: http://www.nlm.nih.gov/medlineplus/ency/article/003212.htm

  Epicanthal folds
  Web site: http://www.nlm.nih.gov/medlineplus/ency/article/003030.htm

Low nasal bridge
Web site: http://www.nlm.nih.gov/medlineplus/ency/article/003056.htm

Microcephaly
Web site: http://www.nlm.nih.gov/medlineplus/ency/article/003272.htm

Micrognathia
Web site: http://www.nlm.nih.gov/medlineplus/ency/article/003306.htm

Restless
Web site: http://www.nlm.nih.gov/medlineplus/ency/article/003212.htm

Simian crease
Web site: http://www.nlm.nih.gov/medlineplus/ency/article/003290.htm

Skeletal (limb) abnormalities
Web site: http://www.nlm.nih.gov/medlineplus/ency/article/003170.htm

- **Diagnostics and Tests for Fetal Alcohol Syndrome**

ECG
Web site: http://www.nlm.nih.gov/medlineplus/ency/article/003868.htm

Echocardiogram
Web site: http://www.nlm.nih.gov/medlineplus/ency/article/003869.htm

Toxicology screen
Web site: http://www.nlm.nih.gov/medlineplus/ency/article/003578.htm

Ultrasound
Web site: http://www.nlm.nih.gov/medlineplus/ency/article/003336.htm

Ultrasound, pregnancy
Web site: http://www.nlm.nih.gov/medlineplus/ency/article/003778.htm

- **Background Topics for Fetal Alcohol Syndrome**

Alcohol abuse
Web site: http://www.nlm.nih.gov/medlineplus/ency/article/001944.htm

Alcohol consumption
Web site: http://www.nlm.nih.gov/medlineplus/ency/article/001944.htm

Alcohol use
Web site: http://www.nlm.nih.gov/medlineplus/ency/article/001944.htm

Alcoholism - support group
Web site: http://www.nlm.nih.gov/medlineplus/ency/article/002199.htm

Head circumference
Web site: http://www.nlm.nih.gov/medlineplus/ency/article/002379.htm

Incidence
Web site: http://www.nlm.nih.gov/medlineplus/ency/article/002387.htm

Intrauterine
Web site: http://www.nlm.nih.gov/medlineplus/ency/article/002389.htm

Stillbirth
Web site: http://www.nlm.nih.gov/medlineplus/ency/article/002304.htm

Support groups
Web site: http://www.nlm.nih.gov/medlineplus/ency/article/002150.htm

Online Dictionary Directories

The following are additional online directories compiled by the National Library of Medicine, including a number of specialized medical dictionaries:

- Medical Dictionaries: Medical & Biological (World Health Organization): **http://www.who.int/hlt/virtuallibrary/English/diction.htm#Medical**

- MEL-Michigan Electronic Library List of Online Health and Medical Dictionaries (Michigan Electronic Library): **http://mel.lib.mi.us/health/health-dictionaries.html**

- Patient Education: Glossaries (DMOZ Open Directory Project): **http://dmoz.org/Health/Education/Patient_Education/Glossaries/**

- Web of Online Dictionaries (Bucknell University): **http://www.yourdictionary.com/diction5.html#medicine**

FETAL ALCOHOL SYNDROME DICTIONARY

The definitions below are derived from official public sources, including the National Institutes of Health [NIH] and the European Union [EU].

Abdomen: That portion of the body that lies between the thorax and the pelvis. [NIH]

Aberrant: Wandering or deviating from the usual or normal course. [EU]

Acceptor: A substance which, while normally not oxidized by oxygen or reduced by hydrogen, can be oxidized or reduced in presence of a substance which is itself undergoing oxidation or reduction. [NIH]

ACE: Angiotensin-coverting enzyme. A drug used to decrease pressure inside blood vessels. [NIH]

Acetaldehyde: A colorless, flammable liquid used in the manufacture of acetic acid, perfumes, and flavors. It is also an intermediate in the metabolism of alcohol. It has a general narcotic action and also causes irritation of mucous membranes. Large doses may cause death from respiratory paralysis. [NIH]

Acetylcholine: A neurotransmitter. Acetylcholine in vertebrates is the major transmitter at neuromuscular junctions, autonomic ganglia, parasympathetic effector junctions, a subset of sympathetic effector junctions, and at many sites in the central nervous system. It is generally not used as an administered drug because it is broken down very rapidly by cholinesterases, but it is useful in some ophthalmological applications. [NIH]

Action Potentials: The electric response of a nerve or muscle to its stimulation. [NIH]

Adaptability: Ability to develop some form of tolerance to conditions extremely different from those under which a living organism evolved. [NIH]

Adaptation: 1. The adjustment of an organism to its environment, or the process by which it enhances such fitness. 2. The normal ability of the eye to adjust itself to variations in the intensity of light; the adjustment to such variations. 3. The decline in the frequency of firing of a neuron, particularly of a receptor, under conditions of constant stimulation. 4. In dentistry, (a) the proper fitting of a denture, (b) the degree of proximity and interlocking of restorative material to a tooth preparation, (c) the exact adjustment of bands to teeth. 5. In microbiology, the adjustment of bacterial physiology to a new environment. [EU]

Adolescence: The period of life beginning with the appearance of secondary sex characteristics and terminating with the cessation of somatic growth. The years usually referred to as adolescence lie between 13 and 18 years of age. [NIH]

Adrenal Medulla: The inner part of the adrenal gland; it synthesizes, stores and releases catecholamines. [NIH]

Adrenergic: Activated by, characteristic of, or secreting epinephrine or substances with similar activity; the term is applied to those nerve fibres that liberate norepinephrine at a synapse when a nerve impulse passes, i.e., the sympathetic fibres. [EU]

Adverse Effect: An unwanted side effect of treatment. [NIH]

Afferent: Concerned with the transmission of neural impulse toward the central part of the nervous system. [NIH]

Affinity: 1. Inherent likeness or relationship. 2. A special attraction for a specific element, organ, or structure. 3. Chemical affinity; the force that binds atoms in molecules; the tendency of substances to combine by chemical reaction. 4. The strength of noncovalent chemical binding between two substances as measured by the dissociation constant of the complex. 5. In immunology, a thermodynamic expression of the strength of interaction between a single antigen-binding site and a single antigenic determinant (and thus of the stereochemical compatibility between them), most accurately applied to interactions among simple, uniform antigenic determinants such as haptens. Expressed as the association constant (K litres mole -1), which, owing to the heterogeneity of affinities in a population of antibody molecules of a given specificity, actually represents an average value (mean intrinsic association constant). 6. The reciprocal of the dissociation constant. [EU]

Agonist: In anatomy, a prime mover. In pharmacology, a drug that has affinity for and stimulates physiologic activity at cell receptors normally stimulated by naturally occurring substances. [EU]

Airway: A device for securing unobstructed passage of air into and out of the lungs during general anesthesia. [NIH]

Airway Obstruction: Any hindrance to the passage of air into and out of the lungs. [NIH]

Alcohol Dehydrogenase: An enzyme that catalyzes reversibly the final step of alcoholic fermentation by reducing an aldehyde to an alcohol. In the case of ethanol, acetaldehyde is reduced to ethanol in the presence of NADH and hydrogen. The enzyme is a zinc protein which acts on primary and secondary alcohols or hemiacetals. EC 1.1.1.1. [NIH]

Aldehyde Dehydrogenase: An enzyme that oxidizes an aldehyde in the presence of NAD+ and water to an acid and NADH. EC 1.2.1.3. Before 1978, it was classified as EC 1.1.1.70. [NIH]

Alexia: The inability to recognize or comprehend written or printed words. [NIH]

Algorithms: A procedure consisting of a sequence of algebraic formulas and/or logical steps to calculate or determine a given task. [NIH]

Alkaline: Having the reactions of an alkali. [EU]

Alkaloid: A member of a large group of chemicals that are made by plants and have nitrogen in them. Some alkaloids have been shown to work against cancer. [NIH]

Allergen: An antigenic substance capable of producing immediate-type hypersensitivity (allergy). [EU]

Alpha-fetoprotein: AFP. A protein normally produced by a developing fetus. AFP levels are usually undetectable in the blood of healthy nonpregnant adults. An elevated level of AFP suggests the presence of either a primary liver cancer or germ cell tumor. [NIH]

Alternative medicine: Practices not generally recognized by the medical community as standard or conventional medical approaches and used instead of standard treatments. Alternative medicine includes the taking of dietary supplements, megadose vitamins, and herbal preparations; the drinking of special teas; and practices such as massage therapy, magnet therapy, spiritual healing, and meditation. [NIH]

Alveoli: Tiny air sacs at the end of the bronchioles in the lungs. [NIH]

Amino Acid Sequence: The order of amino acids as they occur in a polypeptide chain. This is referred to as the primary structure of proteins. It is of fundamental importance in determining protein conformation. [NIH]

Amino Acids: Organic compounds that generally contain an amino (-NH2) and a carboxyl (-COOH) group. Twenty alpha-amino acids are the subunits which are polymerized to form proteins. [NIH]

Amino Acids: Organic compounds that generally contain an amino (-NH2) and a carboxyl (-COOH) group. Twenty alpha-amino acids are the subunits which are polymerized to form proteins. [NIH]

Amphetamines: Analogs or derivatives of amphetamine. Many are sympathomimetics and central nervous system stimulators causing excitation, vasopression, bronchodilation, and to varying degrees, anorexia, analepsis, nasal decongestion, and some smooth muscle relaxation. [NIH]

Amplification: The production of additional copies of a chromosomal DNA sequence, found as either intrachromosomal or extrachromosomal DNA. [NIH]

Ampulla: A sac-like enlargement of a canal or duct. [NIH]

Anaesthesia: Loss of feeling or sensation. Although the term is used for loss of tactile sensibility, or of any of the other senses, it is applied especially to loss of the sensation of pain, as it is induced to permit performance of surgery or other painful procedures. [EU]

Anal: Having to do with the anus, which is the posterior opening of the large bowel. [NIH]

Analgesic: An agent that alleviates pain without causing loss of consciousness. [EU]

Analogous: Resembling or similar in some respects, as in function or appearance, but not in origin or development;. [EU]

Anatomical: Pertaining to anatomy, or to the structure of the organism. [EU]

Anesthesia: A state characterized by loss of feeling or sensation. This depression of nerve function is usually the result of pharmacologic action and is induced to allow performance of surgery or other painful procedures. [NIH]

Animal model: An animal with a disease either the same as or like a disease in humans. Animal models are used to study the development and progression of diseases and to test new treatments before they are given to humans. Animals with transplanted human cancers or other tissues are called xenograft models. [NIH]

Anomalies: Birth defects; abnormalities. [NIH]

Anophthalmia: Absence of an eye or eyes in the newborn due to failure of development of the optic cup or to disappearance of the eyes after partial development. [NIH]

Antagonism: Interference with, or inhibition of, the growth of a living organism by another living organism, due either to creation of unfavorable conditions (e. g. exhaustion of food supplies) or to production of a specific antibiotic substance (e. g. penicillin). [NIH]

Anthropometry: The technique that deals with the measurement of the size, weight, and proportions of the human or other primate body. [NIH]

Antibacterial: A substance that destroys bacteria or suppresses their growth or reproduction. [EU]

Antibiotic: A drug used to treat infections caused by bacteria and other microorganisms. [NIH]

Antibodies: Immunoglobulin molecules having a specific amino acid sequence by virtue of which they interact only with the antigen that induced their synthesis in cells of the lymphoid series (especially plasma cells), or with an antigen closely related to it. [NIH]

Antibody: A type of protein made by certain white blood cells in response to a foreign substance (antigen). Each antibody can bind to only a specific antigen. The purpose of this binding is to help destroy the antigen. Antibodies can work in several ways, depending on the nature of the antigen. Some antibodies destroy antigens directly. Others make it easier for white blood cells to destroy the antigen. [NIH]

Anticoagulant: A drug that helps prevent blood clots from forming. Also called a blood thinner. [NIH]

Antigen: Any substance which is capable, under appropriate conditions, of inducing a specific immune response and of reacting with the products of that response, that is, with specific antibody or specifically sensitized T-lymphocytes, or both. Antigens may be soluble substances, such as toxins and foreign proteins, or particulate, such as bacteria and tissue cells; however, only the portion of the protein or polysaccharide molecule known as the antigenic determinant (q.v.) combines with antibody or a specific receptor on a lymphocyte. Abbreviated Ag. [EU]

Anti-inflammatory: Having to do with reducing inflammation. [NIH]

Antioxidant: A substance that prevents damage caused by free radicals. Free radicals are highly reactive chemicals that often contain oxygen. They are produced when molecules are split to give products that have unpaired electrons. This process is called oxidation. [NIH]

Anus: The opening of the rectum to the outside of the body. [NIH]

Apolipoproteins: The protein components of lipoproteins which remain after the lipids to which the proteins are bound have been removed. They play an important role in lipid transport and metabolism. [NIH]

Apoptosis: One of the two mechanisms by which cell death occurs (the other being the pathological process of necrosis). Apoptosis is the mechanism responsible for the physiological deletion of cells and appears to be intrinsically programmed. It is characterized by distinctive morphologic changes in the nucleus and cytoplasm, chromatin cleavage at regularly spaced sites, and the endonucleolytic cleavage of genomic DNA (DNA fragmentation) at internucleosomal sites. This mode of cell death serves as a balance to mitosis in regulating the size of animal tissues and in mediating pathologic processes associated with tumor growth. [NIH]

Applicability: A list of the commodities to which the candidate method can be applied as presented or with minor modifications. [NIH]

Aqueous: Having to do with water. [NIH]

Arachidonic Acid: An unsaturated, essential fatty acid. It is found in animal and human fat as well as in the liver, brain, and glandular organs, and is a constituent of animal phosphatides. It is formed by the synthesis from dietary linoleic acid and is a precursor in the biosynthesis of prostaglandins, thromboxanes, and leukotrienes. [NIH]

Arginine: An essential amino acid that is physiologically active in the L-form. [NIH]

Aromatic: Having a spicy odour. [EU]

Arterial: Pertaining to an artery or to the arteries. [EU]

Arteries: The vessels carrying blood away from the heart. [NIH]

Aspartate: A synthetic amino acid. [NIH]

Aspiration: The act of inhaling. [NIH]

Assay: Determination of the amount of a particular constituent of a mixture, or of the biological or pharmacological potency of a drug. [EU]

Astrocytes: The largest and most numerous neuroglial cells in the brain and spinal cord. Astrocytes (from "star" cells) are irregularly shaped with many long processes, including those with "end feet" which form the glial (limiting) membrane and directly and indirectly contribute to the blood brain barrier. They regulate the extracellular ionic and chemical environment, and "reactive astrocytes" (along with microglia) respond to injury. Astrocytes have high- affinity transmitter uptake systems, voltage-dependent and transmitter-gated ion channels, and can release transmitter, but their role in signaling (as in many other functions) is not well understood. [NIH]

Ataxia: Impairment of the ability to perform smoothly coordinated voluntary movements. This condition may affect the limbs, trunk, eyes, pharnyx, larnyx, and other structures.

Ataxia may result from impaired sensory or motor function. Sensory ataxia may result from posterior column injury or peripheral nerve diseases. Motor ataxia may be associated with cerebellar diseases; cerebral cortex diseases; thalamic diseases; basal ganglia diseases; injury to the red nucleus; and other conditions. [NIH]

Atrial: Pertaining to an atrium. [EU]

Atrioventricular: Pertaining to an atrium of the heart and to a ventricle. [EU]

Atrium: A chamber; used in anatomical nomenclature to designate a chamber affording entrance to another structure or organ. Usually used alone to designate an atrium of the heart. [EU]

Attenuated: Strain with weakened or reduced virulence. [NIH]

Auditory: Pertaining to the sense of hearing. [EU]

Autoantibodies: Antibodies that react with self-antigens (autoantigens) of the organism that produced them. [NIH]

Autoantigens: Endogenous tissue constituents that have the ability to interact with autoantibodies and cause an immune response. [NIH]

Autonomic: Self-controlling; functionally independent. [EU]

Autonomic Nervous System: The enteric, parasympathetic, and sympathetic nervous systems taken together. Generally speaking, the autonomic nervous system regulates the internal environment during both peaceful activity and physical or emotional stress. Autonomic activity is controlled and integrated by the central nervous system, especially the hypothalamus and the solitary nucleus, which receive information relayed from visceral afferents; these and related central and sensory structures are sometimes (but not here) considered to be part of the autonomic nervous system itself. [NIH]

Axonal: Condition associated with metabolic derangement of the entire neuron and is manifest by degeneration of the distal portion of the nerve fiber. [NIH]

Axons: Nerve fibers that are capable of rapidly conducting impulses away from the neuron cell body. [NIH]

Bacteria: Unicellular prokaryotic microorganisms which generally possess rigid cell walls, multiply by cell division, and exhibit three principal forms: round or coccal, rodlike or bacillary, and spiral or spirochetal. [NIH]

Bactericidal: Substance lethal to bacteria; substance capable of killing bacteria. [NIH]

Basal Ganglia: Large subcortical nuclear masses derived from the telencephalon and located in the basal regions of the cerebral hemispheres. [NIH]

Basal Ganglia Diseases: Diseases of the basal ganglia including the putamen; globus pallidus; claustrum; amygdala; and caudate nucleus. Dyskinesias (most notably involuntary movements and alterations of the rate of movement) represent the primary clinical manifestations of these disorders. Common etiologies include cerebrovascular disease; neurodegenerative diseases; and craniocerebral trauma. [NIH]

Base: In chemistry, the nonacid part of a salt; a substance that combines with acids to form salts; a substance that dissociates to give hydroxide ions in aqueous solutions; a substance whose molecule or ion can combine with a proton (hydrogen ion); a substance capable of donating a pair of electrons (to an acid) for the formation of a coordinate covalent bond. [EU]

Behavioral Symptoms: Observable manifestions of impaired psychological functioning. [NIH]

Beta-Endorphin: A peptide consisting of amino acid sequence 61-91 of the endogenous pituitary hormone beta-lipotropin. The first four amino acids show a common tetrapeptide sequence with methionine- and leucine enkephalin. The compound shows opiate-like activity. Injection of beta-endorphin induces a profound analgesia of the whole body for several hours. This action is reversed after administration of naloxone. [NIH]

Bilateral: Affecting both the right and left side of body. [NIH]

Bile: An emulsifying agent produced in the liver and secreted into the duodenum. Its composition includes bile acids and salts, cholesterol, and electrolytes. It aids digestion of fats in the duodenum. [NIH]

Bile Ducts: Tubes that carry bile from the liver to the gallbladder for storage and to the small intestine for use in digestion. [NIH]

Biliary: Having to do with the liver, bile ducts, and/or gallbladder. [NIH]

Biliary Atresia: Atresia of the biliary tract, most commonly of the extrahepatic bile ducts. [NIH]

Biliary Tract: The gallbladder and its ducts. [NIH]

Binding Sites: The reactive parts of a macromolecule that directly participate in its specific combination with another molecule. [NIH]

Bioassay: Determination of the relative effective strength of a substance (as a vitamin, hormone, or drug) by comparing its effect on a test organism with that of a standard preparation. [NIH]

Biochemical: Relating to biochemistry; characterized by, produced by, or involving chemical reactions in living organisms. [EU]

Biological therapy: Treatment to stimulate or restore the ability of the immune system to fight infection and disease. Also used to lessen side effects that may be caused by some cancer treatments. Also known as immunotherapy, biotherapy, or biological response modifier (BRM) therapy. [NIH]

Biomarkers: Substances sometimes found in an increased amount in the blood, other body fluids, or tissues and that may suggest the presence of some types of cancer. Biomarkers include CA 125 (ovarian cancer), CA 15-3 (breast cancer), CEA (ovarian, lung, breast, pancreas, and GI tract cancers), and PSA (prostate cancer). Also called tumor markers. [NIH]

Biosynthesis: The building up of a chemical compound in the physiologic processes of a living organism. [EU]

Biotechnology: Body of knowledge related to the use of organisms, cells or cell-derived constituents for the purpose of developing products which are technically, scientifically and clinically useful. Alteration of biologic function at the molecular level (i.e., genetic engineering) is a central focus; laboratory methods used include transfection and cloning technologies, sequence and structure analysis algorithms, computer databases, and gene and protein structure function analysis and prediction. [NIH]

Blastocyst: The mammalian embryo in the post-morula stage in which a fluid-filled cavity, enclosed primarily by trophoblast, contains an inner cell mass which becomes the embryonic disc. [NIH]

Blood Coagulation: The process of the interaction of blood coagulation factors that results in an insoluble fibrin clot. [NIH]

Blood Platelets: Non-nucleated disk-shaped cells formed in the megakaryocyte and found in the blood of all mammals. They are mainly involved in blood coagulation. [NIH]

Blood pressure: The pressure of blood against the walls of a blood vessel or heart chamber. Unless there is reference to another location, such as the pulmonary artery or one of the heart chambers, it refers to the pressure in the systemic arteries, as measured, for example, in the forearm. [NIH]

Blood vessel: A tube in the body through which blood circulates. Blood vessels include a network of arteries, arterioles, capillaries, venules, and veins. [NIH]

Blot: To transfer DNA, RNA, or proteins to an immobilizing matrix such as nitrocellulose. [NIH]

Body Fluids: Liquid components of living organisms. [NIH]

Bone Marrow: The soft tissue filling the cavities of bones. Bone marrow exists in two types, yellow and red. Yellow marrow is found in the large cavities of large bones and consists mostly of fat cells and a few primitive blood cells. Red marrow is a hematopoietic tissue and is the site of production of erythrocytes and granular leukocytes. Bone marrow is made up of a framework of connective tissue containing branching fibers with the frame being filled with marrow cells. [NIH]

Bowel: The long tube-shaped organ in the abdomen that completes the process of digestion. There is both a small and a large bowel. Also called the intestine. [NIH]

Bradykinin: A nonapeptide messenger that is enzymatically produced from kallidin in the blood where it is a potent but short-lived agent of arteriolar dilation and increased capillary permeability. Bradykinin is also released from mast cells during asthma attacks, from gut walls as a gastrointestinal vasodilator, from damaged tissues as a pain signal, and may be a neurotransmitter. [NIH]

Brain Stem: The part of the brain that connects the cerebral hemispheres with the spinal cord. It consists of the mesencephalon, pons, and medulla oblongata. [NIH]

Branch: Most commonly used for branches of nerves, but applied also to other structures. [NIH]

Breeding: The science or art of changing the constitution of a population of plants or animals through sexual reproduction. [NIH]

Butyric Acid: A four carbon acid, CH3CH2CH2COOH, with an unpleasant odor that occurs in butter and animal fat as the glycerol ester. [NIH]

Calcineurin: A calcium- and calmodulin-binding protein present in highest concentrations in the central nervous system. Calcineurin is composed of two subunits. A catalytic subunit, calcineurin A, and a regulatory subunit, calcineurin B, with molecular weights of about 60 kD and 19 kD, respectively. Calcineurin has been shown to dephosphorylate a number of phosphoproteins including histones, myosin light chain, and the regulatory subunit of cAMP-dependent protein kinase. It is involved in the regulation of signal transduction and is the target of an important class of immunophilin-immunosuppressive drug complexes in T-lymphocytes that act by inhibiting T-cell activation. EC 3.1.3.-. [NIH]

Calcium: A basic element found in nearly all organized tissues. It is a member of the alkaline earth family of metals with the atomic symbol Ca, atomic number 20, and atomic weight 40. Calcium is the most abundant mineral in the body and combines with phosphorus to form calcium phosphate in the bones and teeth. It is essential for the normal functioning of nerves and muscles and plays a role in blood coagulation (as factor IV) and in many enzymatic processes. [NIH]

Calcium Signaling: Signal transduction mechanisms whereby calcium mobilization (from outside the cell or from intracellular storage pools) to the cytoplasm is triggered by external stimuli. Calcium signals are often seen to propagate as waves, oscillations, spikes or puffs. The calcium acts as an intracellular messenger by activating calcium-responsive proteins. [NIH]

Callus: A callosity or hard, thick skin; the bone-like reparative substance that is formed round the edges and fragments of broken bone. [NIH]

Calmodulin: A heat-stable, low-molecular-weight activator protein found mainly in the brain and heart. The binding of calcium ions to this protein allows this protein to bind to cyclic nucleotide phosphodiesterases and to adenyl cyclase with subsequent activation. Thereby this protein modulates cyclic AMP and cyclic GMP levels. [NIH]

Carbon Dioxide: A colorless, odorless gas that can be formed by the body and is necessary for the respiration cycle of plants and animals. [NIH]

Carcinogenesis: The process by which normal cells are transformed into cancer cells. [NIH]

Carcinogenic: Producing carcinoma. [EU]

Carcinogens: Substances that increase the risk of neoplasms in humans or animals. Both genotoxic chemicals, which affect DNA directly, and nongenotoxic chemicals, which induce neoplasms by other mechanism, are included. [NIH]

Cardiac: Having to do with the heart. [NIH]

Cardiovascular: Having to do with the heart and blood vessels. [NIH]

Cardiovascular System: The heart and the blood vessels by which blood is pumped and circulated through the body. [NIH]

Carotene: The general name for a group of pigments found in green, yellow, and leafy vegetables, and yellow fruits. The pigments are fat-soluble, unsaturated aliphatic hydrocarbons functioning as provitamins and are converted to vitamin A through enzymatic processes in the intestinal wall. [NIH]

Case report: A detailed report of the diagnosis, treatment, and follow-up of an individual patient. Case reports also contain some demographic information about the patient (for example, age, gender, ethnic origin). [NIH]

Case series: A group or series of case reports involving patients who were given similar treatment. Reports of case series usually contain detailed information about the individual patients. This includes demographic information (for example, age, gender, ethnic origin) and information on diagnosis, treatment, response to treatment, and follow-up after treatment. [NIH]

Caspase: Enzyme released by the cell at a crucial stage in apoptosis in order to shred all cellular proteins. [NIH]

Catecholamine: A group of chemical substances manufactured by the adrenal medulla and secreted during physiological stress. [NIH]

Catheterization: Use or insertion of a tubular device into a duct, blood vessel, hollow organ, or body cavity for injecting or withdrawing fluids for diagnostic or therapeutic purposes. It differs from intubation in that the tube here is used to restore or maintain patency in obstructions. [NIH]

Caudal: Denoting a position more toward the cauda, or tail, than some specified point of reference; same as inferior, in human anatomy. [EU]

Causal: Pertaining to a cause; directed against a cause. [EU]

Cell: The individual unit that makes up all of the tissues of the body. All living things are made up of one or more cells. [NIH]

Cell Adhesion: Adherence of cells to surfaces or to other cells. [NIH]

Cell Adhesion Molecules: Surface ligands, usually glycoproteins, that mediate cell-to-cell adhesion. Their functions include the assembly and interconnection of various vertebrate systems, as well as maintenance of tissue integration, wound healing, morphogenic movements, cellular migrations, and metastasis. [NIH]

Cell Count: A count of the number of cells of a specific kind, usually measured per unit volume of sample. [NIH]

Cell Death: The termination of the cell's ability to carry out vital functions such as metabolism, growth, reproduction, responsiveness, and adaptability. [NIH]

Cell Differentiation: Progressive restriction of the developmental potential and increasing specialization of function which takes place during the development of the embryo and leads to the formation of specialized cells, tissues, and organs. [NIH]

Cell Division: The fission of a cell. [NIH]

Cell membrane: Cell membrane = plasma membrane. The structure enveloping a cell, enclosing the cytoplasm, and forming a selective permeability barrier; it consists of lipids, proteins, and some carbohydrates, the lipids thought to form a bilayer in which integral proteins are embedded to varying degrees. [EU]

Cell Movement: The movement of cells from one location to another. [NIH]

Cell proliferation: An increase in the number of cells as a result of cell growth and cell division. [NIH]

Cell Size: The physical dimensions of a cell. It refers mainly to changes in dimensions correlated with physiological or pathological changes in cells. [NIH]

Cell Survival: The span of viability of a cell characterized by the capacity to perform certain functions such as metabolism, growth, reproduction, some form of responsiveness, and adaptability. [NIH]

Central Nervous System: The main information-processing organs of the nervous system, consisting of the brain, spinal cord, and meninges. [NIH]

Cerebellar: Pertaining to the cerebellum. [EU]

Cerebellum: Part of the metencephalon that lies in the posterior cranial fossa behind the brain stem. It is concerned with the coordination of movement. [NIH]

Cerebral: Of or pertaining of the cerebrum or the brain. [EU]

Cerebrum: The largest part of the brain. It is divided into two hemispheres, or halves, called the cerebral hemispheres. The cerebrum controls muscle functions of the body and also controls speech, emotions, reading, writing, and learning. [NIH]

Character: In current usage, approximately equivalent to personality. The sum of the relatively fixed personality traits and habitual modes of response of an individual. [NIH]

Child Psychiatry: The medical science that deals with the origin, diagnosis, prevention, and treatment of mental disorders in children. [NIH]

Cholesterol: The principal sterol of all higher animals, distributed in body tissues, especially the brain and spinal cord, and in animal fats and oils. [NIH]

Cholesterol Esters: Fatty acid esters of cholesterol which constitute about two-thirds of the cholesterol in the plasma. The accumulation of cholesterol esters in the arterial intima is a characteristic feature of atherosclerosis. [NIH]

Chromatin: The material of chromosomes. It is a complex of DNA, histones, and nonhistone proteins (chromosomal proteins, non-histone) found within the nucleus of a cell. [NIH]

Chromosomal: Pertaining to chromosomes. [EU]

Chromosome: Part of a cell that contains genetic information. Except for sperm and eggs, all human cells contain 46 chromosomes. [NIH]

Chromosome Abnormalities: Defects in the structure or number of chromosomes resulting in structural aberrations or manifesting as disease. [NIH]

Chronic: A disease or condition that persists or progresses over a long period of time. [NIH]

Chylomicrons: A class of lipoproteins that carry dietary cholesterol and triglycerides from the small intestines to the tissues. [NIH]

Circadian: Repeated more or less daily, i. e. on a 23- to 25-hour cycle. [NIH]

Circadian Rhythm: The regular recurrence, in cycles of about 24 hours, of biological processes or activities, such as sensitivity to drugs and stimuli, hormone secretion, sleeping, feeding, etc. This rhythm seems to be set by a 'biological clock' which seems to be set by recurring daylight and darkness. [NIH]

CIS: Cancer Information Service. The CIS is the National Cancer Institute's link to the public, interpreting and explaining research findings in a clear and understandable manner, and providing personalized responses to specific questions about cancer. Access the CIS by calling 1-800-4-CANCER, or by using the Web site at http://cis.nci.nih.gov. [NIH]

Clamp: A u-shaped steel rod used with a pin or wire for skeletal traction in the treatment of certain fractures. [NIH]

Cleft Palate: Congenital fissure of the soft and/or hard palate, due to faulty fusion. [NIH]

Clinical Medicine: The study and practice of medicine by direct examination of the patient. [NIH]

Clinical study: A research study in which patients receive treatment in a clinic or other medical facility. Reports of clinical studies can contain results for single patients (case reports) or many patients (case series or clinical trials). [NIH]

Clinical trial: A research study that tests how well new medical treatments or other interventions work in people. Each study is designed to test new methods of screening, prevention, diagnosis, or treatment of a disease. [NIH]

Cloning: The production of a number of genetically identical individuals; in genetic engineering, a process for the efficient replication of a great number of identical DNA molecules. [NIH]

Coca: Any of several South American shrubs of the Erythroxylon genus (and family) that yield cocaine; the leaves are chewed with alum for CNS stimulation. [NIH]

Cocaine: An alkaloid ester extracted from the leaves of plants including coca. It is a local anesthetic and vasoconstrictor and is clinically used for that purpose, particularly in the eye, ear, nose, and throat. It also has powerful central nervous system effects similar to the amphetamines and is a drug of abuse. Cocaine, like amphetamines, acts by multiple mechanisms on brain catecholaminergic neurons; the mechanism of its reinforcing effects is thought to involve inhibition of dopamine uptake. [NIH]

Cochlea: The part of the internal ear that is concerned with hearing. It forms the anterior part of the labyrinth, is conical, and is placed almost horizontally anterior to the vestibule. [NIH]

Cofactor: A substance, microorganism or environmental factor that activates or enhances the action of another entity such as a disease-causing agent. [NIH]

Cognition: Intellectual or mental process whereby an organism becomes aware of or obtains knowledge. [NIH]

Cohort Studies: Studies in which subsets of a defined population are identified. These groups may or may not be exposed to factors hypothesized to influence the probability of the occurrence of a particular disease or other outcome. Cohorts are defined populations which, as a whole, are followed in an attempt to determine distinguishing subgroup characteristics. [NIH]

Collagen: A polypeptide substance comprising about one third of the total protein in mammalian organisms. It is the main constituent of skin, connective tissue, and the organic substance of bones and teeth. Different forms of collagen are produced in the body but all consist of three alpha-polypeptide chains arranged in a triple helix. Collagen is differentiated from other fibrous proteins, such as elastin, by the content of proline, hydroxyproline, and hydroxylysine; by the absence of tryptophan; and particularly by the high content of polar groups which are responsible for its swelling properties. [NIH]

Colloidal: Of the nature of a colloid. [EU]

Coloboma: Congenital anomaly in which some of the structures of the eye are absent due to incomplete fusion of the fetal intraocular fissure during gestation. [NIH]

Complement: A term originally used to refer to the heat-labile factor in serum that causes immune cytolysis, the lysis of antibody-coated cells, and now referring to the entire functionally related system comprising at least 20 distinct serum proteins that is the effector not only of immune cytolysis but also of other biologic functions. Complement activation occurs by two different sequences, the classic and alternative pathways. The proteins of the classic pathway are termed 'components of complement' and are designated by the symbols C1 through C9. C1 is a calcium-dependent complex of three distinct proteins C1q, C1r and C1s. The proteins of the alternative pathway (collectively referred to as the properdin system) and complement regulatory proteins are known by semisystematic or trivial names. Fragments resulting from proteolytic cleavage of complement proteins are designated with lower-case letter suffixes, e.g., C3a. Inactivated fragments may be designated with the suffix 'i', e.g. C3bi. Activated components or complexes with biological activity are designated by a bar over the symbol e.g. C1 or C4b,2a. The classic pathway is activated by the binding of C1 to classic pathway activators, primarily antigen-antibody complexes containing IgM, IgG1, IgG3; C1q binds to a single IgM molecule or two adjacent IgG molecules. The alternative pathway can be activated by IgA immune complexes and also by nonimmunologic materials including bacterial endotoxins, microbial polysaccharides, and cell walls. Activation of the classic pathway triggers an enzymatic cascade involving C1, C4, C2 and C3; activation of the alternative pathway triggers a cascade involving C3 and factors B, D and P. Both result in the cleavage of C5 and the formation of the membrane attack complex. Complement activation also results in the formation of many biologically active complement fragments that act as anaphylatoxins, opsonins, or chemotactic factors. [EU]

Complementary and alternative medicine: CAM. Forms of treatment that are used in addition to (complementary) or instead of (alternative) standard treatments. These practices are not considered standard medical approaches. CAM includes dietary supplements, megadose vitamins, herbal preparations, special teas, massage therapy, magnet therapy, spiritual healing, and meditation. [NIH]

Complementary medicine: Practices not generally recognized by the medical community as standard or conventional medical approaches and used to enhance or complement the standard treatments. Complementary medicine includes the taking of dietary supplements, megadose vitamins, and herbal preparations; the drinking of special teas; and practices such as massage therapy, magnet therapy, spiritual healing, and meditation. [NIH]

Computational Biology: A field of biology concerned with the development of techniques for the collection and manipulation of biological data, and the use of such data to make biological discoveries or predictions. This field encompasses all computational methods and theories applicable to molecular biology and areas of computer-based techniques for solving biological problems including manipulation of models and datasets. [NIH]

Computed tomography: CT scan. A series of detailed pictures of areas inside the body, taken from different angles; the pictures are created by a computer linked to an x-ray machine. Also called computerized tomography and computerized axial tomography (CAT) scan. [NIH]

Computerized axial tomography: A series of detailed pictures of areas inside the body, taken from different angles; the pictures are created by a computer linked to an x-ray machine. Also called CAT scan, computed tomography (CT scan), or computerized tomography. [NIH]

Computerized tomography: A series of detailed pictures of areas inside the body, taken from different angles; the pictures are created by a computer linked to an x-ray machine. Also called computerized axial tomography (CAT) scan and computed tomography (CT scan). [NIH]

Conception: The onset of pregnancy, marked by implantation of the blastocyst; the formation of a viable zygote. [EU]

Conduction: The transfer of sound waves, heat, nervous impulses, or electricity. [EU]

Cones: One type of specialized light-sensitive cells (photoreceptors) in the retina that provide sharp central vision and color vision. [NIH]

Conjunctiva: The mucous membrane that lines the inner surface of the eyelids and the anterior part of the sclera. [NIH]

Connective Tissue: Tissue that supports and binds other tissues. It consists of connective tissue cells embedded in a large amount of extracellular matrix. [NIH]

Connective Tissue: Tissue that supports and binds other tissues. It consists of connective tissue cells embedded in a large amount of extracellular matrix. [NIH]

Consciousness: Sense of awareness of self and of the environment. [NIH]

Constriction: The act of constricting. [NIH]

Consumption: Pulmonary tuberculosis. [NIH]

Continuum: An area over which the vegetation or animal population is of constantly changing composition so that homogeneous, separate communities cannot be distinguished. [NIH]

Contraindications: Any factor or sign that it is unwise to pursue a certain kind of action or treatment, e. g. giving a general anesthetic to a person with pneumonia. [NIH]

Control group: In a clinical trial, the group that does not receive the new treatment being studied. This group is compared to the group that receives the new treatment, to see if the new treatment works. [NIH]

Coordination: Muscular or motor regulation or the harmonious cooperation of muscles or groups of muscles, in a complex action or series of actions. [NIH]

Cor: The muscular organ that maintains the circulation of the blood. c. adiposum a heart that has undergone fatty degeneration or that has an accumulation of fat around it; called also fat or fatty, heart. c. arteriosum the left side of the heart, so called because it contains oxygenated (arterial) blood. c. biloculare a congenital anomaly characterized by failure of formation of the atrial and ventricular septums, the heart having only two chambers, a single atrium and a single ventricle, and a common atrioventricular valve. c. bovinum (L. 'ox heart') a greatly enlarged heart due to a hypertrophied left ventricle; called also c. taurinum and bucardia. c. dextrum (L. 'right heart') the right atrium and ventricle. c. hirsutum, c. villosum. c. mobile (obs.) an abnormally movable heart. c. pendulum a heart so movable that it seems to be hanging by the great blood vessels. c. pseudotriloculare biatriatum a congenital cardiac anomaly in which the heart functions as a three-chambered heart because of tricuspid atresia, the right ventricle being extremely small or rudimentary and the right atrium greatly dilated. Blood passes from the right to the left atrium and thence disease due to pulmonary hypertension secondary to disease of the lung, or its blood vessels, with hypertrophy of the right ventricle. [EU]

Coronary: Encircling in the manner of a crown; a term applied to vessels; nerves, ligaments, etc. The term usually denotes the arteries that supply the heart muscle and, by extension, a pathologic involvement of them. [EU]

Coronary Thrombosis: Presence of a thrombus in a coronary artery, often causing a myocardial infarction. [NIH]

Corpus: The body of the uterus. [NIH]

Corpus Callosum: Broad plate of dense myelinated fibers that reciprocally interconnect regions of the cortex in all lobes with corresponding regions of the opposite hemisphere. The corpus callosum is located deep in the longitudinal fissure. [NIH]

Cortex: The outer layer of an organ or other body structure, as distinguished from the internal substance. [EU]

Cortical: Pertaining to or of the nature of a cortex or bark. [EU]

Cortices: The outer layer of an organ; used especially of the cerebrum and cerebellum. [NIH]

Corticosteroids: Hormones that have antitumor activity in lymphomas and lymphoid leukemias; in addition, corticosteroids (steroids) may be used for hormone replacement and for the management of some of the complications of cancer and its treatment. [NIH]

Cranial: Pertaining to the cranium, or to the anterior (in animals) or superior (in humans) end of the body. [EU]

Craniofacial Abnormalities: Congenital structural deformities, malformations, or other abnormalities of the cranium and facial bones. [NIH]

Cross-Sectional Studies: Studies in which the presence or absence of disease or other health-related variables are determined in each member of the study population or in a representative sample at one particular time. This contrasts with longitudinal studies which are followed over a period of time. [NIH]

Cues: Signals for an action; that specific portion of a perceptual field or pattern of stimuli to which a subject has learned to respond. [NIH]

Curative: Tending to overcome disease and promote recovery. [EU]

Cyclic: Pertaining to or occurring in a cycle or cycles; the term is applied to chemical compounds that contain a ring of atoms in the nucleus. [EU]

Cyclopia: Elements of the two eyes fused into one median eye in the center of the forehead of a fetal monster. [NIH]

Cytokine: Small but highly potent protein that modulates the activity of many cell types, including T and B cells. [NIH]

Cytoplasm: The protoplasm of a cell exclusive of that of the nucleus; it consists of a continuous aqueous solution (cytosol) and the organelles and inclusions suspended in it (phaneroplasm), and is the site of most of the chemical activities of the cell. [EU]

Cytoskeleton: The network of filaments, tubules, and interconnecting filamentous bridges which give shape, structure, and organization to the cytoplasm. [NIH]

Cytotoxic: Cell-killing. [NIH]

Data Collection: Systematic gathering of data for a particular purpose from various sources, including questionnaires, interviews, observation, existing records, and electronic devices. The process is usually preliminary to statistical analysis of the data. [NIH]

Databases, Bibliographic: Extensive collections, reputedly complete, of references and citations to books, articles, publications, etc., generally on a single subject or specialized subject area. Databases can operate through automated files, libraries, or computer disks.

The concept should be differentiated from factual databases which is used for collections of data and facts apart from bibliographic references to them. [NIH]

Day Care: Institutional health care of patients during the day. The patients return home at night. [NIH]

Decidua: The epithelial lining of the endometrium that is formed before the fertilized ovum reaches the uterus. The fertilized ovum embeds in the decidua. If the ovum is not fertilized, the decidua is shed during menstruation. [NIH]

Decision Making: The process of making a selective intellectual judgment when presented with several complex alternatives consisting of several variables, and usually defining a course of action or an idea. [NIH]

Deletion: A genetic rearrangement through loss of segments of DNA (chromosomes), bringing sequences, which are normally separated, into close proximity. [NIH]

Delusions: A false belief regarding the self or persons or objects outside the self that persists despite the facts, and is not considered tenable by one's associates. [NIH]

Dementia: An acquired organic mental disorder with loss of intellectual abilities of sufficient severity to interfere with social or occupational functioning. The dysfunction is multifaceted and involves memory, behavior, personality, judgment, attention, spatial relations, language, abstract thought, and other executive functions. The intellectual decline is usually progressive, and initially spares the level of consciousness. [NIH]

Dendrites: Extensions of the nerve cell body. They are short and branched and receive stimuli from other neurons. [NIH]

Dendritic: 1. Branched like a tree. 2. Pertaining to or possessing dendrites. [EU]

Density: The logarithm to the base 10 of the opacity of an exposed and processed film. [NIH]

Dental Hygienists: Persons trained in an accredited school or dental college and licensed by the state in which they reside to provide dental prophylaxis under the direction of a licensed dentist. [NIH]

Dentate Gyrus: Gray matter situated above the gyrus hippocampi. It is composed of three layers. The molecular layer is continuous with the hippocampus in the hippocampal fissure. The granular layer consists of closely arranged spherical or oval neurons, called granule cells, whose axons pass through the polymorphic layer ending on the dendrites of pyramidal cells in the hippocampus. [NIH]

Dentition: The teeth in the dental arch; ordinarily used to designate the natural teeth in position in their alveoli. [EU]

Depolarization: The process or act of neutralizing polarity. In neurophysiology, the reversal of the resting potential in excitable cell membranes when stimulated, i.e., the tendency of the cell membrane potential to become positive with respect to the potential outside the cell. [EU]

Dermal: Pertaining to or coming from the skin. [NIH]

Desensitization: The prevention or reduction of immediate hypersensitivity reactions by administration of graded doses of allergen; called also hyposensitization and immunotherapy. [EU]

Detoxification: Treatment designed to free an addict from his drug habit. [EU]

Dextroamphetamine: The d-form of amphetamine. It is a central nervous system stimulant and a sympathomimetic. It has also been used in the treatment of narcolepsy and of attention deficit disorders and hyperactivity in children. Dextroamphetamine has multiple mechanisms of action including blocking uptake of adrenergics and dopamine, stimulating release of monamines, and inhibiting monoamine oxidase. It is also a drug of abuse and a psychotomimetic. [NIH]

Diagnostic procedure: A method used to identify a disease. [NIH]

Diencephalon: The paired caudal parts of the prosencephalon from which the thalamus, hypothalamus, epithalamus, and subthalamus are derived. [NIH]

Digestion: The process of breakdown of food for metabolism and use by the body. [NIH]

Dilatation: The act of dilating. [NIH]

Dimerization: The process by which two molecules of the same chemical composition form a condensation product or polymer. [NIH]

Direct: 1. Straight; in a straight line. 2. Performed immediately and without the intervention of subsidiary means. [EU]

Disinfectant: An agent that disinfects; applied particularly to agents used on inanimate objects. [EU]

Dissociation: 1. The act of separating or state of being separated. 2. The separation of a molecule into two or more fragments (atoms, molecules, ions, or free radicals) produced by the absorption of light or thermal energy or by solvation. 3. In psychology, a defense mechanism in which a group of mental processes are segregated from the rest of a person's mental activity in order to avoid emotional distress, as in the dissociative disorders (q.v.), or in which an idea or object is segregated from its emotional significance; in the first sense it is roughly equivalent to splitting, in the second, to isolation. 4. A defect of mental integration in which one or more groups of mental processes become separated off from normal consciousness and, thus separated, function as a unitary whole. [EU]

Distal: Remote; farther from any point of reference; opposed to proximal. In dentistry, used to designate a position on the dental arch farther from the median line of the jaw. [EU]

Dopamine: An endogenous catecholamine and prominent neurotransmitter in several systems of the brain. In the synthesis of catecholamines from tyrosine, it is the immediate precursor to norepinephrine and epinephrine. Dopamine is a major transmitter in the extrapyramidal system of the brain, and important in regulating movement. A family of dopaminergic receptor subtypes mediate its action. Dopamine is used pharmacologically for its direct (beta adrenergic agonist) and indirect (adrenergic releasing) sympathomimetic effects including its actions as an inotropic agent and as a renal vasodilator. [NIH]

Dopamine Agonists: Drugs that bind to and activate dopamine receptors. [NIH]

Dorsal: 1. Pertaining to the back or to any dorsum 2. Denoting a position more toward the back surface than some other object of reference; same as posterior in human anatomy; superior in the anatomy of quadrupeds. [EU]

Dorsum: A plate of bone which forms the posterior boundary of the sella turcica. [NIH]

Drinking Behavior: Behaviors associated with the ingesting of water and other liquids; includes rhythmic patterns of drinking (time intervals - onset and duration), frequency and satiety. [NIH]

Drosophila: A genus of small, two-winged flies containing approximately 900 described species. These organisms are the most extensively studied of all genera from the standpoint of genetics and cytology. [NIH]

Drug Interactions: The action of a drug that may affect the activity, metabolism, or toxicity of another drug. [NIH]

Drug Tolerance: Progressive diminution of the susceptibility of a human or animal to the effects of a drug, resulting from its continued administration. It should be differentiated from drug resistance wherein an organism, disease, or tissue fails to respond to the intended effectiveness of a chemical or drug. It should also be differentiated from maximum tolerated dose and no-observed-adverse-effect level. [NIH]

Duodenum: The first part of the small intestine. [NIH]

Dyslexia: Partial alexia in which letters but not words may be read, or in which words may be read but not understood. [NIH]

Dysplasia: Cells that look abnormal under a microscope but are not cancer. [NIH]

Ectoderm: The outer of the three germ layers of the embryo. [NIH]

Ectopic: Pertaining to or characterized by ectopia. [EU]

Effector: It is often an enzyme that converts an inactive precursor molecule into an active second messenger. [NIH]

Effector cell: A cell that performs a specific function in response to a stimulus; usually used to describe cells in the immune system. [NIH]

Efficacy: The extent to which a specific intervention, procedure, regimen, or service produces a beneficial result under ideal conditions. Ideally, the determination of efficacy is based on the results of a randomized control trial. [NIH]

Elective: Subject to the choice or decision of the patient or physician; applied to procedures that are advantageous to the patient but not urgent. [EU]

Electrolyte: A substance that dissociates into ions when fused or in solution, and thus becomes capable of conducting electricity; an ionic solute. [EU]

Electrons: Stable elementary particles having the smallest known negative charge, present in all elements; also called negatrons. Positively charged electrons are called positrons. The numbers, energies and arrangement of electrons around atomic nuclei determine the chemical identities of elements. Beams of electrons are called cathode rays or beta rays, the latter being a high-energy biproduct of nuclear decay. [NIH]

Electrophoresis: An electrochemical process in which macromolecules or colloidal particles with a net electric charge migrate in a solution under the influence of an electric current. [NIH]

Electrophysiological: Pertaining to electrophysiology, that is a branch of physiology that is concerned with the electric phenomena associated with living bodies and involved in their functional activity. [EU]

Embryo: The prenatal stage of mammalian development characterized by rapid morphological changes and the differentiation of basic structures. [NIH]

Embryo Transfer: Removal of a mammalian embryo from one environment and replacement in the same or a new environment. The embryo is usually in the pre-nidation phase, i.e., a blastocyst. The process includes embryo or blastocyst transplantation or transfer after in vitro fertilization and transfer of the inner cell mass of the blastocyst. It is not used for transfer of differentiated embryonic tissue, e.g., germ layer cells. [NIH]

Embryogenesis: The process of embryo or embryoid formation, whether by sexual (zygotic) or asexual means. In asexual embryogenesis embryoids arise directly from the explant or on intermediary callus tissue. In some cases they arise from individual cells (somatic cell embryoge). [NIH]

Empirical: A treatment based on an assumed diagnosis, prior to receiving confirmatory laboratory test results. [NIH]

Endocrine System: The system of glands that release their secretions (hormones) directly into the circulatory system. In addition to the endocrine glands, included are the chromaffin system and the neurosecretory systems. [NIH]

Endorphin: Opioid peptides derived from beta-lipotropin. Endorphin is the most potent naturally occurring analgesic agent. It is present in pituitary, brain, and peripheral tissues. [NIH]

Endoscope: A thin, lighted tube used to look at tissues inside the body. [NIH]

Endoscopic: A technique where a lateral-view endoscope is passed orally to the duodenum for visualization of the ampulla of Vater. [NIH]

Endothelial cell: The main type of cell found in the inside lining of blood vessels, lymph vessels, and the heart. [NIH]

Endothelium: A layer of epithelium that lines the heart, blood vessels (endothelium, vascular), lymph vessels (endothelium, lymphatic), and the serous cavities of the body. [NIH]

Endothelium-derived: Small molecule that diffuses to the adjacent muscle layer and relaxes it. [NIH]

Enkephalin: A natural opiate painkiller, in the hypothalamus. [NIH]

Entorhinal Cortex: Cortex where the signals are combined with those from other sensory systems. [NIH]

Environmental Health: The science of controlling or modifying those conditions, influences, or forces surrounding man which relate to promoting, establishing, and maintaining health. [NIH]

Enzymatic: Phase where enzyme cuts the precursor protein. [NIH]

Enzyme: A protein that speeds up chemical reactions in the body. [NIH]

Epidemiologic Studies: Studies designed to examine associations, commonly, hypothesized causal relations. They are usually concerned with identifying or measuring the effects of risk factors or exposures. The common types of analytic study are case-control studies, cohort studies, and cross-sectional studies. [NIH]

Epidemiological: Relating to, or involving epidemiology. [EU]

Epinephrine: The active sympathomimetic hormone from the adrenal medulla in most species. It stimulates both the alpha- and beta- adrenergic systems, causes systemic vasoconstriction and gastrointestinal relaxation, stimulates the heart, and dilates bronchi and cerebral vessels. It is used in asthma and cardiac failure and to delay absorption of local anesthetics. [NIH]

Epiphyseal: Pertaining to or of the nature of an epiphysis. [EU]

Epiphyses: The head of a long bone that is separated from the shaft by the epiphyseal plate until bone growth stops. At that time, the plate disappears and the head and shaft are united. [NIH]

Epithelial: Refers to the cells that line the internal and external surfaces of the body. [NIH]

Erythrocytes: Red blood cells. Mature erythrocytes are non-nucleated, biconcave disks containing hemoglobin whose function is to transport oxygen. [NIH]

Estradiol: The most potent mammalian estrogenic hormone. It is produced in the ovary, placenta, testis, and possibly the adrenal cortex. [NIH]

Ethanol: A clear, colorless liquid rapidly absorbed from the gastrointestinal tract and distributed throughout the body. It has bactericidal activity and is used often as a topical disinfectant. It is widely used as a solvent and preservative in pharmaceutical preparations as well as serving as the primary ingredient in alcoholic beverages. [NIH]

Eukaryotic Cells: Cells of the higher organisms, containing a true nucleus bounded by a nuclear membrane. [NIH]

Evoke: The electric response recorded from the cerebral cortex after stimulation of a peripheral sense organ. [NIH]

Evoked Potentials: The electric response evoked in the central nervous system by stimulation of sensory receptors or some point on the sensory pathway leading from the receptor to the cortex. The evoked stimulus can be auditory, somatosensory, or visual, although other modalities have been reported. Event-related potentials is sometimes used synonymously with evoked potentials but is often associated with the execution of a motor, cognitive, or psychophysiological task, as well as with the response to a stimulus. [NIH]

Excitability: Property of a cardiac cell whereby, when the cell is depolarized to a critical level (called threshold), the membrane becomes permeable and a regenerative inward current causes an action potential. [NIH]

Excitation: An act of irritation or stimulation or of responding to a stimulus; the addition of energy, as the excitation of a molecule by absorption of photons. [EU]

Excitatory: When cortical neurons are excited, their output increases and each new input they receive while they are still excited raises their output markedly. [NIH]

Excitotoxicity: Excessive exposure to glutamate or related compounds can kill brain neurons, presumably by overstimulating them. [NIH]

Exhaustion: The feeling of weariness of mind and body. [NIH]

Exogenous: Developed or originating outside the organism, as exogenous disease. [EU]

Exostoses: Benign hypertrophy that projects outward from the surface of bone, often containing a cartilaginous component. [NIH]

Extracellular: Outside a cell or cells. [EU]

Extracellular Matrix: A meshwork-like substance found within the extracellular space and in association with the basement membrane of the cell surface. It promotes cellular proliferation and provides a supporting structure to which cells or cell lysates in culture dishes adhere. [NIH]

Extraction: The process or act of pulling or drawing out. [EU]

Extrapyramidal: Outside of the pyramidal tracts. [EU]

Extremity: A limb; an arm or leg (membrum); sometimes applied specifically to a hand or foot. [EU]

Facial: Of or pertaining to the face. [EU]

Failure to Thrive: A condition in which an infant or child's weight gain and growth are far below usual levels for age. [NIH]

Family Planning: Programs or services designed to assist the family in controlling reproduction by either improving or diminishing fertility. [NIH]

Fat: Total lipids including phospholipids. [NIH]

Fatty acids: A major component of fats that are used by the body for energy and tissue development. [NIH]

Febrile: Pertaining to or characterized by fever. [EU]

Fermentation: An enzyme-induced chemical change in organic compounds that takes place in the absence of oxygen. The change usually results in the production of ethanol or lactic acid, and the production of energy. [NIH]

Fertilization in Vitro: Fertilization of an egg outside the body when the egg is normally fertilized in the body. [NIH]

Fetal Alcohol Syndrome: A disorder occurring in children born to alcoholic women who continue to drink heavily during pregnancy. Common abnormalities are growth deficiency (prenatal and postnatal), altered morphogenesis, mental deficiency, and characteristic facies - small eyes and flattened nasal bridge. Fine motor dysfunction and tremulousness are observed in the newborn. [NIH]

Fetal Death: Death of the young developing in utero. [NIH]

Fetal Development: Morphologic and physiologic growth and development of the mammalian embryo or fetus. [NIH]

Fetoprotein: Transabdominal aspiration of fluid from the amniotic sac with a view to detecting increases of alpha-fetoprotein in maternal blood during pregnancy, as this is an important indicator of open neural tube defects in the fetus. [NIH]

Fetus: The developing offspring from 7 to 8 weeks after conception until birth. [NIH]

Fibroblast Growth Factor: Peptide isolated from the pituitary gland and from the brain. It is a potent mitogen which stimulates growth of a variety of mesodermal cells including chondrocytes, granulosa, and endothelial cells. The peptide may be active in wound healing and animal limb regeneration. [NIH]

Fibroblasts: Connective tissue cells which secrete an extracellular matrix rich in collagen and other macromolecules. [NIH]

Fibrosis: Any pathological condition where fibrous connective tissue invades any organ, usually as a consequence of inflammation or other injury. [NIH]

Fissure: Any cleft or groove, normal or otherwise; especially a deep fold in the cerebral cortex which involves the entire thickness of the brain wall. [EU]

Fixation: 1. The act or operation of holding, suturing, or fastening in a fixed position. 2. The condition of being held in a fixed position. 3. In psychiatry, a term with two related but distinct meanings : (1) arrest of development at a particular stage, which like regression (return to an earlier stage), if temporary is a normal reaction to setbacks and difficulties but if protracted or frequent is a cause of developmental failures and emotional problems, and (2) a close and suffocating attachment to another person, especially a childhood figure, such as one's mother or father. Both meanings are derived from psychoanalytic theory and refer to 'fixation' of libidinal energy either in a specific erogenous zone, hence fixation at the oral, anal, or phallic stage, or in a specific object, hence mother or father fixation. 4. The use of a fixative (q.v.) to preserve histological or cytological specimens. 5. In chemistry, the process whereby a substance is removed from the gaseous or solution phase and localized, as in carbon dioxide fixation or nitrogen fixation. 6. In ophthalmology, direction of the gaze so that the visual image of the object falls on the fovea centralis. 7. In film processing, the chemical removal of all undeveloped salts of the film emulsion, leaving only the developed silver to form a permanent image. [EU]

Flow Cytometry: Technique using an instrument system for making, processing, and displaying one or more measurements on individual cells obtained from a cell suspension. Cells are usually stained with one or more fluorescent dyes specific to cell components of interest, e.g., DNA, and fluorescence of each cell is measured as it rapidly transverses the excitation beam (laser or mercury arc lamp). Fluorescence provides a quantitative measure of various biochemical and biophysical properties of the cell, as well as a basis for cell sorting. Other measurable optical parameters include light absorption and light scattering, the latter being applicable to the measurement of cell size, shape, density, granularity, and stain uptake. [NIH]

Fluorescence: The property of emitting radiation while being irradiated. The radiation emitted is usually of longer wavelength than that incident or absorbed, e.g., a substance can be irradiated with invisible radiation and emit visible light. X-ray fluorescence is used in diagnosis. [NIH]

Fluorescent Dyes: Dyes that emit light when exposed to light. The wave length of the emitted light is usually longer than that of the incident light. Fluorochromes are substances that cause fluorescence in other substances, i.e., dyes used to mark or label other compounds with fluorescent tags. They are used as markers in biochemistry and immunology. [NIH]

Fold: A plication or doubling of various parts of the body. [NIH]

Fossa: A cavity, depression, or pit. [NIH]

Frontal Lobe: The anterior part of the cerebral hemisphere. [NIH]

Fura-2: A fluorescent calcium chelating agent which is used to study intracellular calcium in many tissues. The fluorescent and chelating properties of Fura-2 aid in the quantitation of endothelial cell injury, in monitoring ATP-dependent calcium uptake by membrane vesicles, and in the determination of the relationship between cytoplasmic free calcium and oxidase activation in rat neutrophils. [NIH]

Gait: Manner or style of walking. [NIH]

Gallbladder: The pear-shaped organ that sits below the liver. Bile is concentrated and stored in the gallbladder. [NIH]

Ganglia: Clusters of multipolar neurons surrounded by a capsule of loosely organized connective tissue located outside the central nervous system. [NIH]

Ganglion: 1. A knot, or knotlike mass. 2. A general term for a group of nerve cell bodies located outside the central nervous system; occasionally applied to certain nuclear groups within the brain or spinal cord, e.g. basal ganglia. 3. A benign cystic tumour occurring on a aponeurosis or tendon, as in the wrist or dorsum of the foot; it consists of a thin fibrous capsule enclosing a clear mucinous fluid. [EU]

Gap Junctions: Connections between cells which allow passage of small molecules and electric current. Gap junctions were first described anatomically as regions of close apposition between cells with a narrow (1-2 nm) gap between cell membranes. The variety in the properties of gap junctions is reflected in the number of connexins, the family of proteins which form the junctions. [NIH]

Gas: Air that comes from normal breakdown of food. The gases are passed out of the body through the rectum (flatus) or the mouth (burp). [NIH]

Gas exchange: Primary function of the lungs; transfer of oxygen from inhaled air into the blood and of carbon dioxide from the blood into the lungs. [NIH]

Gastric: Having to do with the stomach. [NIH]

Gastrin: A hormone released after eating. Gastrin causes the stomach to produce more acid. [NIH]

Gastrointestinal: Refers to the stomach and intestines. [NIH]

Gastrointestinal tract: The stomach and intestines. [NIH]

Gelatin: A product formed from skin, white connective tissue, or bone collagen. It is used as a protein food adjuvant, plasma substitute, hemostatic, suspending agent in pharmaceutical preparations, and in the manufacturing of capsules and suppositories. [NIH]

Gene: The functional and physical unit of heredity passed from parent to offspring. Genes are pieces of DNA, and most genes contain the information for making a specific protein. [NIH]

Gene Expression: The phenotypic manifestation of a gene or genes by the processes of gene action. [NIH]

General practitioner: A medical practitioner who does not specialize in a particular branch of medicine or limit his practice to a specific class of diseases. [NIH]

Genetics: The biological science that deals with the phenomena and mechanisms of heredity. [NIH]

Genomics: The systematic study of the complete DNA sequences (genome) of organisms. [NIH]

Genotype: The genetic constitution of the individual; the characterization of the genes. [NIH]

Gestation: The period of development of the young in viviparous animals, from the time of fertilization of the ovum until birth. [EU]

Gestational: Psychosis attributable to or occurring during pregnancy. [NIH]

Gland: An organ that produces and releases one or more substances for use in the body. Some glands produce fluids that affect tissues or organs. Others produce hormones or participate in blood production. [NIH]

Glucocorticoid: A compound that belongs to the family of compounds called corticosteroids (steroids). Glucocorticoids affect metabolism and have anti-inflammatory and immunosuppressive effects. They may be naturally produced (hormones) or synthetic (drugs). [NIH]

Glucose: D-Glucose. A primary source of energy for living organisms. It is naturally occurring and is found in fruits and other parts of plants in its free state. It is used therapeutically in fluid and nutrient replacement. [NIH]

Glutamate: Excitatory neurotransmitter of the brain. [NIH]

Glycerol: A trihydroxy sugar alcohol that is an intermediate in carbohydrate and lipid metabolism. It is used as a solvent, emollient, pharmaceutical agent, and sweetening agent. [NIH]

Glycerophospholipids: Derivatives of phosphatidic acid in which the hydrophobic regions are composed of two fatty acids and a polar alcohol is joined to the C-3 position of glycerol through a phosphodiester bond. They are named according to their polar head groups, such as phosphatidylcholine and phosphatidylethanolamine. [NIH]

Glycine: A non-essential amino acid. It is found primarily in gelatin and silk fibroin and used therapeutically as a nutrient. It is also a fast inhibitory neurotransmitter. [NIH]

Glycoprotein: A protein that has sugar molecules attached to it. [NIH]

Governing Board: The group in which legal authority is vested for the control of health-related institutions and organizations. [NIH]

Graft: Healthy skin, bone, or other tissue taken from one part of the body and used to replace diseased or injured tissue removed from another part of the body. [NIH]

Gramicidin: Antibiotic mixture that is one of the two principle components of tyrothricin from Bacillus brevis. Gramicidin C or S is a cyclic, ten-amino acid polypeptide and gramicidins A, B, D, etc., seem to be linear polypeptides. The mixture is used topically for gram-positive organisms. It is toxic to blood, liver, kidneys, meninges, and the olfactory apparatus. [NIH]

Gram-positive: Retaining the stain or resisting decolorization by alcohol in Gram's method of staining, a primary characteristic of bacteria whose cell wall is composed of a thick layer of peptidologlycan with attached teichoic acids. [EU]

Granule: A small pill made from sucrose. [EU]

Granulocytes: Leukocytes with abundant granules in the cytoplasm. They are divided into three groups: neutrophils, eosinophils, and basophils. [NIH]

Growth: The progressive development of a living being or part of an organism from its earliest stage to maturity. [NIH]

Growth factors: Substances made by the body that function to regulate cell division and cell survival. Some growth factors are also produced in the laboratory and used in biological therapy. [NIH]

Guanylate Cyclase: An enzyme that catalyzes the conversion of GTP to 3',5'-cyclic GMP and pyrophosphate. It also acts on ITP and dGTP. (From Enzyme Nomenclature, 1992) EC 4.6.1.2. [NIH]

Habitual: Of the nature of a habit; according to habit; established by or repeated by force of habit, customary. [EU]

Haptens: Small antigenic determinants capable of eliciting an immune response only when coupled to a carrier. Haptens bind to antibodies but by themselves cannot elicit an antibody response. [NIH]

Health Resources: Available manpower, facilities, revenue, equipment, and supplies to produce requisite health care and services. [NIH]

Hearing Disorders: Conditions that impair the transmission or perception of auditory impulses and information from the level of the ear to the temporal cortices, including the sensorineural pathways. [NIH]

Heartbeat: One complete contraction of the heart. [NIH]

Hemostasis: The process which spontaneously arrests the flow of blood from vessels carrying blood under pressure. It is accomplished by contraction of the vessels, adhesion and aggregation of formed blood elements, and the process of blood or plasma coagulation. [NIH]

Hereditary: Of, relating to, or denoting factors that can be transmitted genetically from one generation to another. [NIH]

Heredity: 1. The genetic transmission of a particular quality or trait from parent to offspring. 2. The genetic constitution of an individual. [EU]

Heterogeneity: The property of one or more samples or populations which implies that they are not identical in respect of some or all of their parameters, e. g. heterogeneity of variance. [NIH]

Hippocampus: A curved elevation of gray matter extending the entire length of the floor of the temporal horn of the lateral ventricle (Dorland, 28th ed). The hippocampus, subiculum, and dentate gyrus constitute the hippocampal formation. Sometimes authors include the entorhinal cortex in the hippocampal formation. [NIH]

Holoprosencephaly: Anterior midline brain, cranial, and facial malformations resulting from the failure of the embryonic prosencephalon to undergo segmentation and cleavage. Alobar prosencephaly is the most severe form and features anophthalmia; cyclopia; severe mental retardation; cleft lip; cleft palate; seizures; and microcephaly. Semilobar holoprosencepaly is characterized by hypotelorism, microphthalmia, coloboma, nasal malformations, and variable degrees of mental retardation. Lobar holoprosencephaly is associated with mild (or absent) facial malformations and intellectual abilities that range from mild mental retardation to normal. Holoprosencephlay is associated with chromosome abnormalities. [NIH]

Homeostasis: The processes whereby the internal environment of an organism tends to remain balanced and stable. [NIH]

Homogeneous: Consisting of or composed of similar elements or ingredients; of a uniform quality throughout. [EU]

Homologous: Corresponding in structure, position, origin, etc., as (a) the feathers of a bird and the scales of a fish, (b) antigen and its specific antibody, (c) allelic chromosomes. [EU]

Hormonal: Pertaining to or of the nature of a hormone. [EU]

Hormone: A substance in the body that regulates certain organs. Hormones such as gastrin help in breaking down food. Some hormones come from cells in the stomach and small intestine. [NIH]

Host: Any animal that receives a transplanted graft. [NIH]

Human Development: Continuous sequential changes which occur in the physiological and psychological functions during the individual's life. [NIH]

Humoral: Of, relating to, proceeding from, or involving a bodily humour - now often used of endocrine factors as opposed to neural or somatic. [EU]

Humour: 1. A normal functioning fluid or semifluid of the body (as the blood, lymph or bile) especially of vertebrates. 2. A secretion that is itself an excitant of activity (as certain hormones). [EU]

Hydrogen: The first chemical element in the periodic table. It has the atomic symbol H, atomic number 1, and atomic weight 1. It exists, under normal conditions, as a colorless, odorless, tasteless, diatomic gas. Hydrogen ions are protons. Besides the common H1 isotope, hydrogen exists as the stable isotope deuterium and the unstable, radioactive isotope tritium. [NIH]

Hydrolysis: The process of cleaving a chemical compound by the addition of a molecule of water. [NIH]

Hydrophobic: Not readily absorbing water, or being adversely affected by water, as a hydrophobic colloid. [EU]

Hypercarbia: Excess of carbon dioxide in the blood. [NIH]

Hypersensitivity: Altered reactivity to an antigen, which can result in pathologic reactions upon subsequent exposure to that particular antigen. [NIH]

Hypertrophy: General increase in bulk of a part or organ, not due to tumor formation, nor to an increase in the number of cells. [NIH]

Hypoplasia: Incomplete development or underdevelopment of an organ or tissue. [EU]

Hypotension: Abnormally low blood pressure. [NIH]

Hypothalamic: Of or involving the hypothalamus. [EU]

Hypothalamus: Ventral part of the diencephalon extending from the region of the optic chiasm to the caudal border of the mammillary bodies and forming the inferior and lateral walls of the third ventricle. [NIH]

Hypoxia: Reduction of oxygen supply to tissue below physiological levels despite adequate perfusion of the tissue by blood. [EU]

Id: The part of the personality structure which harbors the unconscious instinctive desires and strivings of the individual. [NIH]

Immune function: Production and action of cells that fight disease or infection. [NIH]

Immune response: The activity of the immune system against foreign substances (antigens). [NIH]

Immune system: The organs, cells, and molecules responsible for the recognition and disposal of foreign ("non-self") material which enters the body. [NIH]

Immunity: Nonsusceptibility to the invasive or pathogenic effects of foreign microorganisms or to the toxic effect of antigenic substances. [NIH]

Immunization: Deliberate stimulation of the host's immune response. Active immunization involves administration of antigens or immunologic adjuvants. Passive immunization involves administration of immune sera or lymphocytes or their extracts (e.g., transfer factor, immune RNA) or transplantation of immunocompetent cell producing tissue (thymus or bone marrow). [NIH]

Immunodeficiency: The decreased ability of the body to fight infection and disease. [NIH]

Immunodeficiency syndrome: The inability of the body to produce an immune response. [NIH]

Immunohistochemistry: Histochemical localization of immunoreactive substances using labeled antibodies as reagents. [NIH]

Immunology: The study of the body's immune system. [NIH]

Immunophilin: A drug for the treatment of Parkinson's disease. [NIH]

Immunosuppressive: Describes the ability to lower immune system responses. [NIH]

Immunotherapy: Manipulation of the host's immune system in treatment of disease. It includes both active and passive immunization as well as immunosuppressive therapy to prevent graft rejection. [NIH]

Impairment: In the context of health experience, an impairment is any loss or abnormality of psychological, physiological, or anatomical structure or function. [NIH]

Implantation: The insertion or grafting into the body of biological, living, inert, or radioactive material. [EU]

In situ: In the natural or normal place; confined to the site of origin without invasion of neighbouring tissues. [EU]

In Situ Hybridization: A technique that localizes specific nucleic acid sequences within intact chromosomes, eukaryotic cells, or bacterial cells through the use of specific nucleic acid-labeled probes. [NIH]

In vitro: In the laboratory (outside the body). The opposite of in vivo (in the body). [NIH]

In vivo: In the body. The opposite of in vitro (outside the body or in the laboratory). [NIH]

Incubation: The development of an infectious disease from the entrance of the pathogen to the appearance of clinical symptoms. [EU]

Incubation period: The period of time likely to elapse between exposure to the agent of the disease and the onset of clinical symptoms. [NIH]

Indicative: That indicates; that points out more or less exactly; that reveals fairly clearly. [EU]

Induction: The act or process of inducing or causing to occur, especially the production of a specific morphogenetic effect in the developing embryo through the influence of evocators or organizers, or the production of anaesthesia or unconsciousness by use of appropriate agents. [EU]

Infancy: The period of complete dependency prior to the acquisition of competence in walking, talking, and self-feeding. [NIH]

Infant Mortality: Perinatal, neonatal, and infant deaths in a given population. [NIH]

Infantile: Pertaining to an infant or to infancy. [EU]

Infarction: A pathological process consisting of a sudden insufficient blood supply to an area, which results in necrosis of that area. It is usually caused by a thrombus, an embolus, or a vascular torsion. [NIH]

Infection: 1. Invasion and multiplication of microorganisms in body tissues, which may be clinically unapparent or result in local cellular injury due to competitive metabolism, toxins, intracellular replication, or antigen-antibody response. The infection may remain localized, subclinical, and temporary if the body's defensive mechanisms are effective. A local infection may persist and spread by extension to become an acute, subacute, or chronic clinical infection or disease state. A local infection may also become systemic when the microorganisms gain access to the lymphatic or vascular system. 2. An infectious disease. [EU]

Inflammation: A pathological process characterized by injury or destruction of tissues caused by a variety of cytologic and chemical reactions. It is usually manifested by typical signs of pain, heat, redness, swelling, and loss of function. [NIH]

Ingestion: Taking into the body by mouth [NIH]

Initiation: Mutation induced by a chemical reactive substance causing cell changes; being a step in a carcinogenic process. [NIH]

Inlay: In dentistry, a filling first made to correspond with the form of a dental cavity and then cemented into the cavity. [NIH]

Inner ear: The labyrinth, comprising the vestibule, cochlea, and semicircular canals. [NIH]

Innervation: 1. The distribution or supply of nerves to a part. 2. The supply of nervous energy or of nerve stimulus sent to a part. [EU]

Inositol: An isomer of glucose that has traditionally been considered to be a B vitamin although it has an uncertain status as a vitamin and a deficiency syndrome has not been identified in man. (From Martindale, The Extra Pharmacopoeia, 30th ed, p1379) Inositol phospholipids are important in signal transduction. [NIH]

Inotropic: Affecting the force or energy of muscular contractions. [EU]

Insecticides: Pesticides designed to control insects that are harmful to man. The insects may be directly harmful, as those acting as disease vectors, or indirectly harmful, as destroyers of crops, food products, or textile fabrics. [NIH]

Insight: The capacity to understand one's own motives, to be aware of one's own psychodynamics, to appreciate the meaning of symbolic behavior. [NIH]

Insulin: A protein hormone secreted by beta cells of the pancreas. Insulin plays a major role in the regulation of glucose metabolism, generally promoting the cellular utilization of glucose. It is also an important regulator of protein and lipid metabolism. Insulin is used as a drug to control insulin-dependent diabetes mellitus. [NIH]

Insulin-dependent diabetes mellitus: A disease characterized by high levels of blood glucose resulting from defects in insulin secretion, insulin action, or both. Autoimmune, genetic, and environmental factors are involved in the development of type I diabetes. [NIH]

Insulin-like: Muscular growth factor. [NIH]

Intensive Care: Advanced and highly specialized care provided to medical or surgical patients whose conditions are life-threatening and require comprehensive care and constant monitoring. It is usually administered in specially equipped units of a health care facility. [NIH]

Intensive Care Units: Hospital units providing continuous surveillance and care to acutely ill patients. [NIH]

Interleukin-1: A soluble factor produced by monocytes, macrophages, and other cells which activates T-lymphocytes and potentiates their response to mitogens or antigens. IL-1 consists of two distinct forms, IL-1 alpha and IL-1 beta which perform the same functions but are distinct proteins. The biological effects of IL-1 include the ability to replace macrophage requirements for T-cell activation. The factor is distinct from interleukin-2. [NIH]

Interleukin-2: Chemical mediator produced by activated T lymphocytes and which regulates the proliferation of T cells, as well as playing a role in the regulation of NK cell activity. [NIH]

Intermittent: Occurring at separated intervals; having periods of cessation of activity. [EU]

Intestinal: Having to do with the intestines. [NIH]

Intestines: The section of the alimentary canal from the stomach to the anus. It includes the large intestine and small intestine. [NIH]

Intoxication: Poisoning, the state of being poisoned. [EU]

Intracellular: Inside a cell. [NIH]

Intracellular Membranes: Membranes of subcellular structures. [NIH]

Intrinsic: Situated entirely within or pertaining exclusively to a part. [EU]

Intubation: Introduction of a tube into a hollow organ to restore or maintain patency if obstructed. It is differentiated from catheterization in that the insertion of a catheter is usually performed for the introducing or withdrawing of fluids from the body. [NIH]

Invasive: 1. Having the quality of invasiveness. 2. Involving puncture or incision of the skin or insertion of an instrument or foreign material into the body; said of diagnostic techniques. [EU]

Ion Channels: Gated, ion-selective glycoproteins that traverse membranes. The stimulus for channel gating can be a membrane potential, drug, transmitter, cytoplasmic messenger, or a mechanical deformation. Ion channels which are integral parts of ionotropic neurotransmitter receptors are not included. [NIH]

Ionizing: Radiation comprising charged particles, e. g. electrons, protons, alpha-particles, etc., having sufficient kinetic energy to produce ionization by collision. [NIH]

Ionophores: Chemical agents that increase the permeability of biological or artificial lipid membranes to specific ions. Most ionophores are relatively small organic molecules that act as mobile carriers within membranes or coalesce to form ion permeable channels across membranes. Many are antibiotics, and many act as uncoupling agents by short-circuiting the proton gradient across mitochondrial membranes. [NIH]

Ions: An atom or group of atoms that have a positive or negative electric charge due to a gain (negative charge) or loss (positive charge) of one or more electrons. Atoms with a positive charge are known as cations; those with a negative charge are anions. [NIH]

Ischemia: Deficiency of blood in a part, due to functional constriction or actual obstruction of a blood vessel. [EU]

Joint: The point of contact between elements of an animal skeleton with the parts that surround and support it. [NIH]

Kb: A measure of the length of DNA fragments, 1 Kb = 1000 base pairs. The largest DNA fragments are up to 50 kilobases long. [NIH]

Labyrinth: The internal ear; the essential part of the organ of hearing. It consists of an osseous and a membranous portion. [NIH]

Lactation: The period of the secretion of milk. [EU]

Language Development: The gradual expansion in complexity and meaning of symbols and sounds as perceived and interpreted by the individual through a maturational and learning process. Stages in development include babbling, cooing, word imitation with cognition, and use of short sentences. [NIH]

Latent: Phoria which occurs at one distance or another and which usually has no troublesome effect. [NIH]

Learning Disorders: Conditions characterized by a significant discrepancy between an individual's perceived level of intellect and their ability to acquire new language and other cognitive skills. These disorders may result from organic or psychological conditions. Relatively common subtypes include dyslexia, dyscalculia, and dysgraphia. [NIH]

Least-Squares Analysis: A principle of estimation in which the estimates of a set of parameters in a statistical model are those quantities minimizing the sum of squared differences between the observed values of a dependent variable and the values predicted by the model. [NIH]

Lectin: A complex molecule that has both protein and sugars. Lectins are able to bind to the outside of a cell and cause biochemical changes in it. Lectins are made by both animals and plants. [NIH]

Lentivirus: A genus of the family Retroviridae consisting of non-oncogenic retroviruses that produce multi-organ diseases characterized by long incubation periods and persistent infection. Lentiviruses are unique in that they contain open reading frames (ORFs) between the pol and env genes and in the 3' env region. Five serogroups are recognized, reflecting the mammalian hosts with which they are associated. HIV-1 is the type species. [NIH]

Lesion: An area of abnormal tissue change. [NIH]

Lethal: Deadly, fatal. [EU]

Leucine: An essential branched-chain amino acid important for hemoglobin formation. [NIH]

Leukocytes: White blood cells. These include granular leukocytes (basophils, eosinophils, and neutrophils) as well as non-granular leukocytes (lymphocytes and monocytes). [NIH]

Leukotrienes: A family of biologically active compounds derived from arachidonic acid by oxidative metabolism through the 5-lipoxygenase pathway. They participate in host defense reactions and pathophysiological conditions such as immediate hypersensitivity and inflammation. They have potent actions on many essential organs and systems, including the cardiovascular, pulmonary, and central nervous system as well as the gastrointestinal tract and the immune system. [NIH]

Library Services: Services offered to the library user. They include reference and circulation. [NIH]

Ligands: A RNA simulation method developed by the MIT. [NIH]

Likelihood Functions: Functions constructed from a statistical model and a set of observed data which give the probability of that data for various values of the unknown model parameters. Those parameter values that maximize the probability are the maximum likelihood estimates of the parameters. [NIH]

Linear Models: Statistical models in which the value of a parameter for a given value of a factor is assumed to be equal to a + bx, where a and b are constants. The models predict a linear regression. [NIH]

Lip: Either of the two fleshy, full-blooded margins of the mouth. [NIH]

Lipid: Fat. [NIH]

Lipid Peroxidation: Peroxidase catalyzed oxidation of lipids using hydrogen peroxide as an electron acceptor. [NIH]

Lipopolysaccharide: Substance consisting of polysaccharide and lipid. [NIH]

Lipoprotein: Any of the lipid-protein complexes in which lipids are transported in the blood; lipoprotein particles consist of a spherical hydrophobic core of triglycerides or cholesterol esters surrounded by an amphipathic monolayer of phospholipids, cholesterol, and apolipoproteins; the four principal classes are high-density, low-density, and very-low-density lipoproteins and chylomicrons. [EU]

Liver: A large, glandular organ located in the upper abdomen. The liver cleanses the blood and aids in digestion by secreting bile. [NIH]

Lobe: A portion of an organ such as the liver, lung, breast, or brain. [NIH]

Lobule: A small lobe or subdivision of a lobe. [NIH]

Localization: The process of determining or marking the location or site of a lesion or disease. May also refer to the process of keeping a lesion or disease in a specific location or site. [NIH]

Localized: Cancer which has not metastasized yet. [NIH]

Locomotion: Movement or the ability to move from one place or another. It can refer to humans, vertebrate or invertebrate animals, and microorganisms. [NIH]

Locomotor: Of or pertaining to locomotion; pertaining to or affecting the locomotive apparatus of the body. [EU]

Logistic Models: Statistical models which describe the relationship between a qualitative dependent variable (that is, one which can take only certain discrete values, such as the presence or absence of a disease) and an independent variable. A common application is in epidemiology for estimating an individual's risk (probability of a disease) as a function of a given risk factor. [NIH]

Longitudinal Studies: Studies in which variables relating to an individual or group of individuals are assessed over a period of time. [NIH]

Long-Term Potentiation: A persistent increase in synaptic efficacy, usually induced by appropriate activation of the same synapses. The phenomenological properties of long-term potentiation suggest that it may be a cellular mechanism of learning and memory. [NIH]

Low-density lipoprotein: Lipoprotein that contains most of the cholesterol in the blood. LDL carries cholesterol to the tissues of the body, including the arteries. A high level of LDL increases the risk of heart disease. LDL typically contains 60 to 70 percent of the total serum cholesterol and both are directly correlated with CHD risk. [NIH]

Lumbar: Pertaining to the loins, the part of the back between the thorax and the pelvis. [EU]

Lymphatic: The tissues and organs, including the bone marrow, spleen, thymus, and lymph nodes, that produce and store cells that fight infection and disease. [NIH]

Lymphatic system: The tissues and organs that produce, store, and carry white blood cells that fight infection and other diseases. This system includes the bone marrow, spleen, thymus, lymph nodes and a network of thin tubes that carry lymph and white blood cells. These tubes branch, like blood vessels, into all the tissues of the body. [NIH]

Lymphocyte: A white blood cell. Lymphocytes have a number of roles in the immune system, including the production of antibodies and other substances that fight infection and diseases. [NIH]

Lymphoid: Referring to lymphocytes, a type of white blood cell. Also refers to tissue in which lymphocytes develop. [NIH]

Macrophage: A type of white blood cell that surrounds and kills microorganisms, removes dead cells, and stimulates the action of other immune system cells. [NIH]

Magnetic Resonance Imaging: Non-invasive method of demonstrating internal anatomy based on the principle that atomic nuclei in a strong magnetic field absorb pulses of radiofrequency energy and emit them as radiowaves which can be reconstructed into computerized images. The concept includes proton spin tomographic techniques. [NIH]

Malformation: A morphologic defect resulting from an intrinsically abnormal developmental process. [EU]

Malignant: Cancerous; a growth with a tendency to invade and destroy nearby tissue and spread to other parts of the body. [NIH]

Malnutrition: A condition caused by not eating enough food or not eating a balanced diet. [NIH]

Manic: Affected with mania. [EU]

Manic-depressive psychosis: One of a group of psychotic reactions, fundamentally marked by severe mood swings and a tendency to remission and recurrence. [NIH]

Manifest: Being the part or aspect of a phenomenon that is directly observable : concretely expressed in behaviour. [EU]

Mastication: The act and process of chewing and grinding food in the mouth. [NIH]

Maternal Exposure: Exposure of the female parent, human or animal, to potentially harmful chemical, physical, or biological agents in the environment or to environmental factors that may include ionizing radiation, pathogenic organisms, or toxic chemicals that may affect offspring. It includes pre-conception maternal exposure. [NIH]

Maxillary: Pertaining to the maxilla : the irregularly shaped bone that with its fellow forms the upper jaw. [EU]

Maxillary Nerve: The intermediate sensory division of the trigeminal (5th cranial) nerve. The maxillary nerve carries general afferents from the intermediate region of the face including the lower eyelid, nose and upper lip, the maxillary teeth, and parts of the dura. [NIH]

Medial: Lying near the midsaggital plane of the body; opposed to lateral. [NIH]

Mediate: Indirect; accomplished by the aid of an intervening medium. [EU]

Mediator: An object or substance by which something is mediated, such as (1) a structure of the nervous system that transmits impulses eliciting a specific response; (2) a chemical substance (transmitter substance) that induces activity in an excitable tissue, such as nerve or muscle; or (3) a substance released from cells as the result of the interaction of antigen with antibody or by the action of antigen with a sensitized lymphocyte. [EU]

MEDLINE: An online database of MEDLARS, the computerized bibliographic Medical Literature Analysis and Retrieval System of the National Library of Medicine. [NIH]

Medullary: Pertaining to the marrow or to any medulla; resembling marrow. [EU]

Meiosis: A special method of cell division, occurring in maturation of the germ cells, by means of which each daughter nucleus receives half the number of chromosomes characteristic of the somatic cells of the species. [NIH]

Melanin: The substance that gives the skin its color. [NIH]

Membrane: A very thin layer of tissue that covers a surface. [NIH]

Membrane Potentials: Ratio of inside versus outside concentration of potassium, sodium, chloride and other ions in diffusible tissues or cells. Also called transmembrane and resting potentials, they are measured by recording electrophysiologic responses in voltage-dependent ionic channels of (e.g.) nerve, muscle and blood cells as well as artificial membranes. [NIH]

Membrane Proteins: Proteins which are found in membranes including cellular and intracellular membranes. They consist of two types, peripheral and integral proteins. They include most membrane-associated enzymes, antigenic proteins, transport proteins, and drug, hormone, and lectin receptors. [NIH]

Memory: Complex mental function having four distinct phases: (1) memorizing or learning,

(2) retention, (3) recall, and (4) recognition. Clinically, it is usually subdivided into immediate, recent, and remote memory. [NIH]

Meninges: The three membranes that cover and protect the brain and spinal cord. [NIH]

Mental deficiency: A condition of arrested or incomplete development of mind from inherent causes or induced by disease or injury. [NIH]

Mental Disorders: Psychiatric illness or diseases manifested by breakdowns in the adaptational process expressed primarily as abnormalities of thought, feeling, and behavior producing either distress or impairment of function. [NIH]

Mental Health: The state wherein the person is well adjusted. [NIH]

Mental Processes: Conceptual functions or thinking in all its forms. [NIH]

Mental Retardation: Refers to sub-average general intellectual functioning which originated during the developmental period and is associated with impairment in adaptive behavior. [NIH]

Mercury: A silver metallic element that exists as a liquid at room temperature. It has the atomic symbol Hg (from hydrargyrum, liquid silver), atomic number 80, and atomic weight 200.59. Mercury is used in many industrial applications and its salts have been employed therapeutically as purgatives, antisyphilitics, disinfectants, and astringents. It can be absorbed through the skin and mucous membranes which leads to mercury poisoning. Because of its toxicity, the clinical use of mercury and mercurials is diminishing. [NIH]

Mesolimbic: Inner brain region governing emotion and drives. [NIH]

Metabolite: Any substance produced by metabolism or by a metabolic process. [EU]

Metabotropic: A glutamate receptor which triggers an increase in production of 2 intracellular messengers: diacylglycerol and inositol 1, 4, 5-triphosphate. [NIH]

Metastasis: The spread of cancer from one part of the body to another. Tumors formed from cells that have spread are called "secondary tumors" and contain cells that are like those in the original (primary) tumor. The plural is metastases. [NIH]

Methionine: A sulfur containing essential amino acid that is important in many body functions. It is a chelating agent for heavy metals. [NIH]

Methylphenidate: A central nervous system stimulant used most commonly in the treatment of attention-deficit disorders in children and for narcolepsy. Its mechanisms appear to be similar to those of dextroamphetamine. [NIH]

MI: Myocardial infarction. Gross necrosis of the myocardium as a result of interruption of the blood supply to the area; it is almost always caused by atherosclerosis of the coronary arteries, upon which coronary thrombosis is usually superimposed. [NIH]

Microbe: An organism which cannot be observed with the naked eye; e. g. unicellular animals, lower algae, lower fungi, bacteria. [NIH]

Microorganism: An organism that can be seen only through a microscope. Microorganisms include bacteria, protozoa, algae, and fungi. Although viruses are not considered living organisms, they are sometimes classified as microorganisms. [NIH]

Microscopy: The application of microscope magnification to the study of materials that cannot be properly seen by the unaided eye. [NIH]

Midwifery: The practice of assisting women in childbirth. [NIH]

Migration: The systematic movement of genes between populations of the same species, geographic race, or variety. [NIH]

Milk Thistle: The plant Silybum marianum in the family Asteraceae containing the bioflavonoid complex silymarin. For centuries this has been used traditionally to treat liver disease. [NIH]

Mitosis: A method of indirect cell division by means of which the two daughter nuclei normally receive identical complements of the number of chromosomes of the somatic cells of the species. [NIH]

Mitotic: Cell resulting from mitosis. [NIH]

Mobility: Capability of movement, of being moved, or of flowing freely. [EU]

Mobilization: The process of making a fixed part or stored substance mobile, as by separating a part from surrounding structures to make it accessible for an operative procedure or by causing release into the circulation for body use of a substance stored in the body. [EU]

Modeling: A treatment procedure whereby the therapist presents the target behavior which the learner is to imitate and make part of his repertoire. [NIH]

Modification: A change in an organism, or in a process in an organism, that is acquired from its own activity or environment. [NIH]

Molecular: Of, pertaining to, or composed of molecules : a very small mass of matter. [EU]

Molecule: A chemical made up of two or more atoms. The atoms in a molecule can be the same (an oxygen molecule has two oxygen atoms) or different (a water molecule has two hydrogen atoms and one oxygen atom). Biological molecules, such as proteins and DNA, can be made up of many thousands of atoms. [NIH]

Monitor: An apparatus which automatically records such physiological signs as respiration, pulse, and blood pressure in an anesthetized patient or one undergoing surgical or other procedures. [NIH]

Monocytes: Large, phagocytic mononuclear leukocytes produced in the vertebrate bone marrow and released into the blood; contain a large, oval or somewhat indented nucleus surrounded by voluminous cytoplasm and numerous organelles. [NIH]

Morphogenesis: The development of the form of an organ, part of the body, or organism. [NIH]

Morphological: Relating to the configuration or the structure of live organs. [NIH]

Morphology: The science of the form and structure of organisms (plants, animals, and other forms of life). [NIH]

Motility: The ability to move spontaneously. [EU]

Motor Cortex: Area of the frontal lobe concerned with primary motor control. It lies anterior to the central sulcus. [NIH]

Motor Skills: Performance of complex motor acts. [NIH]

Mucosa: A mucous membrane, or tunica mucosa. [EU]

Mucositis: A complication of some cancer therapies in which the lining of the digestive system becomes inflamed. Often seen as sores in the mouth. [NIH]

Mutagenesis: Process of generating genetic mutations. It may occur spontaneously or be induced by mutagens. [NIH]

Mutagens: Chemical agents that increase the rate of genetic mutation by interfering with the function of nucleic acids. A clastogen is a specific mutagen that causes breaks in chromosomes. [NIH]

Myelin: The fatty substance that covers and protects nerves. [NIH]

Myelin Sheath: The lipid-rich sheath investing many axons in both the central and peripheral nervous systems. The myelin sheath is an electrical insulator and allows faster and more energetically efficient conduction of impulses. The sheath is formed by the cell membranes of glial cells (Schwann cells in the peripheral and oligodendroglia in the central nervous system). Deterioration of the sheath in demyelinating diseases is a serious clinical problem. [NIH]

Myocardium: The muscle tissue of the heart composed of striated, involuntary muscle known as cardiac muscle. [NIH]

Myosin: Chief protein in muscle and the main constituent of the thick filaments of muscle fibers. In conjunction with actin, it is responsible for the contraction and relaxation of muscles. [NIH]

Naloxone: A specific opiate antagonist that has no agonist activity. It is a competitive antagonist at mu, delta, and kappa opioid receptors. [NIH]

Narcolepsy: A condition of unknown cause characterized by a periodic uncontrollable tendency to fall asleep. [NIH]

Narcotic: 1. Pertaining to or producing narcosis. 2. An agent that produces insensibility or stupor, applied especially to the opioids, i.e. to any natural or synthetic drug that has morphine-like actions. [EU]

Necrosis: A pathological process caused by the progressive degradative action of enzymes that is generally associated with severe cellular trauma. It is characterized by mitochondrial swelling, nuclear flocculation, uncontrolled cell lysis, and ultimately cell death. [NIH]

Need: A state of tension or dissatisfaction felt by an individual that impels him to action toward a goal he believes will satisfy the impulse. [NIH]

Neonatal: Pertaining to the first four weeks after birth. [EU]

Neonatal period: The first 4 weeks after birth. [NIH]

Nerve: A cordlike structure of nervous tissue that connects parts of the nervous system with other tissues of the body and conveys nervous impulses to, or away from, these tissues. [NIH]

Nerve Growth Factor: Nerve growth factor is the first of a series of neurotrophic factors that were found to influence the growth and differentiation of sympathetic and sensory neurons. It is comprised of alpha, beta, and gamma subunits. The beta subunit is responsible for its growth stimulating activity. [NIH]

Nervous System: The entire nerve apparatus composed of the brain, spinal cord, nerves and ganglia. [NIH]

Networks: Pertaining to a nerve or to the nerves, a meshlike structure of interlocking fibers or strands. [NIH]

Neural: 1. Pertaining to a nerve or to the nerves. 2. Situated in the region of the spinal axis, as the neutral arch. [EU]

Neural Crest: A strip of specialized ectoderm flanking each side of the embryonal neural plate, which after the closure of the neural tube, forms a column of isolated cells along the dorsal aspect of the neural tube. Most of the cranial and all of the spinal sensory ganglion cells arise by differentiation of neural crest cells. [NIH]

Neural Pathways: Neural tracts connecting one part of the nervous system with another. [NIH]

Neural tube defects: These defects include problems stemming from fetal development of the spinal cord, spine, brain, and skull, and include birth defects such as spina bifida, anencephaly, and encephalocele. Neural tube defects occur early in pregnancy at about 4 to 6 weeks, usually before a woman knows she is pregnant. Many babies with neural tube defects have difficulty walking and with bladder and bowel control. [NIH]

Neuroanatomy: Study of the anatomy of the nervous system as a specialty or discipline. [NIH]

Neuroendocrine: Having to do with the interactions between the nervous system and the endocrine system. Describes certain cells that release hormones into the blood in response to stimulation of the nervous system. [NIH]

Neurology: A medical specialty concerned with the study of the structures, functions, and diseases of the nervous system. [NIH]

Neuromuscular: Pertaining to muscles and nerves. [EU]

Neuromuscular Junction: The synapse between a neuron and a muscle. [NIH]

Neuronal: Pertaining to a neuron or neurons (= conducting cells of the nervous system). [EU]

Neuronal Plasticity: The capacity of the nervous system to change its reactivity as the result of successive activations. [NIH]

Neurons: The basic cellular units of nervous tissue. Each neuron consists of a body, an axon, and dendrites. Their purpose is to receive, conduct, and transmit impulses in the nervous system. [NIH]

Neuropharmacology: The branch of pharmacology dealing especially with the action of drugs upon various parts of the nervous system. [NIH]

Neurophysiology: The scientific discipline concerned with the physiology of the nervous system. [NIH]

Neuropsychological Tests: Tests designed to assess neurological function associated with certain behaviors. They are used in diagnosing brain dysfunction or damage and central nervous system disorders or injury. [NIH]

Neuropsychology: A branch of psychology which investigates the correlation between experience or behavior and the basic neurophysiological processes. The term neuropsychology stresses the dominant role of the nervous system. It is a more narrowly defined field than physiological psychology or psychophysiology. [NIH]

Neurotoxic: Poisonous or destructive to nerve tissue. [EU]

Neurotoxicity: The tendency of some treatments to cause damage to the nervous system. [NIH]

Neurotoxins: Toxic substances from microorganisms, plants or animals that interfere with the functions of the nervous system. Most venoms contain neurotoxic substances. Myotoxins are included in this concept. [NIH]

Neurotransmitters: Endogenous signaling molecules that alter the behavior of neurons or effector cells. Neurotransmitter is used here in its most general sense, including not only messengers that act directly to regulate ion channels, but also those that act through second messenger systems, and those that act at a distance from their site of release. Included are neuromodulators, neuroregulators, neuromediators, and neurohumors, whether or not acting at synapses. [NIH]

Neutrophils: Granular leukocytes having a nucleus with three to five lobes connected by slender threads of chromatin, and cytoplasm containing fine inconspicuous granules and stainable by neutral dyes. [NIH]

Nitric Oxide: A free radical gas produced endogenously by a variety of mammalian cells. It is synthesized from arginine by a complex reaction, catalyzed by nitric oxide synthase. Nitric oxide is endothelium-derived relaxing factor. It is released by the vascular endothelium and mediates the relaxation induced by some vasodilators such as acetylcholine and bradykinin. It also inhibits platelet aggregation, induces disaggregation of aggregated platelets, and inhibits platelet adhesion to the vascular endothelium. Nitric oxide activates cytosolic guanylate cyclase and thus elevates intracellular levels of cyclic GMP. [NIH]

Norepinephrine: Precursor of epinephrine that is secreted by the adrenal medulla and is a widespread central and autonomic neurotransmitter. Norepinephrine is the principal transmitter of most postganglionic sympathetic fibers and of the diffuse projection system in the brain arising from the locus ceruleus. It is also found in plants and is used pharmacologically as a sympathomimetic. [NIH]

Nuclear: A test of the structure, blood flow, and function of the kidneys. The doctor injects a mildly radioactive solution into an arm vein and uses x-rays to monitor its progress through the kidneys. [NIH]

Nuclei: A body of specialized protoplasm found in nearly all cells and containing the chromosomes. [NIH]

Nucleic acid: Either of two types of macromolecule (DNA or RNA) formed by polymerization of nucleotides. Nucleic acids are found in all living cells and contain the information (genetic code) for the transfer of genetic information from one generation to the next. [NIH]

Nucleus: A body of specialized protoplasm found in nearly all cells and containing the chromosomes. [NIH]

Nucleus Accumbens: Collection of pleomorphic cells in the caudal part of the anterior horn of the lateral ventricle, in the region of the olfactory tubercle, lying between the head of the caudate nucleus and the anterior perforated substance. It is part of the so-called ventral striatum, a composite structure considered part of the basal ganglia. [NIH]

Obstetrics: A medical-surgical specialty concerned with management and care of women during pregnancy, parturition, and the puerperium. [NIH]

Occupational Therapy: The field concerned with utilizing craft or work activities in the rehabilitation of patients. Occupational therapy can also refer to the activities themselves. [NIH]

Ocular: 1. Of, pertaining to, or affecting the eye. 2. Eyepiece. [EU]

Oligodendroglia: A class of neuroglial (macroglial) cells in the central nervous system. Oligodendroglia may be called interfascicular, perivascular, or perineuronal satellite cells according to their location. The most important recognized function of these cells is the formation of the insulating myelin sheaths of axons in the central nervous system. [NIH]

Oncogenic: Chemical, viral, radioactive or other agent that causes cancer; carcinogenic. [NIH]

Open Reading Frames: Reading frames where successive nucleotide triplets can be read as codons specifying amino acids and where the sequence of these triplets is not interrupted by stop codons. [NIH]

Operon: The genetic unit consisting of a feedback system under the control of an operator gene, in which a structural gene transcribes its message in the form of mRNA upon blockade of a repressor produced by a regulator gene. Included here is the attenuator site of bacterial operons where transcription termination is regulated. [NIH]

Ophthalmic: Pertaining to the eye. [EU]

Opportunistic Infections: An infection caused by an organism which becomes pathogenic under certain conditions, e.g., during immunosuppression. [NIH]

Opsin: A visual pigment protein found in the retinal rods. It combines with retinaldehyde to form rhodopsin. [NIH]

Optic Chiasm: The X-shaped structure formed by the meeting of the two optic nerves. At the optic chiasm the fibers from the medial part of each retina cross to project to the other side of the brain while the lateral retinal fibers continue on the same side. As a result each half of the brain receives information about the contralateral visual field from both eyes. [NIH]

Oral Manifestations: Disorders of the mouth attendant upon non-oral disease or injury. [NIH]

Organelles: Specific particles of membrane-bound organized living substances present in eukaryotic cells, such as the mitochondria; the golgi apparatus; endoplasmic reticulum; lysomomes; plastids; and vacuoles. [NIH]

Otitis: Inflammation of the ear, which may be marked by pain, fever, abnormalities of hearing, hearing loss, tinnitus, and vertigo. [EU]

Otitis Media: Inflammation of the middle ear. [NIH]

Ovary: Either of the paired glands in the female that produce the female germ cells and secrete some of the female sex hormones. [NIH]

Overexpress: An excess of a particular protein on the surface of a cell. [NIH]

Ovulation: The discharge of a secondary oocyte from a ruptured graafian follicle. [NIH]

Ovum: A female germ cell extruded from the ovary at ovulation. [NIH]

Oxidation: The act of oxidizing or state of being oxidized. Chemically it consists in the increase of positive charges on an atom or the loss of negative charges. Most biological oxidations are accomplished by the removal of a pair of hydrogen atoms (dehydrogenation) from a molecule. Such oxidations must be accompanied by reduction of an acceptor molecule. Univalent o. indicates loss of one electron; divalent o., the loss of two electrons. [EU]

Oxidative Stress: A disturbance in the prooxidant-antioxidant balance in favor of the former, leading to potential damage. Indicators of oxidative stress include damaged DNA bases, protein oxidation products, and lipid peroxidation products (Sies, Oxidative Stress, 1991, pxv-xvi). [NIH]

Palliative: 1. Affording relief, but not cure. 2. An alleviating medicine. [EU]

Pancreas: A mixed exocrine and endocrine gland situated transversely across the posterior abdominal wall in the epigastric and hypochondriac regions. The endocrine portion is comprised of the Islets of Langerhans, while the exocrine portion is a compound acinar gland that secretes digestive enzymes. [NIH]

Parietal: 1. Of or pertaining to the walls of a cavity. 2. Pertaining to or located near the parietal bone, as the parietal lobe. [EU]

Parietal Lobe: Upper central part of the cerebral hemisphere. [NIH]

Parturition: The act or process of given birth to a child. [EU]

Patch: A piece of material used to cover or protect a wound, an injured part, etc.: a patch over the eye. [NIH]

Pathogen: Any disease-producing microorganism. [EU]

Pathogenesis: The cellular events and reactions that occur in the development of disease. [NIH]

Pathologic: 1. Indicative of or caused by a morbid condition. 2. Pertaining to pathology (= branch of medicine that treats the essential nature of the disease, especially the structural and functional changes in tissues and organs of the body caused by the disease). [EU]

Pathologic Processes: The abnormal mechanisms and forms involved in the dysfunctions of tissues and organs. [NIH]

Pathophysiology: Altered functions in an individual or an organ due to disease. [NIH]

Patient Advocacy: Promotion and protection of the rights of patients, frequently through a legal process. [NIH]

Patient Education: The teaching or training of patients concerning their own health needs. [NIH]

Pediatrics: A medical specialty concerned with maintaining health and providing medical care to children from birth to adolescence. [NIH]

Penicillin: An antibiotic drug used to treat infection. [NIH]

Peptide: Any compound consisting of two or more amino acids, the building blocks of proteins. Peptides are combined to make proteins. [NIH]

Perception: The ability quickly and accurately to recognize similarities and differences among presented objects, whether these be pairs of words, pairs of number series, or multiple sets of these or other symbols such as geometric figures. [NIH]

Perfusion: Bathing an organ or tissue with a fluid. In regional perfusion, a specific area of the body (usually an arm or a leg) receives high doses of anticancer drugs through a blood vessel. Such a procedure is performed to treat cancer that has not spread. [NIH]

Perinatal: Pertaining to or occurring in the period shortly before and after birth; variously defined as beginning with completion of the twentieth to twenty-eighth week of gestation and ending 7 to 28 days after birth. [EU]

Peripheral Nerves: The nerves outside of the brain and spinal cord, including the autonomic, cranial, and spinal nerves. Peripheral nerves contain non-neuronal cells and connective tissue as well as axons. The connective tissue layers include, from the outside to the inside, the epineurium, the perineurium, and the endoneurium. [NIH]

Peripheral Nervous System: The nervous system outside of the brain and spinal cord. The peripheral nervous system has autonomic and somatic divisions. The autonomic nervous system includes the enteric, parasympathetic, and sympathetic subdivisions. The somatic nervous system includes the cranial and spinal nerves and their ganglia and the peripheral sensory receptors. [NIH]

Perivascular: Situated around a vessel. [EU]

Peroneal Nerve: The lateral of the two terminal branches of the sciatic nerve. The peroneal (or fibular) nerve provides motor and sensory innervation to parts of the leg and foot. [NIH]

Pesticides: Chemicals used to destroy pests of any sort. The concept includes fungicides (industrial fungicides), insecticides, rodenticides, etc. [NIH]

PH: The symbol relating the hydrogen ion (H+) concentration or activity of a solution to that of a given standard solution. Numerically the pH is approximately equal to the negative logarithm of H+ concentration expressed in molarity. pH 7 is neutral; above it alkalinity increases and below it acidity increases. [EU]

Phagocytosis: The engulfing of microorganisms, other cells, and foreign particles by phagocytic cells. [NIH]

Pharmacologic: Pertaining to pharmacology or to the properties and reactions of drugs. [EU]

Phenotype: The outward appearance of the individual. It is the product of interactions between genes and between the genotype and the environment. This includes the killer phenotype, characteristic of yeasts. [NIH]

Phenylalanine: An aromatic amino acid that is essential in the animal diet. It is a precursor of melanin, dopamine, noradrenalin, and thyroxine. [NIH]

Phospholipases: A class of enzymes that catalyze the hydrolysis of phosphoglycerides or glycerophosphatidates. EC 3.1.-. [NIH]

Phospholipids: Lipids containing one or more phosphate groups, particularly those derived from either glycerol (phosphoglycerides; glycerophospholipids) or sphingosine (sphingolipids). They are polar lipids that are of great importance for the structure and function of cell membranes and are the most abundant of membrane lipids, although not stored in large amounts in the system. [NIH]

Phosphorus: A non-metallic element that is found in the blood, muscles, nevers, bones, and teeth, and is a component of adenosine triphosphate (ATP; the primary energy source for the body's cells.) [NIH]

Phosphorylated: Attached to a phosphate group. [NIH]

Phosphorylation: The introduction of a phosphoryl group into a compound through the formation of an ester bond between the compound and a phosphorus moiety. [NIH]

Phosphotyrosine: An amino acid that occurs in endogenous proteins. Tyrosine phosphorylation and dephosphorylation plays a role in cellular signal transduction and possibly in cell growth control and carcinogenesis. [NIH]

Physical Therapy: The restoration of function and the prevention of disability following disease or injury with the use of light, heat, cold, water, electricity, ultrasound, and exercise. [NIH]

Physiologic: Having to do with the functions of the body. When used in the phrase "physiologic age," it refers to an age assigned by general health, as opposed to calendar age. [NIH]

Physiology: The science that deals with the life processes and functions of organismus, their cells, tissues, and organs. [NIH]

Pigments: Any normal or abnormal coloring matter in plants, animals, or micro-organisms. [NIH]

Pilot study: The initial study examining a new method or treatment. [NIH]

Pituitary Gland: A small, unpaired gland situated in the sella turcica tissue. It is connected to the hypothalamus by a short stalk. [NIH]

Placenta: A highly vascular fetal organ through which the fetus absorbs oxygen and other nutrients and excretes carbon dioxide and other wastes. It begins to form about the eighth day of gestation when the blastocyst adheres to the decidua. [NIH]

Plants: Multicellular, eukaryotic life forms of the kingdom Plantae. They are characterized by a mainly photosynthetic mode of nutrition; essentially unlimited growth at localized regions of cell divisions (meristems); cellulose within cells providing rigidity; the absence of organs of locomotion; absense of nervous and sensory systems; and an alteration of haploid and diploid generations. [NIH]

Plasma: The clear, yellowish, fluid part of the blood that carries the blood cells. The proteins that form blood clots are in plasma. [NIH]

Plasma cells: A type of white blood cell that produces antibodies. [NIH]

Plasticity: In an individual or a population, the capacity for adaptation: a) through gene changes (genetic plasticity) or b) through internal physiological modifications in response to changes of environment (physiological plasticity). [NIH]

Platelet Activation: A series of progressive, overlapping events triggered by exposure of the platelets to subendothelial tissue. These events include shape change, adhesiveness, aggregation, and release reactions. When carried through to completion, these events lead to the formation of a stable hemostatic plug. [NIH]

Platelet Aggregation: The attachment of platelets to one another. This clumping together can be induced by a number of agents (e.g., thrombin, collagen) and is part of the mechanism leading to the formation of a thrombus. [NIH]

Platelets: A type of blood cell that helps prevent bleeding by causing blood clots to form. Also called thrombocytes. [NIH]

Plexus: A network or tangle; a general term for a network of lymphatic vessels, nerves, or veins. [EU]

Polymerase: An enzyme which catalyses the synthesis of DNA using a single DNA strand as a template. The polymerase copies the template in the 5'-3'direction provided that sufficient quantities of free nucleotides, dATP and dTTP are present. [NIH]

Polymers: Compounds formed by the joining of smaller, usually repeating, units linked by covalent bonds. These compounds often form large macromolecules (e.g., polypeptides, proteins, plastics). [NIH]

Polymorphic: Occurring in several or many forms; appearing in different forms at different stages of development. [EU]

Polypeptide: A peptide which on hydrolysis yields more than two amino acids; called tripeptides, tetrapeptides, etc. according to the number of amino acids contained. [EU]

Polysaccharide: A type of carbohydrate. It contains sugar molecules that are linked together chemically. [NIH]

Pontine: A brain region involved in the detection and processing of taste. [NIH]

Post partum: After childbirth, or after delivery. [EU]

Posterior: Situated in back of, or in the back part of, or affecting the back or dorsal surface of the body. In lower animals, it refers to the caudal end of the body. [EU]

Postnatal: Occurring after birth, with reference to the newborn. [EU]

Postsynaptic: Nerve potential generated by an inhibitory hyperpolarizing stimulation. [NIH]

Potassium: An element that is in the alkali group of metals. It has an atomic symbol K, atomic number 19, and atomic weight 39.10. It is the chief cation in the intracellular fluid of muscle and other cells. Potassium ion is a strong electrolyte and it plays a significant role in the regulation of fluid volume and maintenance of the water-electrolyte balance. [NIH]

Potentiates: A degree of synergism which causes the exposure of the organism to a harmful substance to worsen a disease already contracted. [NIH]

Potentiation: An overall effect of two drugs taken together which is greater than the sum of the effects of each drug taken alone. [NIH]

Practice Guidelines: Directions or principles presenting current or future rules of policy for the health care practitioner to assist him in patient care decisions regarding diagnosis, therapy, or related clinical circumstances. The guidelines may be developed by government agencies at any level, institutions, professional societies, governing boards, or by the convening of expert panels. The guidelines form a basis for the evaluation of all aspects of health care and delivery. [NIH]

Preclinical: Before a disease becomes clinically recognizable. [EU]

Precursor: Something that precedes. In biological processes, a substance from which another, usually more active or mature substance is formed. In clinical medicine, a sign or symptom that heralds another. [EU]

Predisposition: A latent susceptibility to disease which may be activated under certain conditions, as by stress. [EU]

Pregnancy Outcome: Results of conception and ensuing pregnancy, including live birth, stillbirth, spontaneous abortion, induced abortion. The outcome may follow natural or artificial insemination or any of the various reproduction techniques, such as embryo transfer or fertilization in vitro. [NIH]

Pregnancy-Specific beta 1-Glycoprotein: A glycoprotein with the electrophoretic mobility of a beta-1 globulin. It is produced by the placental trophoblast and secreted into the maternal bloodstream during pregnancy. It can be detected 18 days after ovulation and its concentration in plasma rises steadily until, at the end of gestation, it reaches 200 mg/ml. It has been proposed as a measure of placental function for fertility control and is a candidate for an early pregnancy test. [NIH]

Prenatal: Existing or occurring before birth, with reference to the fetus. [EU]

Prenatal Care: Care provided the pregnant woman in order to prevent complications, and decrease the incidence of maternal and prenatal mortality. [NIH]

Presynaptic: Situated proximal to a synapse, or occurring before the synapse is crossed. [EU]

Prevalence: The total number of cases of a given disease in a specified population at a designated time. It is differentiated from incidence, which refers to the number of new cases in the population at a given time. [NIH]

Probe: An instrument used in exploring cavities, or in the detection and dilatation of strictures, or in demonstrating the potency of channels; an elongated instrument for exploring or sounding body cavities. [NIH]

Problem Solving: A learning situation involving more than one alternative from which a selection is made in order to attain a specific goal. [NIH]

Progression: Increase in the size of a tumor or spread of cancer in the body. [NIH]

Progressive: Advancing; going forward; going from bad to worse; increasing in scope or severity. [EU]

Projection: A defense mechanism, operating unconsciously, whereby that which is emotionally unacceptable in the self is rejected and attributed (projected) to others. [NIH]

Promoter: A chemical substance that increases the activity of a carcinogenic process. [NIH]

Prone: Having the front portion of the body downwards. [NIH]

Proneness: Susceptibility to accidents due to human factors. [NIH]

Prophase: The first phase of cell division, in which the chromosomes become visible, the nucleus starts to lose its identity, the spindle appears, and the centrioles migrate toward opposite poles. [NIH]

Prophylaxis: An attempt to prevent disease. [NIH]

Prosencephalon: The part of the brain developed from the most rostral of the three primary vesicles of the embryonic neural tube and consisting of the diencephalon and telencephalon. [NIH]

Prostaglandin: Any of a group of components derived from unsaturated 20-carbon fatty acids, primarily arachidonic acid, via the cyclooxygenase pathway that are extremely potent mediators of a diverse group of physiologic processes. The abbreviation for prostaglandin is PG; specific compounds are designated by adding one of the letters A through I to indicate the type of substituents found on the hydrocarbon skeleton and a subscript (1, 2 or 3) to indicate the number of double bonds in the hydrocarbon skeleton e.g., PGE2. The predominant naturally occurring prostaglandins all have two double bonds and are synthesized from arachidonic acid (5,8,11,14-eicosatetraenoic acid) by the pathway shown in the illustration. The 1 series and 3 series are produced by the same pathway with fatty acids having one fewer double bond (8,11,14-eicosatrienoic acid or one more double bond (5,8,11,14,17-eicosapentaenoic acid) than arachidonic acid. The subscript a or ß indicates the configuration at C-9 (a denotes a substituent below the plane of the ring, ß, above the plane). The naturally occurring PGF's have the a configuration, e.g., PGF2a. All of the prostaglandins act by binding to specific cell-surface receptors causing an increase in the level of the intracellular second messenger cyclic AMP (and in some cases cyclic GMP also). The effect produced by the cyclic AMP increase depends on the specific cell type. In some cases there is also a positive feedback effect. Increased cyclic AMP increases prostaglandin synthesis leading to further increases in cyclic AMP. [EU]

Prostaglandins A: (13E,15S)-15-Hydroxy-9-oxoprosta-10,13-dien-1-oic acid (PGA(1)); (5Z,13E,15S)-15-hydroxy-9-oxoprosta-5,10,13-trien-1-oic acid (PGA(2)); (5Z,13E,15S,17Z)-15-hydroxy-9-oxoprosta-5,10,13,17-tetraen-1-oic acid (PGA(3)). A group of naturally occurring secondary prostaglandins derived from PGE. PGA(1) and PGA(2) as well as their 19-hydroxy derivatives are found in many organs and tissues. [NIH]

Prostate: A gland in males that surrounds the neck of the bladder and the urethra. It secretes a substance that liquifies coagulated semen. It is situated in the pelvic cavity behind the lower part of the pubic symphysis, above the deep layer of the triangular ligament, and rests upon the rectum. [NIH]

Protein C: A vitamin-K dependent zymogen present in the blood, which, upon activation by thrombin and thrombomodulin exerts anticoagulant properties by inactivating factors Va and VIIIa at the rate-limiting steps of thrombin formation. [NIH]

Protein Kinases: A family of enzymes that catalyze the conversion of ATP and a protein to ADP and a phosphoprotein. EC 2.7.1.37. [NIH]

Protein S: The vitamin K-dependent cofactor of activated protein C. Together with protein C, it inhibits the action of factors VIIIa and Va. A deficiency in protein S can lead to recurrent venous and arterial thrombosis. [NIH]

Protein Subunits: Single chains of amino acids that are the units of a multimeric protein. They can be identical or non-identical subunits. [NIH]

Proteins: Polymers of amino acids linked by peptide bonds. The specific sequence of amino acids determines the shape and function of the protein. [NIH]

Protocol: The detailed plan for a clinical trial that states the trial's rationale, purpose, drug or vaccine dosages, length of study, routes of administration, who may participate, and other aspects of trial design. [NIH]

Proximal: Nearest; closer to any point of reference; opposed to distal. [EU]

Psychiatry: The medical science that deals with the origin, diagnosis, prevention, and treatment of mental disorders. [NIH]

Psychic: Pertaining to the psyche or to the mind; mental. [EU]

Psychology: The science dealing with the study of mental processes and behavior in man and animals. [NIH]

Psychomotor: Pertaining to motor effects of cerebral or psychic activity. [EU]

Psychopathology: The study of significant causes and processes in the development of mental illness. [NIH]

Psychophysiology: The study of the physiological basis of human and animal behavior. [NIH]

Psychosis: A mental disorder characterized by gross impairment in reality testing as evidenced by delusions, hallucinations, markedly incoherent speech, or disorganized and agitated behaviour without apparent awareness on the part of the patient of the incomprehensibility of his behaviour; the term is also used in a more general sense to refer to mental disorders in which mental functioning is sufficiently impaired as to interfere grossly with the patient's capacity to meet the ordinary demands of life. Historically, the term has been applied to many conditions, e.g. manic-depressive psychosis, that were first described in psychotic patients, although many patients with the disorder are not judged psychotic. [EU]

Public Health: Branch of medicine concerned with the prevention and control of disease and disability, and the promotion of physical and mental health of the population on the international, national, state, or municipal level. [NIH]

Public Policy: A course or method of action selected, usually by a government, from among alternatives to guide and determine present and future decisions. [NIH]

Puerperium: Period from delivery of the placenta until return of the reproductive organs to their normal nonpregnant morphologic state. In humans, the puerperium generally lasts for six to eight weeks. [NIH]

Pulmonary: Relating to the lungs. [NIH]

Pulmonary hypertension: Abnormally high blood pressure in the arteries of the lungs. [NIH]

Pulse: The rhythmical expansion and contraction of an artery produced by waves of pressure caused by the ejection of blood from the left ventricle of the heart as it contracts. [NIH]

Purines: A series of heterocyclic compounds that are variously substituted in nature and are known also as purine bases. They include adenine and guanine, constituents of nucleic acids, as well as many alkaloids such as caffeine and theophylline. Uric acid is the metabolic end product of purine metabolism. [NIH]

Pyramidal Cells: Projection neurons in the cerebral cortex and the hippocampus. Pyramidal cells have a pyramid-shaped soma with the apex and an apical dendrite pointed toward the pial surface and other dendrites and an axon emerging from the base. The axons may have local collaterals but also project outside their cortical region. [NIH]

Quality of Life: A generic concept reflecting concern with the modification and enhancement of life attributes, e.g., physical, political, moral and social environment. [NIH]

Race: A population within a species which exhibits general similarities within itself, but is both discontinuous and distinct from other populations of that species, though not sufficiently so as to achieve the status of a taxon. [NIH]

Radiation: Emission or propagation of electromagnetic energy (waves/rays), or the waves/rays themselves; a stream of electromagnetic particles (electrons, neutrons, protons, alpha particles) or a mixture of these. The most common source is the sun. [NIH]

Radioactive: Giving off radiation. [NIH]

Radioisotope: An unstable element that releases radiation as it breaks down. Radioisotopes can be used in imaging tests or as a treatment for cancer. [NIH]

Randomized: Describes an experiment or clinical trial in which animal or human subjects are assigned by chance to separate groups that compare different treatments. [NIH]

Randomized clinical trial: A study in which the participants are assigned by chance to separate groups that compare different treatments; neither the researchers nor the participants can choose which group. Using chance to assign people to groups means that the groups will be similar and that the treatments they receive can be compared objectively. At the time of the trial, it is not known which treatment is best. It is the patient's choice to be in a randomized trial. [NIH]

Reactive Oxygen Species: Reactive intermediate oxygen species including both radicals and non-radicals. These substances are constantly formed in the human body and have been shown to kill bacteria and inactivate proteins, and have been implicated in a number of diseases. Scientific data exist that link the reactive oxygen species produced by inflammatory phagocytes to cancer development. [NIH]

Reality Testing: The individual's objective evaluation of the external world and the ability to differentiate adequately between it and the internal world; considered to be a primary ego function. [NIH]

Receptor: A molecule inside or on the surface of a cell that binds to a specific substance and causes a specific physiologic effect in the cell. [NIH]

Receptors, Serotonin: Cell-surface proteins that bind serotonin and trigger intracellular changes which influence the behavior of cells. Several types of serotonin receptors have been recognized which differ in their pharmacology, molecular biology, and mode of action. [NIH]

Recombinant: A cell or an individual with a new combination of genes not found together in either parent; usually applied to linked genes. [EU]

Recombinant Proteins: Proteins prepared by recombinant DNA technology. [NIH]

Recurrence: The return of a sign, symptom, or disease after a remission. [NIH]

Red Nucleus: A pinkish-yellow portion of the midbrain situated in the rostral mesencephalic tegmentum. It receives a large projection from the contralateral half of the cerebellum via the superior cerebellar peduncle and a projection from the ipsilateral motor cortex. [NIH]

Refer: To send or direct for treatment, aid, information, de decision. [NIH]

Reflex: An involuntary movement or exercise of function in a part, excited in response to a stimulus applied to the periphery and transmitted to the brain or spinal cord. [NIH]

Refraction: A test to determine the best eyeglasses or contact lenses to correct a refractive error (myopia, hyperopia, or astigmatism). [NIH]

Refractory: Not readily yielding to treatment. [EU]

Regeneration: The natural renewal of a structure, as of a lost tissue or part. [EU]

Regimen: A treatment plan that specifies the dosage, the schedule, and the duration of treatment. [NIH]

Regression Analysis: Procedures for finding the mathematical function which best describes the relationship between a dependent variable and one or more independent variables. In linear regression (see linear models) the relationship is constrained to be a straight line and least-squares analysis is used to determine the best fit. In logistic regression (see logistic models) the dependent variable is qualitative rather than continuously variable and likelihood functions are used to find the best relationship. In multiple regression the dependent variable is considered to depend on more than a single independent variable. [NIH]

Rehabilitative: Instruction of incapacitated individuals or of those affected with some mental disorder, so that some or all of their lost ability may be regained. [NIH]

Repressor: Any of the specific allosteric protein molecules, products of regulator genes, which bind to the operator of operons and prevent RNA polymerase from proceeding into the operon to transcribe messenger RNA. [NIH]

Reproduction Techniques: Methods pertaining to the generation of new individuals. [NIH]

Research Design: A plan for collecting and utilizing data so that desired information can be obtained with sufficient precision or so that an hypothesis can be tested properly. [NIH]

Respiration: The act of breathing with the lungs, consisting of inspiration, or the taking into the lungs of the ambient air, and of expiration, or the expelling of the modified air which contains more carbon dioxide than the air taken in (Blakiston's Gould Medical Dictionary, 4th ed.). This does not include tissue respiration (= oxygen consumption) or cell respiration (= cell respiration). [NIH]

Respiratory distress syndrome: A lung disease that occurs primarily in premature infants; the newborn must struggle for each breath and blueing of its skin reflects the baby's inability to get enough oxygen. [NIH]

Respiratory Paralysis: Complete or severe weakness of the muscles of respiration. This condition may be associated with motor neuron diseases; peripheral nerve disorders; neuromuscular junction diseases; spinal cord diseases; injury to the phrenic nerve; and other disorders. [NIH]

Respiratory Physiology: Functions and activities of the respiratory tract as a whole or of any of its parts. [NIH]

Respiratory System: The tubular and cavernous organs and structures, by means of which pulmonary ventilation and gas exchange between ambient air and the blood are brought about. [NIH]

Restoration: Broad term applied to any inlay, crown, bridge or complete denture which restores or replaces loss of teeth or oral tissues. [NIH]

Retina: The ten-layered nervous tissue membrane of the eye. It is continuous with the optic nerve and receives images of external objects and transmits visual impulses to the brain. Its outer surface is in contact with the choroid and the inner surface with the vitreous body. The outer-most layer is pigmented, whereas the inner nine layers are transparent. [NIH]

Retinal: 1. Pertaining to the retina. 2. The aldehyde of retinol, derived by the oxidative enzymatic splitting of absorbed dietary carotene, and having vitamin A activity. In the retina, retinal combines with opsins to form visual pigments. One isomer, 11-cis retinal combines with opsin in the rods (scotopsin) to form rhodopsin, or visual purple. Another, all-trans retinal (trans-r.); visual yellow; xanthopsin) results from the bleaching of rhodopsin by light, in which the 11-cis form is converted to the all-trans form. Retinal also combines with opsins in the cones (photopsins) to form the three pigments responsible for colour vision. Called also retinal, and retinene1. [EU]

Retinoid: Vitamin A or a vitamin A-like compound. [NIH]

Retinol: Vitamin A. It is essential for proper vision and healthy skin and mucous membranes. Retinol is being studied for cancer prevention; it belongs to the family of drugs called retinoids. [NIH]

Ribose: A pentose active in biological systems usually in its D-form. [NIH]

Risk factor: A habit, trait, condition, or genetic alteration that increases a person's chance of developing a disease. [NIH]

Rod: A reception for vision, located in the retina. [NIH]

Rodenticides: Substances used to destroy or inhibit the action of rats, mice, or other rodents. [NIH]

Ryanodine: Insecticidal alkaloid isolated from Ryania speciosa; proposed as a myocardial depressant. [NIH]

Satellite: Applied to a vein which closely accompanies an artery for some distance; in cytogenetics, a chromosomal agent separated by a secondary constriction from the main body of the chromosome. [NIH]

Schizoid: Having qualities resembling those found in greater degree in schizophrenics; a person of schizoid personality. [NIH]

Schizophrenia: A mental disorder characterized by a special type of disintegration of the personality. [NIH]

Schizotypal Personality Disorder: A personality disorder in which there are oddities of thought (magical thinking, paranoid ideation, suspiciousness), perception (illusions, depersonalization), speech (digressive, vague, overelaborate), and behavior (inappropriate affect in social interactions, frequently social isolation) that are not severe enough to characterize schizophrenia. [NIH]

Sciatic Nerve: A nerve which originates in the lumbar and sacral spinal cord (L4 to S3) and supplies motor and sensory innervation to the lower extremity. The sciatic nerve, which is the main continuation of the sacral plexus, is the largest nerve in the body. It has two major branches, the tibial nerve and the peroneal nerve. [NIH]

Sclerosis: A pathological process consisting of hardening or fibrosis of an anatomical structure, often a vessel or a nerve. [NIH]

Screening: Checking for disease when there are no symptoms. [NIH]

Second Messenger Systems: Systems in which an intracellular signal is generated in response to an intercellular primary messenger such as a hormone or neurotransmitter. They are intermediate signals in cellular processes such as metabolism, secretion, contraction, phototransduction, and cell growth. Examples of second messenger systems are the adenyl cyclase-cyclic AMP system, the phosphatidylinositol diphosphate-inositol triphosphate system, and the cyclic GMP system. [NIH]

Secretion: 1. The process of elaborating a specific product as a result of the activity of a gland; this activity may range from separating a specific substance of the blood to the elaboration of a new chemical substance. 2. Any substance produced by secretion. [EU]

Secretory: Secreting; relating to or influencing secretion or the secretions. [NIH]

Sedative: 1. Allaying activity and excitement. 2. An agent that allays excitement. [EU]

Segmentation: The process by which muscles in the intestines move food and wastes through the body. [NIH]

Seizures: Clinical or subclinical disturbances of cortical function due to a sudden, abnormal, excessive, and disorganized discharge of brain cells. Clinical manifestations include abnormal motor, sensory and psychic phenomena. Recurrent seizures are usually referred to as epilepsy or "seizure disorder." [NIH]

Semicircular canal: Three long canals of the bony labyrinth of the ear, forming loops and opening into the vestibule by five openings. [NIH]

Sensitization: 1. Administration of antigen to induce a primary immune response; priming; immunization. 2. Exposure to allergen that results in the development of hypersensitivity. 3. The coating of erythrocytes with antibody so that they are subject to lysis by complement in the presence of homologous antigen, the first stage of a complement fixation test. [EU]

Sepsis: The presence of bacteria in the bloodstream. [NIH]

Serine: A non-essential amino acid occurring in natural form as the L-isomer. It is synthesized from glycine or threonine. It is involved in the biosynthesis of purines, pyrimidines, and other amino acids. [NIH]

Serotonin: A biochemical messenger and regulator, synthesized from the essential amino acid L-tryptophan. In humans it is found primarily in the central nervous system, gastrointestinal tract, and blood platelets. Serotonin mediates several important physiological functions including neurotransmission, gastrointestinal motility, hemostasis, and cardiovascular integrity. Multiple receptor families (receptors, serotonin) explain the broad physiological actions and distribution of this biochemical mediator. [NIH]

Serous: Having to do with serum, the clear liquid part of blood. [NIH]

Serum: The clear liquid part of the blood that remains after blood cells and clotting proteins have been removed. [NIH]

Sex Characteristics: Those characteristics that dstinguish one sex from the other. The primary sex characteristics are the ovaries and testes and their related hormones. Secondary sex characteristics are those which are masculine or feminine but not directly related to reproduction. [NIH]

Shock: The general bodily disturbance following a severe injury; an emotional or moral upset occasioned by some disturbing or unexpected experience; disruption of the circulation, which can upset all body functions: sometimes referred to as circulatory shock. [NIH]

Side effect: A consequence other than the one(s) for which an agent or measure is used, as the adverse effects produced by a drug, especially on a tissue or organ system other than the one sought to be benefited by its administration. [EU]

Signal Transduction: The intercellular or intracellular transfer of information (biological activation/inhibition) through a signal pathway. In each signal transduction system, an activation/inhibition signal from a biologically active molecule (hormone, neurotransmitter) is mediated via the coupling of a receptor/enzyme to a second messenger system or to an ion channel. Signal transduction plays an important role in activating cellular functions, cell differentiation, and cell proliferation. Examples of signal transduction systems are the GABA-postsynaptic receptor-calcium ion channel system, the receptor-mediated T-cell activation pathway, and the receptor-mediated activation of phospholipases. Those coupled to membrane depolarization or intracellular release of calcium include the receptor-mediated activation of cytotoxic functions in granulocytes and the synaptic potentiation of protein kinase activation. Some signal transduction pathways may be part of larger signal transduction pathways; for example, protein kinase activation is part of the platelet activation signal pathway. [NIH]

Silymarin: A mixture of flavonoids extracted from seeds of the milk thistle, Silybum marianum. It consists primarily of three isomers: silicristin, silidianin, and silybin, its major component. Silymarin displays antioxidant and membrane stabilizing activity. It protects various tissues and organs against chemical injury, and shows potential as an antihepatoxic agent. [NIH]

Skeletal: Having to do with the skeleton (boney part of the body). [NIH]

Skeleton: The framework that supports the soft tissues of vertebrate animals and protects many of their internal organs. The skeletons of vertebrates are made of bone and/or cartilage. [NIH]

Skull: The skeleton of the head including the bones of the face and the bones enclosing the brain. [NIH]

Small intestine: The part of the digestive tract that is located between the stomach and the large intestine. [NIH]

Social Environment: The aggregate of social and cultural institutions, forms, patterns, and processes that influence the life of an individual or community. [NIH]

Social Problems: Situations affecting a significant number of people, that are believed to be sources of difficulty or threaten the stability of the community, and that require programs of amelioration. [NIH]

Socioeconomic Factors: Social and economic factors that characterize the individual or group within the social structure. [NIH]

Sodium: An element that is a member of the alkali group of metals. It has the atomic symbol Na, atomic number 11, and atomic weight 23. With a valence of 1, it has a strong affinity for oxygen and other nonmetallic elements. Sodium provides the chief cation of the extracellular body fluids. Its salts are the most widely used in medicine. (From Dorland, 27th ed) Physiologically the sodium ion plays a major role in blood pressure regulation, maintenance of fluid volume, and electrolyte balance. [NIH]

Soft tissue: Refers to muscle, fat, fibrous tissue, blood vessels, or other supporting tissue of the body. [NIH]

Solvent: 1. Dissolving; effecting a solution. 2. A liquid that dissolves or that is capable of dissolving; the component of a solution that is present in greater amount. [EU]

Somatic: 1. Pertaining to or characteristic of the soma or body. 2. Pertaining to the body wall in contrast to the viscera. [EU]

Somatosensory Cortex: Area of the parietal lobe concerned with receiving general sensations. It lies posterior to the central sulcus. [NIH]

Sound wave: An alteration of properties of an elastic medium, such as pressure, particle displacement, or density, that propagates through the medium, or a superposition of such alterations. [NIH]

Specialist: In medicine, one who concentrates on 1 special branch of medical science. [NIH]

Species: A taxonomic category subordinate to a genus (or subgenus) and superior to a subspecies or variety, composed of individuals possessing common characters distinguishing them from other categories of individuals of the same taxonomic level. In taxonomic nomenclature, species are designated by the genus name followed by a Latin or Latinized adjective or noun. [EU]

Specificity: Degree of selectivity shown by an antibody with respect to the number and types of antigens with which the antibody combines, as well as with respect to the rates and the extents of these reactions. [NIH]

Spectrum: A charted band of wavelengths of electromagnetic vibrations obtained by refraction and diffraction. By extension, a measurable range of activity, such as the range of bacteria affected by an antibiotic (antibacterial s.) or the complete range of manifestations of a disease. [EU]

Sperm: The fecundating fluid of the male. [NIH]

Spinal cord: The main trunk or bundle of nerves running down the spine through holes in the spinal bone (the vertebrae) from the brain to the level of the lower back. [NIH]

Spinal Nerves: The 31 paired peripheral nerves formed by the union of the dorsal and ventral spinal roots from each spinal cord segment. The spinal nerve plexuses and the spinal roots are also included. [NIH]

Spleen: An organ that is part of the lymphatic system. The spleen produces lymphocytes, filters the blood, stores blood cells, and destroys old blood cells. It is located on the left side of the abdomen near the stomach. [NIH]

Spontaneous Abortion: The non-induced birth of an embryo or of fetus prior to the stage of viability at about 20 weeks of gestation. [NIH]

Steel: A tough, malleable, iron-based alloy containing up to, but no more than, two percent carbon and often other metals. It is used in medicine and dentistry in implants and instrumentation. [NIH]

Stem Cells: Relatively undifferentiated cells of the same lineage (family type) that retain the ability to divide and cycle throughout postnatal life to provide cells that can become specialized and take the place of those that die or are lost. [NIH]

Steroids: Drugs used to relieve swelling and inflammation. [NIH]

Stillbirth: The birth of a dead fetus or baby. [NIH]

Stimulant: 1. Producing stimulation; especially producing stimulation by causing tension on muscle fibre through the nervous tissue. 2. An agent or remedy that produces stimulation. [EU]

Stimulus: That which can elicit or evoke action (response) in a muscle, nerve, gland or other excitable issue, or cause an augmenting action upon any function or metabolic process. [NIH]

Stomach: An organ of digestion situated in the left upper quadrant of the abdomen between the termination of the esophagus and the beginning of the duodenum. [NIH]

Stress: Forcibly exerted influence; pressure. Any condition or situation that causes strain or tension. Stress may be either physical or psychologic, or both. [NIH]

Stria: 1. A streak, or line. 2. A narrow bandlike structure; a general term for such longitudinal collections of nerve fibres in the brain. [EU]

Stromal: Large, veil-like cell in the bone marrow. [NIH]

Stromal Cells: Connective tissue cells of an organ found in the loose connective tissue. These are most often associated with the uterine mucosa and the ovary as well as the hematopoietic system and elsewhere. [NIH]

Styrene: A colorless, toxic liquid with a strong aromatic odor. It is used to make rubbers, polymers and copolymers, and polystyrene plastics. [NIH]

Subacute: Somewhat acute; between acute and chronic. [EU]

Subclinical: Without clinical manifestations; said of the early stage(s) of an infection or other disease or abnormality before symptoms and signs become apparent or detectable by clinical examination or laboratory tests, or of a very mild form of an infection or other disease or abnormality. [EU]

Subiculum: A region of the hippocampus that projects to other areas of the brain. [NIH]

Subspecies: A category intermediate in rank between species and variety, based on a smaller number of correlated characters than are used to differentiate species and generally conditioned by geographical and/or ecological occurrence. [NIH]

Substance P: An eleven-amino acid neurotransmitter that appears in both the central and peripheral nervous systems. It is involved in transmission of pain, causes rapid contractions of the gastrointestinal smooth muscle, and modulates inflammatory and immune responses. [NIH]

Substrate: A substance upon which an enzyme acts. [EU]

Sudden death: Cardiac arrest caused by an irregular heartbeat. The term "death" is somewhat misleading, because some patients survive. [NIH]

Supplementation: Adding nutrients to the diet. [NIH]

Support group: A group of people with similar disease who meet to discuss how better to cope with their cancer and treatment. [NIH]

Suppression: A conscious exclusion of disapproved desire contrary with repression, in which the process of exclusion is not conscious. [NIH]

Suprachiasmatic Nucleus: An ovoid densely packed collection of small cells of the anterior hypothalamus lying close to the midline in a shallow impression of the optic chiasm. [NIH]

Surfactant: A fat-containing protein in the respiratory passages which reduces the surface tension of pulmonary fluids and contributes to the elastic properties of pulmonary tissue.

[NIH]

Sympathomimetic: 1. Mimicking the effects of impulses conveyed by adrenergic postganglionic fibres of the sympathetic nervous system. 2. An agent that produces effects similar to those of impulses conveyed by adrenergic postganglionic fibres of the sympathetic nervous system. Called also adrenergic. [EU]

Synapses: Specialized junctions at which a neuron communicates with a target cell. At classical synapses, a neuron's presynaptic terminal releases a chemical transmitter stored in synaptic vesicles which diffuses across a narrow synaptic cleft and activates receptors on the postsynaptic membrane of the target cell. The target may be a dendrite, cell body, or axon of another neuron, or a specialized region of a muscle or secretory cell. Neurons may also communicate through direct electrical connections which are sometimes called electrical synapses; these are not included here but rather in gap junctions. [NIH]

Synapsis: The pairing between homologous chromosomes of maternal and paternal origin during the prophase of meiosis, leading to the formation of gametes. [NIH]

Synaptic: Pertaining to or affecting a synapse (= site of functional apposition between neurons, at which an impulse is transmitted from one neuron to another by electrical or chemical means); pertaining to synapsis (= pairing off in point-for-point association of homologous chromosomes from the male and female pronuclei during the early prophase of meiosis). [EU]

Synaptic Vesicles: Membrane-bound compartments which contain transmitter molecules. Synaptic vesicles are concentrated at presynaptic terminals. They actively sequester transmitter molecules from the cytoplasm. In at least some synapses, transmitter release occurs by fusion of these vesicles with the presynaptic membrane, followed by exocytosis of their contents. [NIH]

Systemic: Affecting the entire body. [NIH]

Telencephalon: Paired anteriolateral evaginations of the prosencephalon plus the lamina terminalis. The cerebral hemispheres are derived from it. Many authors consider cerebrum a synonymous term to telencephalon, though a minority include diencephalon as part of the cerebrum (Anthoney, 1994). [NIH]

Temporal: One of the two irregular bones forming part of the lateral surfaces and base of the skull, and containing the organs of hearing. [NIH]

Teratogen: A substance which, through immediate, prolonged or repeated contact with the skin may involve a risk of subsequent non-hereditable birth defects in offspring. [NIH]

Teratogenesis: Production of monstrous growths or fetuses. [NIH]

Teratogenic: Tending to produce anomalies of formation, or teratism (= anomaly of formation or development : condition of a monster). [EU]

Teratogenicity: The power to cause abnormal development. [NIH]

Testis: Either of the paired male reproductive glands that produce the male germ cells and the male hormones. [NIH]

Testosterone: A hormone that promotes the development and maintenance of male sex characteristics. [NIH]

Thalamic: Cell that reaches the lateral nucleus of amygdala. [NIH]

Thalamic Diseases: Disorders of the centrally located thalamus, which integrates a wide range of cortical and subcortical information. Manifestations include sensory loss, movement disorders; ataxia, pain syndromes, visual disorders, a variety of neuropsychological conditions, and coma. Relatively common etiologies include cerebrovascular disorders; craniocerebral trauma; brain neoplasms; brain hypoxia;

intracranial hemorrhages; and infectious processes. [NIH]

Thalamus: Paired bodies containing mostly gray substance and forming part of the lateral wall of the third ventricle of the brain. The thalamus represents the major portion of the diencephalon and is commonly divided into cellular aggregates known as nuclear groups. [NIH]

Therapeutics: The branch of medicine which is concerned with the treatment of diseases, palliative or curative. [NIH]

Third Ventricle: A narrow cleft inferior to the corpus callosum, within the diencephalon, between the paired thalami. Its floor is formed by the hypothalamus, its anterior wall by the lamina terminalis, and its roof by ependyma. It communicates with the fourth ventricle by the cerebral aqueduct, and with the lateral ventricles by the interventricular foramina. [NIH]

Threonine: An essential amino acid occurring naturally in the L-form, which is the active form. It is found in eggs, milk, gelatin, and other proteins. [NIH]

Threshold: For a specified sensory modality (e. g. light, sound, vibration), the lowest level (absolute threshold) or smallest difference (difference threshold, difference limen) or intensity of the stimulus discernible in prescribed conditions of stimulation. [NIH]

Thrombin: An enzyme formed from prothrombin that converts fibrinogen to fibrin. (Dorland, 27th ed) EC 3.4.21.5. [NIH]

Thrombomodulin: A cell surface glycoprotein of endothelial cells that binds thrombin and serves as a cofactor in the activation of protein C and its regulation of blood coagulation. [NIH]

Thrombosis: The formation or presence of a blood clot inside a blood vessel. [NIH]

Thromboxanes: Physiologically active compounds found in many organs of the body. They are formed in vivo from the prostaglandin endoperoxides and cause platelet aggregation, contraction of arteries, and other biological effects. Thromboxanes are important mediators of the actions of polyunsaturated fatty acids transformed by cyclooxygenase. [NIH]

Thymidine: A chemical compound found in DNA. Also used as treatment for mucositis. [NIH]

Thymus: An organ that is part of the lymphatic system, in which T lymphocytes grow and multiply. The thymus is in the chest behind the breastbone. [NIH]

Thyroid: A gland located near the windpipe (trachea) that produces thyroid hormone, which helps regulate growth and metabolism. [NIH]

Tibial Nerve: The medial terminal branch of the sciatic nerve. The tibial nerve fibers originate in lumbar and sacral spinal segments (L4 to S2). They supply motor and sensory innervation to parts of the calf and foot. [NIH]

Tinnitus: Sounds that are perceived in the absence of any external noise source which may take the form of buzzing, ringing, clicking, pulsations, and other noises. Objective tinnitus refers to noises generated from within the ear or adjacent structures that can be heard by other individuals. The term subjective tinnitus is used when the sound is audible only to the affected individual. Tinnitus may occur as a manifestation of cochlear diseases; vestibulocochlear nerve diseases; intracranial hypertension; craniocerebral trauma; and other conditions. [NIH]

Tissue: A group or layer of cells that are alike in type and work together to perform a specific function. [NIH]

Tolerance: 1. The ability to endure unusually large doses of a drug or toxin. 2. Acquired drug tolerance; a decreasing response to repeated constant doses of a drug or the need for increasing doses to maintain a constant response. [EU]

Tomography: Imaging methods that result in sharp images of objects located on a chosen plane and blurred images located above or below the plane. [NIH]

Tonic: 1. Producing and restoring the normal tone. 2. Characterized by continuous tension. 3. A term formerly used for a class of medicinal preparations believed to have the power of restoring normal tone to tissue. [EU]

Topical: On the surface of the body. [NIH]

Toxic: Having to do with poison or something harmful to the body. Toxic substances usually cause unwanted side effects. [NIH]

Toxicity: The quality of being poisonous, especially the degree of virulence of a toxic microbe or of a poison. [EU]

Toxicology: The science concerned with the detection, chemical composition, and pharmacologic action of toxic substances or poisons and the treatment and prevention of toxic manifestations. [NIH]

Toxins: Specific, characterizable, poisonous chemicals, often proteins, with specific biological properties, including immunogenicity, produced by microbes, higher plants, or animals. [NIH]

Traction: The act of pulling. [NIH]

Transduction: The transfer of genes from one cell to another by means of a viral (in the case of bacteria, a bacteriophage) vector or a vector which is similar to a virus particle (pseudovirion). [NIH]

Transfection: The uptake of naked or purified DNA into cells, usually eukaryotic. It is analogous to bacterial transformation. [NIH]

Translational: The cleavage of signal sequence that directs the passage of the protein through a cell or organelle membrane. [NIH]

Transmitter: A chemical substance which effects the passage of nerve impulses from one cell to the other at the synapse. [NIH]

Trauma: Any injury, wound, or shock, must frequently physical or structural shock, producing a disturbance. [NIH]

Tricuspid Atresia: Absence of the orifice between the right atrium and ventricle, with the presence of an atrial defect through which all the systemic venous return reaches the left heart. As a result, there is left ventricular hypertrophy because the right ventricle is absent or not functional. [NIH]

Trigeminal: Cranial nerve V. It is sensory for the eyeball, the conjunctiva, the eyebrow, the skin of face and scalp, the teeth, the mucous membranes in the mouth and nose, and is motor to the muscles of mastication. [NIH]

Trigeminal Nerve: The 5th and largest cranial nerve. The trigeminal nerve is a mixed motor and sensory nerve. The larger sensory part forms the ophthalmic, mandibular, and maxillary nerves which carry afferents sensitive to external or internal stimuli from the skin, muscles, and joints of the face and mouth and from the teeth. Most of these fibers originate from cells of the trigeminal ganglion and project to the trigeminal nucleus of the brain stem. The smaller motor part arises from the brain stem trigeminal motor nucleus and innervates the muscles of mastication. [NIH]

Trophic: Of or pertaining to nutrition. [EU]

Trophoblast: The outer layer of cells of the blastocyst which works its way into the endometrium during ovum implantation and grows rapidly, later combining with mesoderm. [NIH]

Tryptophan: An essential amino acid that is necessary for normal growth in infants and for nitrogen balance in adults. It is a precursor serotonin and niacin. [NIH]

Tuberculosis: Any of the infectious diseases of man and other animals caused by species of Mycobacterium. [NIH]

Tumor marker: A substance sometimes found in an increased amount in the blood, other body fluids, or tissues and which may mean that a certain type of cancer is in the body. Examples of tumor markers include CA 125 (ovarian cancer), CA 15-3 (breast cancer), CEA (ovarian, lung, breast, pancreas, and gastrointestinal tract cancers), and PSA (prostate cancer). Also called biomarker. [NIH]

Tyrosine: A non-essential amino acid. In animals it is synthesized from phenylalanine. It is also the precursor of epinephrine, thyroid hormones, and melanin. [NIH]

Tyrothricin: A polypeptide antibiotic mixture obtained from Bacillus brevis. It consists of a mixture of three tyrocidines (60%) and several gramicidins (20%) and is very toxic to blood, liver, kidneys, meninges, and the olfactory apparatus. It is used topically. [NIH]

Unconditioned: An inborn reflex common to all members of a species. [NIH]

Unconscious: Experience which was once conscious, but was subsequently rejected, as the "personal unconscious". [NIH]

Uncoupling Agents: Chemical agents that uncouple oxidation from phosphorylation in the metabolic cycle so that ATP synthesis does not occur. Included here are those ionophores that disrupt electron transfer by short-circuiting the proton gradient across mitochondrial membranes. [NIH]

Uterus: The small, hollow, pear-shaped organ in a woman's pelvis. This is the organ in which a fetus develops. Also called the womb. [NIH]

Vaccine: A substance or group of substances meant to cause the immune system to respond to a tumor or to microorganisms, such as bacteria or viruses. [NIH]

Vascular: Pertaining to blood vessels or indicative of a copious blood supply. [EU]

Vasoactive: Exerting an effect upon the calibre of blood vessels. [EU]

Vasoactive Intestinal Peptide: A highly basic, single-chain polypeptide isolated from the intestinal mucosa. It has a wide range of biological actions affecting the cardiovascular, gastrointestinal, and respiratory systems. It is also found in several parts of the central and peripheral nervous systems and is a neurotransmitter. [NIH]

Vasodilator: An agent that widens blood vessels. [NIH]

Vector: Plasmid or other self-replicating DNA molecule that transfers DNA between cells in nature or in recombinant DNA technology. [NIH]

Vein: Vessel-carrying blood from various parts of the body to the heart. [NIH]

Venoms: Poisonous animal secretions forming fluid mixtures of many different enzymes, toxins, and other substances. These substances are produced in specialized glands and secreted through specialized delivery systems (nematocysts, spines, fangs, etc.) for disabling prey or predator. [NIH]

Venous: Of or pertaining to the veins. [EU]

Ventilation: 1. In respiratory physiology, the process of exchange of air between the lungs and the ambient air. Pulmonary ventilation (usually measured in litres per minute) refers to the total exchange, whereas alveolar ventilation refers to the effective ventilation of the alveoli, in which gas exchange with the blood takes place. 2. In psychiatry, verbalization of one's emotional problems. [EU]

Ventral: 1. Pertaining to the belly or to any venter. 2. Denoting a position more toward the belly surface than some other object of reference; same as anterior in human anatomy. [EU]

Ventral Tegmental Area: A region in the mesencephalon which is dorsomedial to the substantia nigra and ventral to the red nucleus. The mesocortical and mesolimbic dopaminergic systems originate here, including an important projection to the nucleus accumbens. Overactivity of the cells in this area has been suspected to contribute to the positive symptoms of schizophrenia. [NIH]

Ventricle: One of the two pumping chambers of the heart. The right ventricle receives oxygen-poor blood from the right atrium and pumps it to the lungs through the pulmonary artery. The left ventricle receives oxygen-rich blood from the left atrium and pumps it to the body through the aorta. [NIH]

Ventricular: Pertaining to a ventricle. [EU]

Verbal Learning: Learning to respond verbally to a verbal stimulus cue. [NIH]

Vertigo: An illusion of movement; a sensation as if the external world were revolving around the patient (objective vertigo) or as if he himself were revolving in space (subjective vertigo). The term is sometimes erroneously used to mean any form of dizziness. [EU]

Vestibular: Pertaining to or toward a vestibule. In dental anatomy, used to refer to the tooth surface directed toward the vestibule of the mouth. [EU]

Vestibule: A small, oval, bony chamber of the labyrinth. The vestibule contains the utricle and saccule, organs which are part of the balancing apparatus of the ear. [NIH]

Veterinary Medicine: The medical science concerned with the prevention, diagnosis, and treatment of diseases in animals. [NIH]

Virulence: The degree of pathogenicity within a group or species of microorganisms or viruses as indicated by case fatality rates and/or the ability of the organism to invade the tissues of the host. [NIH]

Virus: Submicroscopic organism that causes infectious disease. In cancer therapy, some viruses may be made into vaccines that help the body build an immune response to, and kill, tumor cells. [NIH]

Visceral: , from viscus a viscus) pertaining to a viscus. [EU]

Visual Perception: The selecting and organizing of visual stimuli based on the individual's past experience. [NIH]

Vitamin A: A substance used in cancer prevention; it belongs to the family of drugs called retinoids. [NIH]

Vitro: Descriptive of an event or enzyme reaction under experimental investigation occurring outside a living organism. Parts of an organism or microorganism are used together with artificial substrates and/or conditions. [NIH]

Vivo: Outside of or removed from the body of a living organism. [NIH]

Weight Gain: Increase in body weight over existing weight. [NIH]

White blood cell: A type of cell in the immune system that helps the body fight infection and disease. White blood cells include lymphocytes, granulocytes, macrophages, and others. [NIH]

Withdrawal: 1. A pathological retreat from interpersonal contact and social involvement, as may occur in schizophrenia, depression, or schizoid avoidant and schizotypal personality disorders. 2. (DSM III-R) A substance-specific organic brain syndrome that follows the cessation of use or reduction in intake of a psychoactive substance that had been regularly used to induce a state of intoxication. [EU]

Wound Healing: Restoration of integrity to traumatized tissue. [NIH]

Xenobiotics: Chemical substances that are foreign to the biological system. They include naturally occurring compounds, drugs, environmental agents, carcinogens, insecticides, etc. [NIH]

Xenograft: The cells of one species transplanted to another species. [NIH]

X-ray: High-energy radiation used in low doses to diagnose diseases and in high doses to treat cancer. [NIH]

Yeasts: A general term for single-celled rounded fungi that reproduce by budding. Brewers' and bakers' yeasts are Saccharomyces cerevisiae; therapeutic dried yeast is dried yeast. [NIH]

Zygote: The fertilized ovum. [NIH]

Zymogen: Inactive form of an enzyme which can then be converted to the active form, usually by excision of a polypeptide, e. g. trypsinogen is the zymogen of trypsin. [NIH]

INDEX

Printed in the United States
80815LV00001B/82